DATE DUE

JUL 0 7 2004	
SEP 2 4 2004	

BRODART   Cat. No. 23-221

Handbook of
Chronic Depression

Medical Psychiatry

Series Editor Emeritus

William A. Frosch, M.D.

Weill Medical College of Cornell University
New York, New York, U.S.A.

Advisory Board

ADDITIONAL VOLUMES IN PREPARATION

Handbook of Chronic Depression

Diagnosis and Therapeutic Management

edited by

Jonathan E. Alpert
Maurizio Fava

*Massachusetts General Hospital
and Harvard Medical School
Boston, Massachusetts, U.S.A.*

MARCEL DEKKER, INC.   NEW YORK · BASEL

Library of Congress Cataloging-in-Publication Data
A catalog record for this book is available from the Library of Congress.

ISBN: 0-8247-4046-7

This book is printed on acid-free paper.

Headquarters
Marcel Dekker, Inc., 270 Madison Avenue, New York, NY 10016, U.S.A.
tel: 212-696-9000; fax: 212-685-4540

Distribution and Customer Service
Marcel Dekker, Inc., Cimarron Road, Monticello, New York 12701, U.S.A.
tel: 800-228-1160; fax: 845-796-1772

Eastern Hemisphere Distribution
Marcel Dekker AG, Hutgasse 4, Postfach 812, CH-4001 Basel, Switzerland
tel: 41-61-260-6300; fax: 41-61-260-6333

World Wide Web
http://www.dekker.com

The publisher offers discounts on this book when ordered in bulk quantities. For more information, write to Special Sales/Professional Marketing at the headquarters address above.

Current printing (last digit):

10 9 8 7 6 5 4 3 2 1

PRINTED IN THE UNITED STATES OF AMERICA

To Wendy, Sam, and Tony
and
Stefania and Giovanni
and our parents
whose love and all too frequent sacrifices are appreciated beyond words
and to our dear friend and colleague
Joyce Root Tedlow, M.D.
whose extraordinary thoughtfulness, insight, and courage will inspire us always

Preface

Our goal as editors of this handbook was to join with respected colleagues with complementary expertise to produce a guide to chronic depression that would be accessible, clinically relevant, and empirically based. The enthusiasm with which we have pursued this project has been fueled by the steadily emerging recognition that chronic depression is not an esoteric subtype of depression, but rather a ubiquitous clinical feature associated with significant morbidity.

Although the majority of controlled depression treatment trials extend over months (1), the burden of depressive disorders is frequently measured in years. Consistent with clinical experience, major epidemiological studies (2–4) and observations from a number of large outcome studies over the past two decades, including the Zurich Follow-Up Study (5), the National Institute of Mental Health Collaborative Depression Study (6), and the Medical Outcomes Study (7), have helped refocus our understanding of major depressive disorder (MDD) from that of an episodic illness to that of a disorder with a strong tendency to persist and/or recur and a propensity to produce long-lasting and pervasive psychosocial and general medical consequences, indeed even when present in diminished intensity as subsyndromal symptoms.

There exists, as yet, no uniform definition of "chronic depression" and there is relatively little work comparing the clinical significance, if any, of different expressions of chronicity (8,9). Hence, the subject is defined broadly in this book, incorporating, in part, the DSM-IV specifiers for chronicity (10), but more generally regarding a depression as chronic when its clinically significant burden of symptoms and/or functional impairment extends over several years. This includes a chronic major depressive episode (≥2 years meeting full MDD criteria), a major depressive episode with incomplete inter-episode recovery, dysthymic disorder, and other protracted subsyndromal depressions, and a major depressive episode superimposed upon dysthymic disorder ["double depression" (11)]. In some clinical instances, persistence of depression is related to absence of or inadequate treatment, although in others it reflects treatment refractoriness or intolerance, and these different sources of chronicity are addressed in the chapters that follow.

The first five chapters of the handbook focus on biopsychosocial factors in chronic depression. Miller, Battle, and Anthony provide an incisive introduction to the definition and assessment of psychosocial functioning in chronic depression as well as theoretical perspectives on psychosocial impairment as antecedents and consequences of depression. Rothschild and Zimmerman explore and illuminate the often hazy and clinically challenging interface between chronic depression and personality pathology. Riso and Klein provide an overview of studies concerning risk factors for chronicity and advance a preliminary model that incorporates these findings and sets the stage for further research. Although few biological studies relate to chronicity per se, Mischoulon, Dougherty, and Fava draw broadly on neuroimaging, neuroendocrine, genetic, electro-encephalographic, and immunological studies to yield current perspectives on the pathophysiology of depression, while Smoller and Perlis focus on the rapidly evolving field of family and genetic studies.

The midsection of the handbook concerns treatment. Howland provides an expert review of the growing literature on the psychopharmacology of dysthymia and double depression, while Keitner and Cardemil describe psychotherapy treatment studies for chronic depression from a variety of perspectives, including cognitive-behavior therapy (CBT), interpersonal psychotherapy (IPT), the cognitive behavioral analysis system of psychotherapy (CBASP), group treatment, and family-based treatment. Maddux and Rapaport extend the discussion of psychopharmacological and psychotherapeutic studies to the treatment of subsyndromal forms of depression. Turning to the prevention of depressive relapse and recurrence, Friedman and Thase review continuation and maintenance treatment studies involving psychotherapy alone and in combination with medications and call attention to areas that require further study, while Petersen, Nierenberg, Ryan, and Alpert review the companion literature on long-term antidepressant therapy for the prevention of relapse and recurrence and address the problem of depressive re-emergence ("breakthrough") during treatment. M. Fava provides an up-to-date discussion of pharmacological treatment tactics and strategies for resistant depression and residual symptoms, while G.A. Fava and Ruini look specifically at psychotherapy of residual symptoms, including a description of a novel approach known as "well-being therapy" (WBT).

Treatment of chronic depression among special populations and in special settings is the agenda of the subsequent four chapters, including an introduction by Nonacs and Cohen to the management of depression during pregnancy, insights about the assessment and treatment of depression in later life by Apfeldorf and Alexopoulos, and a comprehensive and thoughtful review of current knowledge about pediatric depression and its treatment by Pilowsky and Weissman. Finally, Rosenstein, Soleymani, and Cai tackle the complexities of treating chronic depression in the setting of concurrent medical illness, including the risks of drug–drug interactions.

Simon and Ludman highlight critical shortcomings and barriers in the treatment of chronic depression and describe how chronic illness management principles could be used to optimize patient care. Zajecka and Beeler focus on improving patient adherence, a major challenge in long term depression treatment, and Kinrys, Simon, Farach, and Pollack provide a detailed and practical guide to the treatment of common antidepressant side effects to enhance both treatment adherence and quality of life for those many individuals requiring long-term pharmacotherapy.

Despite the growing recognition of depression as a chronic disorder for which management rather than cure is frequently the most accurate model, perhaps nowhere has the gap been more obvious between clinical practice and research than when it comes to the long-term management of depression. Our fond hope is that this book, by providing a synthesis of current research findings and clinical strategies for addressing chronic depression, helps bridge this gap.

Jonathan E. Alpert
Maurizio Fava

REFERENCES

1. Geddes JR, Carney SM, Davies C, Furukawa TA, Kupfer DJ, Frank E, Goodwin GM. Relapse prevention with antidepressant drug treatment in depressive disorders: a systematic review. Lancet 2003; 361(9358): 653–661.
2. Robins L, Regier DA, eds. Psychiatric Disorders in America: The Epidemiological Catchment Area Study. New York: Free Press, 1991.

3. Kessler RC, McGonagle KA, Zhao S. Lifetime and 12-month prevalence of DSM-III-R psychiatric disorders in the United States: results from the National Comorbidity Survey. Arch Gen Psychiatry 1994; 51:8–19.

4. Kessler RC, Berglund P, Demler O, Jin R, Koretz D, Merikangas KR, Rush AJ, Walters EE, Wang PS. The epidemiology of major depressive disorder: results from the National Comorbidity Survey Replication (NCS-R). JAMA 2003; 289(23):3095–3105.

5. Angst J, Kupfer DJ, Rosenbaum JF. Recovery from depression: risk or reality? Acta Psychiatr Scand 1996; 93:413–419.

6. Keller MB, Boland RJ. Implication of failing to achieve successful long-term maintenance treatment of recurrent unipolar major depression. Biol Psychiatry 1998; 44:348–360.

7. Wells KB, Stewart A, Hays RD. The functioning and well-being of depressed patients: results from the Medical Outcomes Study. JAMA 1989; 262:914–919.

8. Kocsis JH, Klein DN, eds. Diagnosis and Treatment of Chronic Depression. New York: Guilford Press, 1995.

9. McCullough JP Jr, Klein DN, Keller MB, Holzer CE III, Davis SM, Kornstein SG, Howland RH, Thase ME, Harrison WM. Comparison of DSM-III-R chronic major depression and major depression superimposed upon dysthymia (double depression): validity of the distinction. J. Abnorm Psychol 2000; 109:419–427.

10. American Psychiatric Association. Diagnostic and Statistical Manual of Mental Disorders. 4th ed. Text Revision. Washington, DC: American Psychiatric Press, 2000.

11. Keller MB, Shapiro RW. "Double depression": superimposition of acute depressive episodes on chronic depressive disorders. Am J Psychiatry 1982; 139:438–442.

Acknowledgments

A book of this kind has many proud parents. We are very grateful to the outstanding group of authors whose expertise and interest in chronic depression are reflected in the superb quality of their contributions. We also know more than anyone the extent to which this book owes its existence to the enthusiasm, perseverance, and creative input of Jinnie Kim, Acquisitions Editor at Marcel Dekker, Inc. We are grateful as well to Barbara Mathieu, Production Editor, and her associates, for helping to keep us on track as we came down to the wire, and to Heidi Montoya and Julie Ryan within our own department for their fine editorial assistance.

We are indebted to our departmental chief, Jerrold F. Rosenbaum, and our colleagues and trainees at the Massachusetts General Hospital for the extraordinarily collaborative and stimulating Department of Psychiatry they have created. We thank our colleagues in the Depression Clinical and Research Program who furnish an inexhaustible source of camaraderie, energy, and humor. In addition to those whose written contributions appear in this volume, it is a pleasure to acknowledge the countless ideas and insights we owe to Drs. Joel Pava, John Worthington, Albert Yeung, Paolo Cassano, Christina Dording, Shamsah Sonawalla, Amy Farabaugh, Joyce Tedlow, Dan Iosifescu, George Papakostas, John Matthews, and Jackie Buchin.

We trained with remarkable individuals, including Jerrold F. Rosenbaum and Donald J. Cohen, whose mark on us, as on many others, is indelible. Their capacity to integrate astute observation, clinical research, and basic science in the service of treatment and their profound generosity as mentors are qualities we recall gratefully and struggle to approximate.

Finally, we thank the patients we have the privilege of treating. We consider them our most important teachers and their contributions to our work cannot be overestimated.

Contents

Contributors

George S. Alexopoulos, M.D. Professor, Department of Psychiatry, Cornell Institute of Geriatric Psychiatry, Joan and Sanford I. Weill Medical College of Cornell University, White Plains, New York, U.S.A.

Jonathan E. Alpert, M.D., Ph.D. Associate Director, Depression Clinical and Research Program, Massachusetts General Hospital, and Assistant Professor, Department of Psychiatry, Harvard Medical School, Boston, Massachusetts, U.S.A.

Jennifer Anthony, Ph.D. Department of Psychiatry, Brown University School of Medicine and Rhode Island Hospital, Providence, Rhode Island, U.S.A.

William Apfeldorf, M.D., Ph.D. Associate Professor, Department of Psychiatry, University of New Mexico School of Medicine, Albuquerque, New Mexico, U.S.A.

Cynthia L. Battle, Ph.D. Department of Psychiatry, Brown University School of Medicine and Butler Hospital, Providence, Rhode Island, U.S.A.

Margaret Beeler   Department of Psychiatry, Rush Medical College and the Women's Board Depression Treatment and Research Center, Rush-Presbyterian–St. Luke's Medical Center, Chicago, Illinois, U.S.A.

Boris Birmaher, M.D.   Professor, Department of Child Psychiatry, Western Psychiatric Institute and Clinic, University of Pittsburgh Medical Center, Pittsburgh, Pennsylvania, U.S.A.

June Cai, M.D.   Assistant Professor, Miriam Hospital and Brown University, Providence, Rhode Island, U.S.A.

Esteban V. Cardemil, M.D., Ph.D.   Assistant Professor, Department of Psychology, Clark University, Worcester, Massachusetts, U.S.A.

Lee S. Cohen, M.D.   Director, Perinatal and Reproductive Psychiatry Clinical Research Program, Clinical Psychopharmacology Unit, Department of Psychiatry, Massachusetts General Hospital, and Associate Professor, Department of Psychiatry, Harvard Medical School, Boston, Massachusetts, U.S.A.

Darin D. Dougherty, M.D.   Assistant Professor, Department of Psychiatry, Massachusetts General Hospital and Harvard Medical School, Boston, Massachusetts, U.S.A.

Frank J. Farach, B.A.   Massachusetts General Hospital and Harvard Medical School, Boston, Massachusetts, U.S.A.

Giovanna A. Fava, M.D.   Professor, Department of Psychology, University of Bologna, Bologna, Italy, and State University of New York at Buffalo, Buffalo, New York, U.S.A.

Maurizio Fava, M.D.   Director, Depression Clinical and Research Program, and Associate Chief of Psychiatry, Massachusetts General Hospital, and Professor of Psychiatry, Harvard Medical School, Boston, Massachusetts, U.S.A.

Edward S. Friedman, M.D.   Medical Director, Depression Treatment and Research Program, Western Psychiatric Institute and Clinic, and Assistant Professor, Department of Psychiatry, University of Pittsburgh Medical Center, Pittsburgh, Pennsylvania, U.S.A.

Robert H. Howland, M.D. Associate Professor, Department of Psychiatry, Western Psychiatric Institute and Clinic, University of Pittsburgh School of Medicine, Pittsburgh, Pennsylvania, U.S.A.

Gabor I. Keitner, M.D., F.R.C.P.(C) Professor, Department of Psychiatry, Brown University, and Director of Adult Psychiatry and Mood Disorders Program, Rhode Island Hospital, Providence, Rhode Island, U.S.A.

Gustavo Kinrys, M.D. Instructor, Department of Psychiatry, Cambridge Hospital and Harvard Medical School, Boston, Massachusetts, U.S.A.

Daniel N. Klein, Ph.D. Professor, Departments of Psychology and Psychiatry, State University of New York at Stony Brook, Stony Brook, New York, U.S.A.

Evette J. Ludman, Ph.D. Research Associate, Center for Health Studies, Group Health Cooperative, Seattle, Washington, U.S.A.

Rachel E. Maddux, B.A. Research Associate, Department of Psychiatry, Cedars-Sinai Medical Center, Los Angeles, California, U.S.A.

Ivan W. Miller, Ph.D. Professor, Department of Psychiatry and Human Behavior, Brown University School of Medicine, and Director, Psychosocial Research Program, Butler Hospital, Providence, Rhode Island, U.S.A.

David Mischoulon, M.D., Ph.D. Director, Alternative Remedy Studies, Depression Clinical and Research Program, and Assistant Professor, Department of Psychiatry, Massachusetts General Hospital and Harvard Medical School, Boston, Massachusetts, U.S.A.

Andrew A. Nierenberg, M.D. Associate Director, Depression Clinical and Research Program, and Medical Director, Bipolar Programs, Massachusetts General Hospital, and Associate Professor, Department of Psychiatry, Harvard Medical School, Boston, Massachusetts, U.S.A.

Ruta Nonacs, M.D., Ph.D. Perinatal and Reproductive Psychiatry Clinical Research Program, Department of Psychiatry, Massachusetts General Hospital, Boston, Massachusetts, U.S.A.

Roy H. Perlis, M.D. Director, Pharmacogenetic Studies, Depression Clinical and Research Program, Massachusetts General Hospital, and Instructor,

Department of Psychiatry, Harvard Medical School, Boston, Massachusetts, U.S.A.

Timothy J. Petersen, Ph.D. Director, Psychotherapy Research, Depression Clinical and Research Program, Massachusetts General Hospital, and Department of Psychiatry, Harvard Medical School, Boston, Massachusetts, U.S.A.

Daniel J. Pilowsky, M.D., M.P.H. Staff Scientist, New York State Psychiatric Institute, Assistant Professor of Psychiatry, College of Physicians and Surgeons, and Assistant Professor of Epidemiology, Mailman School of Public Health, Columbia University, New York, New York, U.S.A.

Mark H. Pollack, M.D. Director, Center for Anxiety and Traumatic Stress Related Disorders, Massachusetts General Hospital, and Associate Professor, Department of Psychiatry, Harvard Medical School, Boston, Massachusetts, U.S.A.

Mark H. Rapaport, M.D. Chairman, Department of Psychiatry, Cedars-Sinai Medical Center, Los Angeles, California, U.S.A.

Lawrence P. Riso, Ph.D. Assistant Professor, Department of Psychology, Georgia State University, Atlanta, Georgia, U.S.A.

Donald L. Rosenstein, M.D. Chief, Psychiatry Consultation-Liaison Service, National Institute of Mental Health, National Institutes of Health, Bethesda, Maryland, U.S.A.

Louis Rothschild, Ph.D. Clinical Psychologist, Department of Psychiatry, Rhode Island Hospital and Brown University School of Medicine, Providence, Rhode Island, U.S.A.

Chiara Ruini, Ph.D. Research Fellow, Department of Psychology, University of Bologna, Bologna, Italy

Julie L. Ryan, B.A. Program Coordinator, Depression Clinical and Research Program, Massachusetts General Hospital, and Department of Psychiatry, Harvard Medical School, Boston, Massachusetts, U.S.A.

Gregory E. Simon, M.D., M.P.H. Investigator, Center for Health Studies, Group Health Cooperative, Seattle, Washington, U.S.A.

Naomi M. Simon, M.D. Associate Director, Center for Anxiety and Traumatic Stress Related Disorders, Massachusetts General Hospital, and Department of Psychiatry, Harvard Medical School, Boston, Massachusetts, U.S.A.

Jordan W. Smoller, M.D., Sc.D. Director, Psychiatric Genetics Program in Mood and Anxiety Disorders, Department of Psychiatry, Massachusetts General Hospital, and Assistant Professor, Department of Psychiatry, Harvard Medical School, Boston, Massachusetts, U.S.A.

Kambiz Soleymani, M.D. Psychiatry Consultation-Liaison Service, National Institute of Mental Health, National Institutes of Health, Bethesda, Maryland, U.S.A.

Michael E. Thase, M.D. Western Psychiatric Institute and Clinic and Professor, Department of Psychiatry, University of Pittsburgh Medical Center, Pittsburgh, Pennsylvania, U.S.A.

Myrna M. Weissman, Ph.D. Professor, Division of Clinical-Genetic Epidemiology, New York State Psychiatric Institute, and Department of Psychiatry, College of Physicians and Surgeons, Columbia University, New York, New York, U.S.A.

John Zajecka, M.D. Department of Psychiatry, Rush Medical College and the Women's Board Depression Treatment and Research Center, Rush-Presbyterian–St. Luke's Medical Center, Chicago, Illinois, U.S.A.

Mark Zimmerman, M.D. Associate Professor of Psychiatry and Human Behavior, Department of Psychiatry, Rhode Island Hospital and Brown University School of Medicine, Providence, Rhode Island, U.S.A.

1

Psychosocial Functioning in Chronic Depression

Ivan W. Miller and Cynthia L. Battle
Brown University School of Medicine
and Butler Hospital
Providence, Rhode Island, U.S.A.

Jennifer Anthony
Brown University School of Medicine
and Rhode Island Hospital
Providence, Rhode Island, U.S.A.

INTRODUCTION

Recent years have seen increased recognition that patients with mood disorders have significant impairments in a number of areas of functioning [1–6]. These nonsymptomatic, or "psychosocial," impairments are found in a number of areas and appear to be quite severe and pervasive [1,3,7–9].

This chapter will review the available empirical findings concerning the psychosocial impairments found in chronically depressed patients. We will begin by defining psychosocial impairments and then briefly review some of the more commonly used scales to assess psychosocial impairment. Following these introductory comments, we will review published studies investigating psychosocial impairments in chronically depressed patients.

1

Finally, we will attempt to put these findings into a theoretical context by reviewing several major theoretical models and their hypotheses regarding psychosocial impairments in depression.

DEFINITIONS OF PSYCHOSOCIAL IMPAIRMENT

As noted above, psychosocial impairments refer to impairments in functioning in areas other than symptoms. A number of areas of functioning are subsumed under the construct of psychosocial functioning. These areas include social/interpersonal functioning, family/marital relationships, work/school performance, physical health status, and leisure/ recreational activities.

The notion of psychosocial impairment is similar to constructs such as quality of life or life satisfaction in that it refers to other aspects of the patient's life beyond the symptoms of the disorder. However, in our view, psychosocial functioning differs from quality of life in two important ways. First, quality of life is a somewhat broader construct than psychosocial functioning. Quality of life reflects the patient's overall perceived satisfaction or quality, which includes both symptoms and other areas. Psychosocial functioning, on the other hand, refers solely to non-symptom areas of functioning. The second difference between quality of life and psychosocial functioning is that quality of life is, almost by definition, a more subjective construct. Who else besides the individual can judge the overall level of life satisfaction? On the other hand, psychosocial impairment is a somewhat less subjective construct, which considers the perspectives of other relevant individuals and to some extent society, as well as those of the patients. For example, a given patient could consider their quality of life quite high if they are not working and are being supported by welfare and their spouse. But from the perspective of the spouse, family, and society, this patient may not be seen as exhibiting optimal psychosocial functioning.

ASSESSMENT OF PSYCHOSOCIAL FUNCTIONING

There are numerous assessment instruments that have been developed to measure one or more aspects of psychosocial functioning. Scales assessing one aspect of psychosocial functioning (e.g., family functioning, work performance) are too numerous to review in this chapter, but it is worth briefly noting the most commonly used scales which measure multiple dimensions of psychosocial functioning. These scales include (1) the Social Adjustment Scale (SAS) [10], (2) Medical Outcomes Study 36-item Short

Form Health Survey (SF-36) [11], and (3) the Sheehan Disability Scale (SDS) [12] and the psychosocial items from the Longitudinal Interval Follow-up Evaluation (LIFE) [13]. Although all of these scales assess multiple aspects of psychosocial functioning, they vary significantly in the domains assessed and in their format.

The SAS was originally designed as an interview-based measure to assess six domains of psychosocial functioning (work, family, marital, parental, economic, social) as well as an overall functioning score. Later studies developed a self-report version of this instrument (SAS-SR) [14], which is more widely used. The SF-36 was designed as a self-report survey instrument to assess "health" [11]. The eight domains measured by the SF-36 include (1) limitations in physical activities because of health problems, (2) limitations in usual role activities because of physical health problems, (3) bodily pain, (4) general health perceptions, (5) energy, (6) limitations in social activities because of physical or emotional problems, (7) limitations in usual role activities because of emotional problems, and (8) overall mental health. The Sheehan Disability Scale consists of three visual analogue items asking patients to rate themselves on work, social life, and home life. The LIFE interview was designed to assess the course of symptoms and functioning over time. The psychosocial items on the LIFE assess similar domains to the SAS. The psychosocial items of the LIFE have recently been combined into an overall scale (LIFE-RIFT) [15] that provides an overall assessment of psychosocial functioning.

Although of all of these scales have reported adequate reliability and validity data, they have important strengths and weaknesses. First, as typically used, all of these scales, except for the LIFE, are self-report instruments. Thus, they measure the patient's *perception* of their psychosocial functioning. Although the patient's perceptions are obviously important, these perceptions may be influenced by the depressed patient's current mood state and level of cognitive distortion. Although interview-based measures of psychosocial functioning do exist (e.g., interview version of SAS, LIFE), these scales are not as widely used.

Second, as noted above, the domains assessed by these scales vary. The SDS assesses the least comprehensive set of domains, whereas the SAS and the LIFE assess a more inclusive set of variables. The SF-36, although assessing a wide range of domains, includes only a few subscales that assess psychosocial functioning (e.g., limitations in social activities because of physical or emotional problems and limitations in usual role activities because of emotional problems).

Finally, these scales differ in their complexity and the time required to complete them. The SDS is the shortest and easiest to complete, requiring only 2–3 min. Conversely, the SAS is quite complex, requires skipping of some items depending upon the subject's employment situation, and typically takes 20–30 min to complete. The LIFE, as an interview, requires a trained evaluator to complete.

In summary, there are multiple measures available to assess psychosocial functioning. Although all measures have adequate reliability and validity data, there are marked differences between them in terms of format, areas assessed, and respondent burden.

PSYCHOSOCIAL IMPAIRMENTS IN CHRONIC DEPRESSION

Empirical studies have supported the notion that patients with chronic depression demonstrate significant impairments in multiple areas of psychosocial functioning including social relationships, family functioning, work performance, and physical health. Although patients with episodic forms of depression demonstrate impairments in these areas as well, it has been suggested that chronically depressed patients demonstrate more severe and longer lasting psychosocial impairments [16]. However, the research in chronic depression is limited. In presenting the research that does exist, we will compare (1) the psychosocial impairments in patients with chronic depression to nonclinical control subjects, (2) the differences in impairments between chronic depression and other forms of depression, and (3) the impairments associated with chronic depression compared to impairments in other medical disorders.

Comparisons with Nonclinical Samples

Social Impairments

Several studies have demonstrated that a high proportion patients with chronic depression have impaired social functioning. Miller et al. [17] reported that 75% of chronically depressed patients were rated has having "poor" or "very poor" functioning on the LIFE, and they have SAS-SR scores more than two standard deviations higher than a community normative sample. This finding was duplicated by Hirschfeld and colleagues [18], who found that the social functioning of chronic depressed individuals was significantly impaired compared to community samples, and that 72% of chronic depressed patients were rated as poor or very poor on the LIFE assessment of social adjustment. Other studies have found similar results. Hays and colleagues [19] demonstrated that patients with double depression had significant impairments in social functioning on the SF-36 compared to the general population. Leader and Klein [20] found that patients diagnosed with double depression were more impaired socially than normal controls on both interview (LIFE) and self-report measures (SAS-SR).

Work Functioning

Depression has consistently been associated with increased disability days from work, excess absenteeism, and decreased productivity at work [21]. It has been estimated that the annual costs of depression in the United States are approximately 43.7 billion dollars [22]. This economic burden is due to (1) direct costs of medical psychiatric and pharmacological care, (2) mortality costs associated with depression-related suicides, and (3) morbidity costs associated with depression in the workplace (e.g., costs of excess absenteeism, reduction in productivity). Miller et al. [17] examined a sample of chronic depressed patients and found that they were significantly impaired in work functioning and employment status compared to community samples, with over 75% of the chronically depressed patients being rated as having work impairment. Again, similar findings were reported by Hirschfeld et al. [18] in another large study of chronically depressed patients, with 62% of the patients being rated has having impaired work performance. The early-onset subtype of chronic depression has been specifically associated with substantial human capital loss, especially for women. Berndt et al. [23] examined the impact of early-onset chronic depression on education, occupational choice, and increased earnings potential compared with data from normal controls in community studies. Women with early-onset chronic depression were shown to have considerable reductions in educational attainment (less likely to graduate from college, less likely to seek postgraduate training) and significant declines in expected future annual earnings.

Marital/Family Functioning

Research has shown that family functioning plays an important role in depressive disorders [8]. Using the Family Assessment Device, a specific measure of family functioning, Keitner et al. [24] reported that patients with chronic forms of depression report severe problems in all areas of their family functioning including problem solving, communication, roles, affective responsiveness, affective involvement, behavior control, and general functioning. Similarly, studies have reported impairments in chronically depressed patients on the marital and family subscales of the SAS-SR [17,18].

Physical Functioning/Health

The data regarding potential impairments in physical functioning are somewhat mixed. Hays and colleagues [19] reported significant impairments in general health and physical functioning of patients with double depression compared to the general population. Similarly, Hirschfeld, et al. [18]

reported impaired physical functioning in a large sample of chronically depressed patients. However, Miller et al. [17] did not find significant differences in physical functioning between chronically depressed patients and community norms.

Comparisons with Other Types of Depression

Social Functioning

The majority of research on chronic depression suggests that impairments in social functioning may be more profound for patients with chronic depression compared with patients with milder forms of depression [16]. Although Miller et al. [25] found no significant differences between inpatients with double depression and those with recurrent episodic depression on the SAS-SR administered during the acute phase of the disorder, Klein et al. [26] found that patients with double depression had significantly greater overall social impairment compared to those with episodic major depression in a 6-month follow-up study. Hays and colleagues [19] found that patients with double depression were more impaired in social functioning than patients with major depression. A study comparing social adjustment of patients with double depression, dysthymia, and episodic depression demonstrated that patients diagnosed with double depression were significantly more impaired than patients diagnosed with dysthymia and episodic major depression [20]. Finally, one study found chronically depressed patients had twice the rate of impaired social support compared to those patients presenting with an index of shorter duration [27]. This finding supports other research which link higher levels of social support to faster recovery from, or a shorter duration of, a depressive episode [28].

Marital/Family Functioning

Although there have been few direct tests of differences in family functioning between chronic and nonchronically depressed patients, there are several studies which are suggestive. In the most direct test, Keitner et al. [24] found that chronically depressed patients viewed their family functioning worse than nonchronically depressed individuals. Similar results were also found in an earlier study by Leader and Klein [20], who reported that double depressives were more impaired in relationships with extended family than patients diagnosed with dysthymia or episodic depression.

Work Functioning

The only available study suggests that patients diagnosed with double depression were significantly more impaired in work functioning compared with dysthymics and episodic major depressives [20].

Physical Functioning/Health

Longitudinal data on patients with various types of depression suggests that individuals with chronic depression show increased medical comorbidity [27]. Compared with patients with episodic major depression, chronically depressed patients have significantly increased health care utilization and comorbid medical conditions [30]. These findings reinforce previous research that suggests that physical illness predicts incomplete recovery, relapse, and chronicity of depression [31]. This relationship tends to be viewed as a bidirectional [32]; in some cases, medical comorbidity can cause depression and in other cases depression can exacerbate the impact of medical comorbidities. Additionally, the deleterious effects of depressive symptoms and medical conditions on functioning have been shown to be additive [6]. In particular, the comorbidity of current depressive and medical conditions increases morbidity, impairments of social functioning, and health care utilization [4].

Comparisons with Medical Disorders

The Medical Outcomes Study compared 1790 adult outpatients with depression (subthreshold depression, major depression, dysthymia, and double depression), diabetes, hypertension, recent myocardial infarction, and congestive heart failure [19]. All types of depressed patients were found to have worse impairments than patients with major chronic medical conditions including diabetes, hypertension, recent myocardial infarction, and/or congestive heart failure. The only medical condition that has been shown to be comparable to depression was current heart conditions. Chronic depression tends to be more debilitating than most other medical conditions in terms of physical functioning (e.g., sports activities, climbing stairs, walking, dressing, and bathing), role functioning (e.g., interference in work, housework, or schoolwork,) and normal social functioning [19]. Additionally, patients with chronic depression tended to have lower overall well-being than patients with chronic medical illness. Although substantial improvements were found in functional status and well-being at 2 years after initial assessment, depressed patients still remained as limited in physical health and more limited in mental health outcomes than were patients with chronic medical conditions [19].

In summary, patients diagnosed with chronic depression demonstrate significant impairments in social, family, work, and physical functioning. Furthermore, chronic depressed patients tend to be more impaired in these areas than nonclinical samples, other types of depressed patients, and patients with major chronic medical conditions.

PSYCHOSOCIAL IMPAIRMENTS IN CHRONIC DEPRESSION AFTER TREATMENT

The studies reviewed in previous sections have demonstrated that patients with chronic depression manifest a wide range of psychosocial impairments. The next question is whether treatment helps alleviate these impairments? A small number of studies have investigated this question. Six studies have investigated changes in psychosocial functioning after pharmacological treatment [17,18,33–36]. The results of these studies have been remarkably similar. As a group, chronically depressed patients treated pharmacologically showed significantly improved psychosocial functioning after treatment. However, the level of psychosocial functioning remains impaired relative to nondepressed norms. Compared to nonresponders, patients whose depressive symptoms respond to antidepressant treatment show larger improvements in psychosocial functioning and appear to approach, but not quite equal, normative functioning.

Only one study has investigated changes in psychosocial functioning among chronically depressed patients after treatment with psychotherapy [18]. This study found equivalent improvements in psychosocial functioning among patients who received pharmacotherapy and psychotherapy; however, similar to the results from analyses of depressive symptoms [37], the study found that chronically depressed patients who received combined pharmacotherapy and psychotherapy had a significantly better level of psychosocial functioning than patients receiving either pharmacotherapy or psychotherapy alone.

Overall the available research indicates that patients with chronic depression have severe and pervasive levels of psychosocial impairments. These impairments improve significantly with treatment (both pharmacological and psychological), but do not return to "normal" levels in a majority of patients.

THEORETICAL PERSPECTIVES ON PSYCHOSOCIAL IMPAIRMENT

In previous sections, we have described the psychosocial correlates and consequences of chronic depression, including disruption in social/interpersonal functioning, family/marital relationships, work/school functioning, and physical health. What are the underlying biopsychosocial mechanisms that are likely to be responsible for the functional impairments observed in chronically depressed patients? Do impairments in psychosocial functioning exist prior to the onset of depression and play an etiological role in the disorder or are they consequences of being depressed for an extended period of time? We now turn to three dominant theories regarding the etiology and maintenance of depression in general—(1) cognitive theory, (2) interpersonal theory, and (3) biological approaches—to understand better the processes that may result in impaired psychosocial functioning when depressive episodes are more chronic in nature. We will first explore the question of whether these difficulties exist before or after an individual becomes chronically depressed.

Distinguishing Antecedents from Consequences of Chronic Depression

In the context of a chronic mood disorder, it is important to recognize that psychosocial impairments could be both possible antecedents and/or possible consequences of the disorder. For example, poor interpersonal and social functioning has been shown to be a risk factor for the development of depression, in general, in terms of both poor marital adjustment [38] and low social support [39] predicting future depression. But impaired social and interpersonal functioning may also be a *consequence* of living with a depressive disorder. For example, a depressed person may gradually deplete their social resources over time [40], or they develop interpersonal friction and inhibited communication patterns with family members that persist after remission of the episode [41]. A related issue is that depressed individuals may have a negative bias [42] which could influence their perception of their own functioning (at work, in the family, with friends) and therefore report levels of impairment that are inaccurately high by objective standards. This bias can further complicate the task of disentangling the association between psychosocial functioning and depression. As such, differentiating between antecedent and consequence variables is extremely difficult. Implementing the large-scale prospective investigations that would be necessary truly to clarify the temporal relation of these variables would be both methodologically challenging and costly. The extant research offers only some indication of the psychosocial variables that precede and result from depression [43]; data regarding functional impairments as antecedents or consequences of chronic forms of depression, in particular, are even more limited. In our view, it seems likely that psychosocial variables are both important antecedents *and* possible consequences of the depression. Theoretical models are needed to guide empirical research and elucidate these issues. The cognitive, interpersonal, and biological theories of depression, described below, each offer a different perspective on how functional impairments may relate to the onset and course of the disorder.

Cognitive Approaches

Cognitive theorists emphasize the role of stable, enduring mental templates, or *schemas*, in organizing and interpreting information about oneself and one's social world. Beck's [44,45] cognitive model of depression focuses specifically on both the "cognitive triad"—persistent negative concepts about oneself, the world, and the future—as well as a biased pattern of information processing that functions to maintain these negative views. The depressed individual may, as a result of early life experience, develop a negative self-schema (e.g., *"I am defective," "I am unlovable"*) which, although continually present, becomes more salient when activated by certain schema-consistent life experiences. Cognitive theorists such as Beck posit that schemas persist because new information is processed in a distorted manner; various types of cognitive distortions (e.g., "all or nothing" thinking, overgeneralization) block the assimilation of disconfirming evidence that could potentially alter the schema. Another prominent cognitive theory is Seligman's [46] learned helplessness model of depression and the reformulated learned helplessness theory [47,48]. This theory posits that some people are more vulnerable to becoming depressed due to their attributional style, or the manner in which they typically perceive the causes of events in their lives. When negative events occur and an individual makes stable, global, and internalized attributions about the reason the events took place, depression may result; a habitual pattern of explaining events in this way is thought to predict more chronic depressive symptoms.

From a cognitive perspective, it follows that depressed individuals would not only experience sadness and psychological distress, but they would also be likely to suffer from psychosocial impairments related to their maladaptive cognitive processes. For example, a rigidly held self-schema of undesirability (*"No one could ever like me for who I am"*) could restrict a depressed person's openness to new social relationships because of fears of rejection by others. Cognitive distortions could also interfere with that individual's ability to integrate contradictory information and take positive steps to change; for example, if an acquaintance invites the depressed person on a social outing, the invitation may be interpreted as being insincere (*"She doesn't really like me—she just feels obligated to invite me"*). When social relations become impaired, the individual may experience a reduction in social support, which may in turn perpetuate their depressive symptoms, confirm their self-view as socially undesirable, and lead to increased hopelessness about the future.

Cognitive factors could also impact functioning at work. For example, a self-schema of defectiveness (*"I am a failure—there is something inherently wrong with me"*) could lead to a lack of motivation and persistence in the individual's job-related or career pursuits, as well as selective attention to failure experiences and disregard of successes. An individual with this view may consistently underestimate his or her abilities, feel reluctant to apply for new jobs, or pursue advanced education because of the notion that failure is inevitable. It is plausible that this type of belief system about one's abilities could similarly lead to decreased effort and poor performance/ productivity on the job, fewer promotions, and a higher rate of sick days. Given a pattern of internalized, global attributions of these negative events, such experiences would only serve to reinforce the individual's negative self-view and sense of hopelessness that things would never change for the better.

Interpersonal Approaches

Interpersonal and interactional models of depression focus on how individuals' depressive symptoms relate to negative social interactions with others. Whereas some theories emphasize the role of depression in causing interpersonal conflict and distress, others conceptualize interpersonal difficulties as predating depression and playing a causal role in the development of the disorder. Although the emphasis may differ, many interpersonal theorists acknowledge the bidirectional influence of interpersonal problems and depression. Lewinsohn's original interpersonal theory [49] posited that depressed individuals experience a lack of positive reinforcement from others due to their deficient social skills, as well as a reduction in their own ability to reinforce others, which results in a reduction in social reciprocity. Coyne [50] proposed an interpersonal theory of depression based on the concept of a escalating depressive cycle: An individual becomes depressed and seeks reassurance in the form of understanding, sympathy, and attention from others; these behaviors eventually become irritating to the depressed person's friends and family members. As a result, over time, the support offered to the depressed person by significant others becomes less sincere. When the depressed person perceives his or her social environment as being less caring and more hostile, the desire for reassurance increases more; however, increased reassurance-seeking behaviors only exacerbate the negative response from others. Finally, a number of theorists have focused specifically on the association between marital relationships and depression (e.g., see Ref. 51); they argue that marital distress significantly increases a person's risk for depression by both lowering the amount of social support available (marital cohesion, intimacy, dependability) and increasing stress and hostility (criticism, blame, verbal aggression).

Functional impairment in social and family relationships is at the core of interpersonal theories of depression whether viewed as a cause or consequence of the disorder. Coyne's theory in particular speaks to the chronicity of depressive symptoms as they relate to cyclical patterns of interpersonal behavior occurring over time and the disruption that depression-related behaviors may have on close relationships. Based on interpersonal theories of depression, social alienation and dysfunction in an individual's most intimate relationships—those with family and partner—result from ongoing negative exchanges. Indeed, empirical studies have consistently shown a strong association between depression and marital distress (e.g. see Refs. 52–54) and depression and overall family functioning [55,56].

From an interactional model of depression, it also follows that depressed individuals would experience difficulty in other settings requiring effective social skills, such as work and school, as depression-linked interpersonal behaviors are not limited to close relationships. Thus, a depressed individual may be more likely to experience interpersonal tension or conflicts with coworkers, a problem that could lead to lowered productivity or even termination of employment. Studies of depressed and nondepressed individuals have supported the notion that interpersonal difficulties are not limited to close relationships. Findings from observational studies have suggested that depressed individuals demonstrate more negative communication patterns during interpersonal interactions (e.g. see Ref. 57); moreover, depressed persons tend to elicit negative responses such as anger and social rejection from others [58].

Biological Approaches

Biological theories of depression have focused primarily on the role of (1) dysregulation of neurotransmitter systems, particularly norepinephrine, serotonin, dopamine, and acetylcholine; (2) dysregulation in hormonal systems, particularly thyroid hormones and the hypothalamic-pituitary-acetylcholine system, and (3) biological rhythm and sleep disturbances, such as irregular circadian or ultradian rhythms. The emphasis of biological models is on understanding the underlying biological processes that create the symptoms of depression. The symptoms are, in turn, seen as driving the functional impairments. Thus, in contrast to cognitive and interpersonal models, the causal mechanisms leading to specific problems in functioning are less explicit.

Another approach that emphasizes biological underpinnings of depression and other psychological disorders has recently been presented by Reiss and colleagues [59]. In their Evocative Model, they posit that genetic and environmental influences have a reciprocal effect that together result in the individual's psychological adjustment and psychopathology. In brief, the model describes a process by which heritable aspects of the individual, such as temperament, evoke particular behavioral response patterns from close friends and family members. These interpersonal patterns affect the individual's adjustment and psychopathology, including level of depressive symptoms. Although this model is not specific to chronic depression, it is an example of a theoretical approach that incorporates genetic influences with social/interpersonal factors. A large-scale twin study examining environmental and genetic influences on maternal adjustment and psychological symptoms found support for the overall model [60].

CONCLUSION

Although there are not a large number of studies investigating psychosocial functioning in chronically depressed patients, the results of existing studies are fairly consistent. Depressed patients with chronic depression manifest significant levels of impairment across many domains of psychosocial functioning, including problems in the areas of (1) family/marriage, (2) work, (3) interpersonal/social relationships, and (4) physical functioning. These impairments appear to be severe and pervasive, and they may be more severe than other types of depressive disorders and than many other types of chronic medical conditions. With treatment, these psychosocial impairments improve, but for many patients do not return to normative levels. Thus, even with a remission of depressive symptoms, many patients with a history of chronic depression continue to manifest significant impairments in important areas of life functioning. Although the severity of these psychosocial deficits is consistent, available research does not allow a determination whether these impairments are the sequelae of chronic depression or whether they are also precipitants. Different theoretical models have differing perspectives on these issues of the possible causality of psychosocial variables, but the large-scale, prospective studies necessary to distinguish between these possibilities have not been conducted.

REFERENCES

1. Coryell W, Scheftner W, Keller M, Endicott J, Maser J. The enduring psychosocial consequences of mania and depression. Am J Psychiatry 150: 720–727, 1993.
2. Hirschfeld R, Montgomery S, Keller M, Kasper S, Schatzberg A, Moller H, Healy D, Valdwin D, Humble M, Versiani M, Montegegro R, Bourgeois M. Social functioning in depression: a review. J Clin Psychiatry 61: 268–275, 2000.
3. Judd L, Akiskal H, Zeller P, Paulus M, Leon A, Maser J, Endicott J, Coryell W, Kunovac J, Mueller T, Rice J, Keller M. Psychosocial disability during the long terms course of unipolar major depressive disorder. Arch Gen Psychiatry 57: 375–382, 2000.

4. Klerman GL. Depressive disorders: Further evidence for increased medical morbidity and impairment of social functioning. Arch Gen Psychiatry 46: 856–999, 1989.
5. Mintz J, Mintz L, Arruda M, Hwang S. Treatments of depression and the functional capacity to work. Arch Gen Psychiatry, 49: 761–768, 1992.
6. Wells KB, Stewart A, Hays RD, Burnam MA, Rogers W, Daniels M, Berry S, Greenfield S, Ware. JAMA 262: 914–919, 1989.
7. Weissman M, Paykel E. The Depressed Woman: A Study of Social Relationships. Chicago: University of Chicago Press, 1974.
8. Keitner GI, Miller IW. Family functioning and major depression: An overview. Am J Psychiatry, 147: 1128–1137, 1990.
9. McCullough J, Roverts W, McCune K, Kaye A, Hampton C. Social adjustment, coping style and clinical course among DSM-III-R community unipolar depressives. Depression 2: 36–42, 1994.
10. Weissman M, Paykel E, Siegel R, and Klerman G. The social role performance of depressed women: comparisons with a normal group. Am J Orthopsychiatry, 41: 390–405, 1971.
11. Ware J and Sherbourne C. The MOS 36-item Short-Form Health Survey (SF-36). Med Care 30: 473–481, 1992.
12. Sheehan D, Harnett-Sheehan K, Raj A. The measurement of disability. Int Clin Psychopharmacol 11, 89–95, 1996.
13. Keller M, Lavori P, Friedman B, Nielsen E, Endicott J. The Longitudinal Follow-up Evaluation. Arch Gen Psychiatry 44: 540–548, 1987.
14. Weissman MM, Bothwell S. Assessment of social adjustment by patient self-report. Arch Gen Psychiatry 33: 1111–1115, 1976.
15. Leon A, Solomon D, Mueller T, Endicott J, Posternak M. A brief assessment of psychosocial functioning of subjects with bipolar I disorder: The LIFE-RIFT. J Nerv Ment Dis 188: 805–812, 2000.
16. Friedman RA. Social impairment in dysthymia. Psychiatr Ann 23: 632–637, 1993.
17. Miller IW, Keitner GI, Schatzberg AF, Klein DN, Thase ME, Rush JA, Markowitz JC, Schlager DS, Kornstein SG, Davis SM, Harrison WM, Keller MB. The treatment of chronic depression. Part III: Psychosocial functioning before and after treatment with sertraline or imipramine. J Clin Psychiatry, 59: 608–619, 1998.
18. Hirshfeld R, Dunner D, Keitner G, Klein D, Koran L, Kornstein S, Markowitz J, Mille, I, Nemeroff C, Ninan P, Rush A, Schatzberg A, Thase M, Trivedi M, Borian F, Crits-Cristoph P, Keller M. Does psychosocial functioning improve independent of depressive symptoms? A comparison of nefazadone, psychotherapy and their combination in the treatment of chronic depression. Biol Psychiatry 51: 123–133, 2002.
19. Hays RD, Wells KB, Sherbourne CD, Rogers W, Spritzer K. Functioning and well-being outcomes of patients with depression compared with chronic general medical illness. Arch Gen Psychiatry, 52: 11–19, 1995.
20. Leader JB, Klein DN. Social adjustment in dysthymia, double depression and episodic major depression. J Affect Disord 37: 91–101, 1996.

21. Broadhead WE, Blazer DG, George LK, Tse CK. Depression, disability days, and days lost from work in prospective epidemiologic survey. JAMA, 264: 2524–2528, 1990.
22. Greenberg PE, Stiglin LE, Finkelstein SN, Berndt ER. The economic burden of depression in 1990. J Clin Psychiatry, 54: 405–418, 1993.
23. Berndt E, Koran L, Finkelstein S, Gelenberg A, Kornstein S, Miller I, Thase M, Trapp G, Keller M. Lost human capital from early-onset chronic depression. Am J Psychiatry, 157: 940–947, 2000.
24. Keitner GI, Ryan CE, Miller IW, Keller MB. Family functioning of chronically depressed patients. Presentation at American Psychiatric Association, New York, May, 1996.
25. Miller IW, Norman WH, Dow MG. Psychosocial characteristics of "double depression." Am J Psychiatry, 143: 1042–1045, 1986.
26. Klein DN, Taylor EB, Harding K, Dickstein S. Double depression and episodic major depression: demographic, familial, personality, and socioenvironmental characteristics and short-term outcome. Am J Psychiatry, 145: 1226–1231, 1988.
27. Hays JC, Krishnan KRR, George LK, Pieper CF, Flint EP, Blazer DG. Psychosocial and physical correlates of chronic depression. Psychiatry Res 72: 149–159, 1997.
28. George LK, Blazer DG, Hughes DC, Fowler N. (1989). Social support and the outcome of major depression. Bri Jo Psychiatry 154, 478–485.
29. Miller IW, McDermut W, Gordon K, Keitner GI, Ryan CE, Norman W. Personality and family functioning in families of depressed patients. J Abnorm Psychol 109: 539–545, 2000.
30. Howland R. Chronic depression. Hosp Commun Psychiatry, 44(7): 633–639, 1993.
31. Sherbourne CD, Hays RD, Wells KB. Personal and psychosocial risk factors for physical and mental health outcomes and course of depression among depressed patients. J Consul Clin Psychol, 63: 345–355, 1995.
32. Katz IR. On the inseparability of mental and physical health in aged persons: Lessons from depression and medical comorbidity Am J Ger Psychiatry, 4: 1–16, 1996.
33. Agosti V, Stewart JW, Quitkin FM. Life satisfaction and psychosocial functioning in chronic depression: Effect of acute treatment with antidepressants. J Affect Disord 23: 35–41, 1991.
34. Friedman R, Markowitz J, Parides M, Kocsis J. Acute response of social functioning in dysthymic patients with desipramine. J Affect Disord 34: 85–88, 1995.
35. Kocsis J. Imipramine and social-vocational adjustment in chronic depression. Am J Psychiatry, 145: 997–999, 1988.
36. Stewart JW, Quitkin FM, McGrath PJ, Rabkin JG, Markowitz JS, Tricamo E, Klein DF. Social functioning in chronic depression: Effect of six weeks of antidepressant treatment. Psychiatry Res 25: 213–222, 1988.
37. Keller M, McCullough J, Klein D, Arnow B, Dunner D, Gelenberg A, Markowitz J, Nemeroff C, Russell J, Thase M, Trivedi M, Zajecka J, Blalock J,

Borian F, Fawcett J, Hirschfeld R, Jody D, Keitner G, Kocsis J, Koran L, Kornstein S, Manber R, Miller I, Ninan P, Rothbaum B, Rush A, Schatzberg A. The acute treatment of chronic major depression: A comparison of nefazodone, cognitive behavioral analysis system of psychotherapy, and their combination. New Engl J Med 342, 1462–1470, 2000.

38. Whisman MA, Bruce ML. Marital distress and incidence of major depressive episode in a community sample. J Abnorm Psychol,, 108: 674–678, 1999.

39. Phifer JF, Murrell SA. Etiologic factors in the onset of depressive symptoms in older adults. J Consult Clin Psychol, 95: 282–291, 1986.

40. Hinrichsen GA, Hernandez NA. Factors associated with recovery from and relapse into major depressive disorder in the elderly. Am J Psychiatry, 150: 1820–1825, 1993.

41. Paykel ES, Weissman MM. Social adjustment and depression: a longitudinal study. Arch Gen Psychiatry, 28: 659–63, 1973.

42. White J, Davison GC, Haaga DA, White K. Cognitive bias in the articulated thoughts of depressed and nondepressed psychiatric patients. T J Nerv Mental Dis 180: 77–81, 1992.

43. Barnett PA, Gotlib IH. Psychosocial functioning and depression: Distinguishing among antecedents, concomitants, and consequences. Psychol Bull, 10: 97–126, 1988.

44. Beck AT. Depression: Clinical, Experimental, and Theoretical Aspects. Philadelphia: University of Pennsylvania Press, 1967.

45. Beck AT, Rush AJ, Shaw BF, Emery G. Cognitive Therapy for Depression. New York: Guilford Press, 1979.

46. Seligman MEP. Helplessness: On Depression, Development, and Death. San Francisco: Freeman, 1975.

47. Abramson LY, Seligman MEP, Teasdale J. Learned helplessness in humans: Critique and reformulation. J Abnorm Psychol, 87: 49–74, 1978.

48. Miller IW, Norman WH. Learned helplessness in humans: A review and attribution theory model. Psychol Bull, 86: 93–118, 1979.

49. Lewinsohn PM. A behavioral approach to depression. In: Friedman RJ, Katz MM (eds). The Psychology of Depression: Contemporary Theory and Research. Washington, DC: Winston, 1974: 157–178.

50. Coyne JC. Toward an interactional description of depression. Psychiatry, 39: 28–40, 1976.

51. Beach SRH, Sandeen EE, O'Leary KD. Depression in Marriage: A Model for Etiology and Treatment. New York: Guilford Press, 1990.

52. Hooley JM, Teasdale JD. Predictors of relapse in unipolar depressives: Expressed emotion, marital distress, and perceived criticism. J Abnorm Psychol, 98: 229–235, 1989.

53. Johnson SL, Jacob T. Marital interactions of depressed men and women. J Consul Clin Psychol, 65:15–23, 1997.

54. Whisman MA. The association between depression and marital dissatisfaction. In: Beach SRH (ed). Marital and Family Processes in Depression: A Scientific Foundation for Clinical Practice. Washington, DC: American Psychological Association, 2001; pp 3–24.

55. Keitner GI, Ryan CE, Miller IW, Zlotnick C. Psychosocial factors and the long-term course of major depression. J Affect Disord 44, 57–67, 1997.

56. Miller IW, Keitner GI, Whisman MA, Ryan CE, Epstein NB, Bishop DS. Depressed patients with dysfunctional families: description and course of illness. J Abnorm Psychol, 101: 637–646, 1992.

57. Hops H, Biglan A, Sherman L, Arthur J, Friedman L, Osteen V. Home observations of family interactions of depressed women. J Consul Clin Psychol, 55:341–346, 1987.

58. Sacco WP, Milana S, Dunn VK. Effect of depression level and length of acquaintance on reaction of others to a request for help. J Pers Soc Psychol, 49:1728–1737, 1985.

59. Reiss D, Pedersen NL, Cederblad M, Lichtenstein P, Hansson K, Neiderhiser JM, Elthammer O. Genetic probes of three theories of maternal: I. Recent evidence and a model. Fam Proc 40:, 247–260, 2001.

60. Reiss D, Cederblad M, Pedersen NL, Lichtenstein P, Elthammer O, Neiderhiser JM, Hansson K. Genetic probes of three theories of maternal: II. Genetic and environmental influences. Fam Proc 40: 261–272, 2001.

2

Interface Between Personality and Depression

Louis Rothschild and Mark Zimmerman
Rhode Island Hospital
and Brown University School of Medicine
Providence, Rhode Island, U.S.A.

INTRODUCTION

When two entities such as personality and depression interact on our collective radar screen, scientific discussion tends to become rather complicated. Discourse pertaining to these entities may be considered to have crossed the threshold of complexity once Schneider challenged Kraepelin's [1] argument that mild chronic depression is in fact a variant of what was then referred to as manic-depressive illness with the suggestion that mild chronic depression is best understood as a problem pertaining to an aberrant personality [2]. Since that time questions of distinctiveness and ubiquity have been applied to taxonomies, methodologies, and theories in the quest to tease apart the relationship between depression and personality.

Amid such questions regarding the relationship between personality and depression is the concern that current knowledge is limited and disproportional. Although there are not yet exhaustive models of depressive subtypes [3], there is even less agreement about the components of a personality disorder than the components of a depressive syndrome [4]. Such inequalities and limitations are amplified when the depressive syndrome in question is chronic major depression, because it may be impossible to distinguish a "long-lasting" state from a trait [5]. In fact, within the discourse that surrounds this intersection, one finds criticism maintaining that theorists have confused chronic depression with personality and then have argued that it is the pathogenesis of depression [4].

Amid such complexity, one would like a firm place to stand, and established classification systems such as the *Diagnostic and Statistical Manual of Mental Disorders* (DSM) [6] afford some promise of terra firma. Accordingly, in the text that follows, the term *Personality Disorder* (PD), found on Axis II since the publication of DSM-III [7], refers to the enduring and maladaptive patterns of pervasive and inflexible inner experience and behavior that deviate markedly from the expectations of the individual's culture and lead to distress or impairment. Additionally, depression refers to disorders characterized by major depressive episodes in the psychiatric nosology. The studies we review and qualitatively evaluate in this chapter categorize mood and personality disorders according to this nomenclature.

This chapter appears in an edited text of discourse on chronic depression. In DSM-IV, the chronic specifier necessitates continuously meeting criteria for a Major Depressive Episode for at least 2 years, and may be applied to a Major Depressive Disorder or to a Bipolar I or II Disorder if a Major Depressive Episode is the most recent type of mood episode [6]. Unfortunately, little research has studied the relationship of PDs and the chronic specifier. Consequently, in order to examine the interface between PDs and depression chronicity, we focus on two types of studies. First, we review studies comparing the clinical characteristics of depressed patients with and without a PD and examine whether personality pathology is associated with indices of chronicity (e.g., recurrence of episodes and duration of the episode). Second, we review studies of the prognostic significance of PDs in the treatment of depression. Thus, the first set of studies represents a retrospective perspective on the relationship between PDs and chronicity and the second set of studies a prospective perspective. Before reviewing these reports, we first review pertinent issues regarding taxonomy and co-occurrence, some of the major methodological issues to be considered in the assessment of PDs, and epidemiological and clinical studies examining the relationships between depression and PD.

TAXONOMY AND CO-OCCURRENCE

The DSM, a conceptual system of human design [8] that has yet to denote the essence of a disorder [9], has been considered comprise arbitrary selections drawn from diverse sources with no explicit theoretical or empirical rationale [10]. The inability to locate discrete disease entities has led to debate regarding issues of diagnostic comorbidity versus symptom overlap. Originally used to refer to a distinct and additional disease entity that existed during the course of a primary disease [11], *comorbidity* is a term often used to capture the presence of both mood and personality disorders in a given patient. However, in regard to this particular inter-section, distinctiveness has been challenged on at least three counts. First, major depressive disorder (MDD) appears to be ubiquitous across person-ality disorders [12]. Second, controversy surrounding the possible inclusion of depressive personality disorder on Axis II has led to a question of the relationship and boundary between Axis I and Axis II [13,14]. And third, overlap between the individual personality disorders listed on Axis II has been considered to represent a failure of discriminant validity that affords a rationale to argue for a dimensional model of personality disorders [15].

The argument has been made that it is misleading to refer to disorders with such overlap as being truly comorbid [16], as these disorders may simply be classes of manageable groups in which distinctiveness is an artifact of the current nosology [17]. The term *co-occurrence* has been introduced in order to avoid the distinctiveness assumption inherent in comorbidity [18], and as it is neutral [19] in its simultaneous avoidance of the nondistinctive assumption found in the use of the term *overlap*, we will adopt the term *co-occurrence* throughout this review.

Although not yet well understood, the factors of co-occurrence that need to be considered are etiology, pathophysiology, and behavior [16]. The etiological level encompasses genes and the environment, whereas the patho-physiological level accounts for biology (e.g., neurotransmitters) and psy-chology (e.g., learned helplessness and object relations). The manner in which these mechanisms have been considered to account for co-occurrence has resulted in the consideration of several models. Models that seek to explain the co-occurrence of depression and personality disorders may be considered to utilize at least one of six possible concepts: independent causes, common cause, spectrum (one is subclinical), predisposition (one is a risk factor for the other), pathoplasty (not casually related but influences the other), or scar (residual effects of one influences the other) [20]. It has been noted that many models may be distinguished in regard to the co-occurrence of depression and personality disorders [21], and the question has been raised if in fact enough is known to move toward an integrative model [22].

Co-occurrence is also a salient factor within personality disorders, as the frequency in which more than one personality disorder is diagnosed in a given patient has led to debate regarding the conceptualization of the PD taxonomy. Recently, varied empirically derived taxonomies of personality disorders have been presented [23,24], and dimensional versus categorical conceptions are discussed [5,25–28]. Although Cattell maintained that the discrete versus dimensional debate is in fact two sides of same coin, as any object may be defined in either conceptualization [29], statistical models now allow researchers to discriminate between categorical and dimensional taxonomies [30]. However, the findings from studies of particular PDs that utilize these models are far from parsimonious [31,32], and there is a need for additional research.

Debate regarding the axis where a PD taxonomy should be located [10,33] illustrates the difficulty met in the attempt to disentangle personality disorders and chronic depression. On the one hand, the suggestion has been made that future editions of DSM circumvent discrete categories with the consideration of a multilevel hierarchical matrix of symptom cluster dimensions in order to account for the variety of psychopathology [19]. However, current discrete categories could well be an important guide in the construction of new taxonomies [34], and constant new starts may not help to refine current concepts [35]. It has also been suggested that better measurement and a common assessment to aggregate data are a necessary precursor that should proceed rising to the challenge of new models [21]. Addressing current methods of assessment utilized in the studies under review sheds light on issues that will remain no matter how the taxonomy may change in the future.

METHODOLOGICAL ISSUES

Research involving the diagnosis of Axis II disorders presents several methodological challenges. Here we discuss a number of important issues that should be addressed when conducting research that involves diagnosing Axis II pathology. A more intricate discussion of these issues as well as an overview of the reliability of measures of personality disorder may be found in an earlier review by Zimmerman [36]. Among the questions that are faced upon deciding to study personality disorders in patients with chronic depression are (1) who should provide the information for determining the presence or absence of a personality disorder, (2) what instrument should be used to make the diagnosis, and (3) when should one attempt to diagnose a personality disorder—when symptomatic on presentation for treatment or after symptom improvement?

For any individual to describe validly his or her normal personality, he or she must be somewhat introspective and aware of the personal and interpersonal impact of his or her behavior, and clinicians and researchers sometimes interview an informant of the patient such as a spouse or family member with the hope of obtaining more accurate information. However, agreement between patients and informants is generally poor (Kappas usually

0.40) [37,38], and informants tend to report more pathology [38]. There are insufficient data to recommend one source of information over the other [36]. In addition to the finding that informants report more pathology, the increased expenditure of time and resources needed to supplement the patient interview with informant information does not appear warranted according to evidence that when personality diagnoses were derived from a combination of patient and informant information, the results were similar to that of patient-only data [39].

A variety of interviews and questionnaires are utilized to assess personality, and these may be differentiated across several features. On occasion, a focal battery of diverse assessment instruments is used [40]. Some measures assess only one or two personality disorders [41,42], whereas others cover all of the DSM disorders [43–48]. Many instruments measure personality disorder constructs that are related, but not identical, to those of the DSM criteria, such as the Personality Assessment Inventory (PAI) [49] and the Millon Clinical Multiaxial Inventory (MCMI) [45]. In contrast, other measures such as the Personality Disorder Examination (PDE) [44], the Structured clinical interview for DSM-IV Personality Disorders (SCID-II) [47], the Diagnostic Interview for Personality Disorders (DIPD) [48], the Personality Diagnostic Questionnaire (PDQ-4+) [46], and the Structured Interview for DSM-IV Personality (SIDP-IV)[43] were explicitly developed to assess DSM criteria.

There is a long history within personality assessment of using paper and pencil tests, while an interview is often the standard assessment procedure in clinical practice. Common to both self-report questionnaires and interviews, direct questions may bias findings by leading to an increase in subject defensiveness [50], and such questions may become mired in the lack of insight that is one of the hallmarks of a personality disorder [51]. Additionally, poor agreement has been found between interview and self-report assessments, and when compared to interviews, self-report questionnaires tend to overdiagnose personality disorders in patient and nonpatient samples [36]. Furthermore, the various assessment instruments use questions that vary to a sufficient degree so that it cannot be assumed that individuals who are rated positive on one measure will be positive on the others [52].

If one decides to employ one of the interview-based measures, several variables such as the amount of clinical experience necessary to use the instrument in a reliable manner, test item construction, and scoring need to be considered. Research comparing different interview techniques is sparse, because it is technically difficult, requiring at least two raters with high levels of test-retest reliability to administer the two instruments under consideration. When the modest short-interval test-retest reliability of these interview measures is considered, it is not surprising that agreement between measures is generally poor to fair [53,54].

The active interaction between a subject and interviewer may well be a foundational property of clinical assessment that goes beyond being the passive observer and recorder of test responses [55]; hence the development of semistructured interviews in which clinical judgment is considered part and parcel of the assessment process. However, this interaction may aid and hinder the assessment process. An interviewer's personality, age, sex, and race may all interact in a manner that affect rapport and thus bias the interview-based evaluation and data collection [36]. The structure of the interview then serves to reduce interviewer variance which self-report scales could be useful in detecting [56].

The amount of clinical experience recommended for interviewer competence also varies among instruments. At one end of the continuum lay interviewers may assess personality pathology [57]. At the other end of the experience continuum is the PDE that was designed for use by experienced psychiatrists, clinical psychologists, or other professionals with comparable training [44]. The authors of the SIDP-IV recommended an intermediate level of experience (i.e., an undergraduate degree in the social sciences, at least 6 months experience interviewing psychiatric patients, and about 1 month of specific training using the SIDP-IV) [43]. Although fully structured interviews require less training to administer, and like more flexible interviews, have been shown to be accurate when respondents are certain as to how questions map onto their circumstances, flexible, semistructured interviewing provides greater accuracy when respondents lack complete certainty in regard to the mapping of questions onto their circumstances [58].

The manner in which questions are grouped and delivered varies among the instruments. Unique to the SCID-II is the concurrent use of a screening questionnaire that is completed by the respondent and reviewed by the interviewer before the interview. The interviewer only inquires about the criteria that are endorsed on the questionnaire. Of the semistructured interviews, the SIDP-IV and PDE group questions thematically by content areas such as interpersonal relationships and emotions. In contrast, the SCID-II and DIPD are organized by diagnosis. The diagnostically organized interview may be more prone to halo effects in which ratings of individual criteria may be influenced by how close an individual is to meeting criteria for a disorder, so thematically organized instruments may be more appropriate for the study of co-occurrence.

Time frame, rating, and scoring vary by assessment instrument. The PDQ instructs the respondent to consider the past several years, whereas the DIPD evaluates the past 2 years prior to the interview. The SCID-II, PDE, and SIDP-IV each consider the past 5 years, although the SCID-II and PDE evaluate attitudes and behaviors, whereas the SIDP-IV asks that the individual focus on their "usual self." On the PDE, the interviewer also inquires about the age of onset of pathological attitudes and behavior, and at least one criterion must be present before age 25 years to diagnose a personality disorder. Thus, the PDE emphasizes persistence and early onset more than the other measures, and it is more concordant with the DSM definition of a personality disorder. The PDE is the only interview accompanied by a detailed item-by-item scoring manual.

Given what is known about negative cognitive bias in depression and mood-state-dependent recall, the time in which a personality disorder assessment is conducted is another factor that warrants consideration. Although there is some evidence suggestive of the stability of higher order personality traits such as neuroticism and extroversion during the course of a depressive illness [59], studies of Axis II pathology tend to find a reduction of symptoms at the conclusion of treatment. Such studies that tested the hypothesis that reported levels of Axis II pathology are greater when someone is in the midst of an episode of major depression have typically administered personality assessment instruments to patients prior to the start of treatment and then again at the conclusion of treatment. The fairly consistent result that less personality pathology is reported following brief treatment when compared to pretreatment levels has been found in several different patient populations including patients with depression [60], eating disorders [61], and anxiety disorders [62]. In addition, the available data suggest that both personality disorder interviews and self-report inventories are susceptible to overreporting bias owing to the acute psychiatric state [63]. These results suggest that symptom abatement be a prerequisite for personality disorder assessment, since personality pathology seems to be overreported during the acute stage of psychiatric illness. On the other hand, despite the inflated rates of personality pathology during acute Axis I illness, conducting a personality assessment during the acute stage of an Axis I disorder generally coincides with the planning of treatment. If such an assessment is to have treatment implications, it should be made early. Moreover, as the review that follows will attest, such assessments have consistent prognostic value.

EPIDEMIOLOGICAL STUDIES OF CO-OCCURRENCE

Owing to the increase in treatment seeking when symptoms are exacerbated by multiple illnesses, rates of multiple diagnoses are generally greater in the clinic than in the community [64]. Findings from nonclinical samples afford a check to what could be a shortsighted generalization of inflated findings obtained with skewed clinical samples (Table 1). In addition, epidemiological research has identified variables that are not typically the

TABLE 1 Epidemiological Studies of Co-Occurrence

Study [Ref.]	Sample	PD measure[a]	Time of assessment	Results and comment[b]
Zimmerman & Coryell, 1989 [71]	797 first-degree relatives of normal controls and patients	DIS SIDP	Initial, cross sectional	Presence of PD is associated with increased incidence of mood disorders. MDD is most strongly associated with avoidant PD.
Heikkinen et al., 1997 [75]	112 suicides	Interview & records	Postmortem	Similar rates of MDD in subjects with and without PD. Interpersonal and job-related problems may proceed suicide in subjects with PD.
Lewinsohn et al., 1997 [68]	299 individuals	PDE	2 points over 5 yrs	Increased levels of personality pathology in young adults who suffered chronic depression.
Daley et al., 1999 [72]	155 adolescent women	PDQ, PDQ-R, & SCID-II	5 points over 3 yrs	Subclinical Axis II symptoms endure and are a risk factor for depression.
Johnson et al., 1999 [67]	717 youths and mothers	DISC-I, DPI Modified PDQ	2 points over 6 yrs	PDs elevate risk for mood disorders and suicidal ideation and behavior during young adulthood.
Kasen et al., 1999 [70]	551 youths	PDQ & SCID-II	4 points over 10 yrs	MDD increased the odds of young adult PD independently of an adolescent diagnosis of PD.
Lenzenweger, 1999 [69]	250 university students	IPDE, MCMI-II	3 points over 4 yrs	Increase in rates of PD when MDD co-occurs. Presence of Axis I disorder did not moderate PD feature changes.
Gustafsson and Jacobsson, 2000 [74]	100 suicides	Interview, reports, records	Postmortem	Greater frequency of PDs in suicide subjects diagnosed with MDD than in suicide subjects in general.

[a] Diagnostic Interview Schedule (DIS), Structured Interview for DSM Personality Disorders (SIDP), Personality Diagnostic Questionnaire (PDQ), Personality Diagnostic Questionnaire - Revised (PDQ-R), Composite International Diagnostic Interview (CIDI), Diagnostic Schedule for Children (DISC-I), Personality Disorder Examination (PDE), Disorganizing Poverty Interview (DPI), International Personality Disorders Examination (IPDE), Millon Clinical Multiaxial Inventory II (MCMI-II).
[b] MDD, Major depressive disorder; PD, personality disorder.

focus of clinical assessment. For example, migration and rapid social change have been considered to be pertinent explanatory variables in regard to evidence that Axis II diagnoses have different prevalence rates in different societies [65].

Interestingly, prevalence rates have not remained constant within American psychiatric epidemiology. Specifically, greater illness rates were found in the National Comorbidity Study when compared to the previously conducted Epidemiological Catchment Area study. In addition to mood disorders, these studies assessed antisocial personality disorder, and the findings of such large-scale studies are important on a number of accounts. Data from the Epidemiological Catchment Area study indicate that the lifetime co-occurrence of psychiatric disorders increases with earlier age of onset in major depressive disorder [57]. What is particularly striking about this finding is that it is unique to major depression as the early age of onset distinction did not occur for anxiety disorders or other mood disorders [57]. According to the National Comorbidity Study data, as the severity of depression increases so does the length of the current episode, the number of past episodes, and the presence of conformist and dependent personality traits [66].

Several longitudinal studies have examined the specific relationship between depression and personality pathology in nonclinical samples. Co-occurrence rates range from 19% of personality disordered subjects presenting with a mood disorder in early adulthood [67] and 21.5% of individuals with major depression also meeting criteria for a personality disorder [68] to 36.4% of young adults with major depression having significant features of personality disorders [69]. The overall findings suggest that a strong relationship exists between mood and personality pathology as the rates of personality pathology increase when depression co-occurs [69,70], and the presence of personality disorders increases the risk of mood disorder co-occurrence [67].

An increase in the incidence of mood disorders has been associated with the presence of PD [71], and longitudinal studies are in a particularly good position to evaluate the status of personality pathology as subjects are followed over a number of years. Subclinical or spectrum model findings suggest that pathological personality traits appear stable over time [69,72]. Although some findings indicate that personality pathology does not appear to be moderated by Axis I disorders [69], other studies find that major depression increases the odds of co-occurring Cluster B and C personality disorders [70], and that chronic depression is associated with an increase in personality pathology [68]. Other findings indicate that pathological traits (especially the odd/eccentric cluster A and the dramatic/emotional Cluster B) are a predisposing risk factor for subsequent depressive episodes [72,73]. Also, the anxious/fearful Cluster C personality disorders appear to elevate risk for suicidal ideation or behavior [67].

Psychiatric epidemiology has a long established tradition in Nordic countries, and postmortem accounts of suicide, which require that a diagnosis be reached by the use of records and interviews of family and clinicians, have been a source of valuable data. When suicides are divided by the presence of major depression or not, personality disorders are more common in those with major depression (38%) than in those who completed suicide but were not diagnosed with major depression (22%) [74]. The rate of major depression within suicides diagnosed with a personality disorder varies, as one study finds 26% [75], whereas another finds 50% [74]. It has been hypothesized that interpersonal and job-related problems may proceed suicide among subjects with personality disorders, as negative life events such as family discord and unemployment were more common among those suicides diagnosed with personality disorders [75].

CLINICAL FINDINGS

As the rate in which major depression and personality disorders co-occur in clinical samples far exceeds the rates found in epidemiological studies, treatment seeking itself is an important factor [76]. In an oft-cited review, Farmer and Nelson-Gray [77] found that rates of personality disorders and major depression co-occurrence ranged from 30 to 70%. A handful of more recent studies continue to support that range as rates have ranged from 19 to 82%[12,52,78–82]. Additionally, multiple PDs are often diagnosed in a single subject. For example, one study found that 32% of depressed subjects presented with a co-occurrence of two or more personality disorders [78]. As these rates of co-occurrence are relatively high and demonstrate significant bandwidth, one might ask what, if anything, is specific to this association.

Claims that personality disorders are ubiquitous to Axis I are not uncommon [12,83]. In addition to finding a lack of specificity in a comparison of remitted patients with mood disorders and schizophrenia, Oulis et al. found no significant differences between personality disorder clusters. Further, the claim that depressive episodes are ubiquitous in regard to co-occurrence within particular personality disorders is supported by findings from another study in which a co-occurrence rate of MDD across PDs is understood to be an effect of the base rate of such co-occurrence [12].

Claims of ubiquity are further supported in the study of particular PDs. In addition to a finding of high odds for co-occurrence of mood and dependent and avoidant cluster C personality disorders, the odds for anxiety, psychotic, and eating disorder co-occurrence are also high for these PDs [18]. Cluster B disorders have been linked to substance-use disorders [84,85], and the relationship of Cluster B to mood disorders is considered to be less specific than the relationship to substance-use disorders [18]. More specifically, borderline personality disorder (BPD) has also been linked to anxiety disorders and disorders characterized by disinhibition such as eating and substance-use disorders in addition to being associated with MDD [86–88].

One might wonder if any case can be made in support of a specific relationship between mood and specific personality disorders, as every personality disorder save histrionic is found to co-occur with depression [78,79,82,89–92]. However, depressive subtype appears to matter, and variables such as recurrence and duration of MDD may be employed in order to subtype chronicity (Table 2).

In regard to recurrence, specific findings exist for Clusters B and C. The co-occurrence of Cluster C disorders with episodes of depression has been strongly associated with the recurrence of depressive episodes following treatment [93]. Another study of psychiatric outpatients suggests that both age of onset and recurrence are pertinent variables for study, as BPD and dependent traits each play a role in recurrent major depression [94].

It might be fair to assume that given adults of the same age, age of onset should be correlated with recurrence and PD, as an earlier age of onset affords an increase in the amount of time in which pathology might occur. The hypothesis that PDs occur with greater frequency in early-onset major depression is supported in some studies [95–97] but not in others [89,98]. Some evidence also implicates so-called double depression, as the co-occurrence of dysthymia with early-onset major depression has been associated with an increase in personality disorders [99].

Depressive episodes of longer duration have been associated with a trend of greater personality disorder frequencies [77], and the chronic specifier holds some promise of specificity. However, little research has studied the co-occurrence of personality disorders and the chronic major depression specifier found in the DSM. At least one study [100] has assessed episode duration as greater or less than 1 year, thereby missing the chronic specifier by a year, whereas other studies have used the distinction of recurrent episodes of major depression with co-occurring dysthymia in order to measure chronicity [78,89,99]. Empirical use of the latter definition has supported the theory that a chronic mood disorder with a progression in severity is associated with disorders of personality, and this finding is intensified for BPD in particular [89]. As both dysthymia and BPD have been implicated in the association between chronic MDD and PD, we turn to a closer examination of BPD and the DSM-IV research criteria for depressive personality disorder (DPD) before reviewing studies of prognostic significance.

Borderline personality disorder commonly co-occurs with a variety of Axis I disorders, and when BPD co-occurs with MDD, MDD is generally

TABLE 2 Retrospective Studies of Chronicity Characteristics

Study [Ref.]	Sample	PD measure[a]	Time of assessment	Results and comment[b]
Alnaes and Torgersen, 1997 [94]	253 adult outpatients	SIDP-I, MCMI-I, BCI	2 points over 6 years for Axis I and initial only for Axis II	Borderline PDs were more frequent in MDD relapse and new MDD groups. Dependency predicted MDD relapse. Avoidant PD predicted new cases of MDD.
Garyfallos et al., 1999 [99]	364 adult outpatients	SCID-II & MMPI	Initial, cross sectional	Early-onset dysthymia showed higher PD rates than episodic MDD. However, patients with double depression had high rates of PD.
Skodol et al., 1999 [89]	571 adult outpatients	DIPD-IV, PSQ	Initial wave, longitudinal study	61.3% of PDs with current mood disorder and 92.6% with lifetime mood disorder. Findings support argument that chronic mood disorder with progression in severity leads to PD.
Kool et al., 2000 [78]	211 adult outpatients	IPDE (self-report version)	Initial, cross sectional	60% of patients with MDD have at least one PD, and 32% have two or more PDs. Relationship found between double depression and schizoid and avoidant PDs.

[a] Structured Clinical Interview for DSM Personality Disorders (SCID-II), Structured Interview for DSM Personality Disorders (SIDP), Millon Clinical Multiaxial Inventory (MCMI-I), Basic Character Inventory (BCI), International Personality Disorder Examination (IPDE), Minnesota Multiphasic Personality Inventory (MMPI), the Diagnostic Interview for Personality Disorders (DIPD-IV), Personality Screening Questionnaire (PSQ).
[b] MDD, major depressive disorder; PD, personality disorder.

chronic [77]. This particular PD serves to illustrate the difficulty in teasing out the relationship between chronic MDD and PD, as debate concerning BPD has evoked both biological and characterological models of co-occurrence. Although some evidence suggests that bipolar disorder and BPD may be discrete diagnoses [101], from a biological position, Akiskal suggests that patients who are diagnosed with BPD or histrionic personality disorder in Cluster B and are also diagnosed with avoidant personality disorder on Cluster C should be suspected as belonging to the bipolar II subtype [102]. Furthermore, Akiskal maintains that a diagnosis of BPD obscures the affective origin of an illness that is indicative of a mood disorder [102]. From this viewpoint, BPD may be understood as a marker of movement from a nonbipolar to a bipolar mood disorder. Akiskal's argument is opposed by another model that maintains that personality may underlie and cause symptom states, and that when depression co-occurs with BPD, it is an interpersonally focused depression that is essentially independent of major depression, as it is of characterological origin [103–105]. According to this model, chronicity would be interpreted as a function of personality.

Like the debate regarding bipolar II and BPD, the mood disorder spectrum is again evoked along characterological and biological lines in debate surrounding DPD [14]. As a personality disorder, DPD is chronic by definition. In addition to being characterized by unhappiness, it comprises beliefs of inadequacy, self-criticism, brooding, negativism, pessimism, and guilt. A fair amount of ink has been spilled to date in controversies regarding the substantial, but incomplete, overlap between DPD, major depression, and dysthymia [89,106–113]. Taxonomic location is debated, as questions exist as to whether or not DPD should be considered to exist between major depression and personality disorders or between major depression and dysthymic disorders [78]. Such debate may be traced back to the placement of personality disorders on Axis II, and the decision to classify depressive character traits as a mood disorder on Axis I in the construct of dysthymia [114,115]. The eventual fate of DPD may serve as a barometer from which to assess the *zeitgeist* in regard to the intersection of personality and chronic depression. For now, the proposal that DPD be considered to be a formal diagnosis found in DSM simply raises issues of the relationship between depression and personality and the taxonomy that should be utilized to represent these co-occurring phenomena [116]. Although the taxonomy is questioned, patients continue to present and require treatment.

PROGNOSTIC SIGNIFICANCE AND TREATMENT

There is general support for the clinical heuristic that when depressive and personality disorders co-occur, one may expect greater severity of depressive symptoms, slower response to treatment, and decreased likelihood of recovery. Indeed, a majority of studies of depressed patients with and without a personality disorder found statistically significant evidence that the presence of a personality disorder is associated with worse outcome [63]. This finding that PD is associated with worse outcome is consistent across type of treatment involved, and has been replicated in several patient populations including inpatients, outpatients, those referred from primary care, and the elderly [117–138]. However, the conclusion that co-occurring PD leads to a poor prognosis for MDD should by no means be considered a universally applicable conclusion, as some, albeit a minority, of studies find PD related to better outcome [117,118], no difference in outcome [119], and mixed results in regard to outcome [120].

As the preponderance of evidence suggests that the co-occurrence of PD and MDD is related to poor prognosis, the challenge of ubiquity is again addressed in clinical research. Simply, the question again arises as to if there is a discernible relationship between specific PDs and MDD. In order to determine the effect of type of PD on treatment response, researchers have compared depressed patients with at least one PD to those without a PD in terms of recovery (Table 3) or compared responders to nonresponders in terms of character pathology (Table 4).

It is often difficult to recruit enough patients with each type of PD to conduct a meaningful analysis [122,139]. In addition to difficulty in obtaining adequate subjects for the general clusters [140], the difficulty increases when one seeks to recruit for particular personality disorders. Despite this difficulty, Clusters A, B, and C are frequently compared on outcome in depression [118,119,124,125,127,129,131,139–141]. A few research groups studying major depression have reported that certain PDs undermine recovery, whereas others seem to enhance recovery. However, no systematic pattern has emerged.

Cluster A and C pathology has been linked to slower improvement or worse outcome in many comparisons of the influence of clusters on outcome in depression when compared to subjects with no PD [124,125,127,129]. More specifically, avoidant and dependent patients have been found to respond slowly [128], yet these particular PDs have also been implicated in treatment success in a subsequent study that associated compulsive and passive-aggressive personality with poor prognosis [130]. A subsequent study found a better outcome for patients rated obsessive-compulsive [120].

No studies found that Cluster B pathology accounted for the differences in outcome between PD and no PD subjects. In fact, patients with a Cluster B diagnosis have been found to exhibit a greater drop in depressive symptomatology compared to those without a Cluster B diagnosis [119]. Analysis of MCMI data suggests that high scores on antisocial and paranoid scales are associated with treatment response [118], and it has been suggested that patients with borderline or antisocial PDs have tended to improve, possibly because depression might function as a motivator toward treatment compliance [85,142]. It has also been suggested that the typically narrow inclusion criteria of most depression treatment studies be altered to include difficult borderline patients that are depressed [143].

Interestingly, one study finds that a Cluster B diagnoses do not change after treatment for depression, but Cluster A and C symptomatology recedes after successful treatment for depression [144]. Peselow et al. suggest that Cluster A and C "traits" may be interwoven with depressive "states," thereby implying that a distinction between chronic depression and personality disorder may be difficult to draw for Clusters A and C. However, there is no convincing evidence that depressed individuals with any particular personality disorder have a better or worse prognosis than depressed subjects with any other disorder.

As significant cluster crossing overlap has been noted in PD diagnosis, it has been suggested that global personality pathology could be a valid predictor of outcome [141]. A recent finding supports this hypothesis in that a diagnosis of PD was not associated with treatment outcome, whereas an increase in the number of PDs diagnosed in a particular patient was associated with worse outcome [145]. The finding that a single PD is not associated with treatment outcome may be considered to aid understanding regarding the failure to implicate a particular PD in prognosis. Additionally, there is support for the conception that higher numbers of PD are associated with worse outcome [124,125,129,141]. This suggests that measures of overall personality pathology have some validity in predicting treatment response.

It has also been noted that depressed patients with personality disorders do demonstrate an overall treatment response, but simply do not improve to the same point or at the same rate as those without a personality disorder [17,146]. Symptoms may remain after short-term treatment [132], and longer term psychotherapy may be most appropriate when a PD co-occurs with MDD [142,145–148]. However, neither acute nor long-term approaches to the treatment of chronic depression have been well studied [149], and a tentative theory suggests that that future research should seek to determine if chronicity itself might account for prognosis [13].

The above review has demonstrated that PDs are associated with greater chronicity in depression. One might predict that personality disordered patients' interpersonal problems would maintain or create circumstances that exacerbate depressive symptomatology. Such patterns of behavior could manifest in the treatment relationship. It has been noted that a failure to establish a working alliance may lead to treatment failures [142],

TABLE 3 Prognostic Comparison of Depressed Patients With and Without PD

Study [Ref.]	Sample	PD measure[a]	Time of assessment[b]	Results and comment[c]
Charney et al., 1981 [121]	64 inpatients	Chart review	NA	Non-PD patients had better response to treatment than PD patients.
Pfohl et al., 1984	78 inpatients	SIDP	Within first week of admission	Non-PD patients more likely to improve on HRSD, BDI, GAS; PD patients less responsive to medication.
Zimmerman et al., 1986 [135]	25 inpatients	SIDP	Within first week of hospitalization	PD patients less likely to recover; PD patients had more hospitalizations and more symptoms during 6-month follow-up.
Pfohl et al., 1987 [141]	78 inpatients	SIDP, PDQ	Within first week of admission	Patients with higher numbers of SIDP or PDQ criteria had poorer outcome at discharge and 6 month follow-up.
Black et al., 1988 [140]	228 inpatients	Chart review	NA	PD patients less likely to recover at discharge and more likely to attempt suicide after discharge.
Pilkonis and Frank, 1988 [129]	119 outpatients	PAF	Upon recovery during acute treatment	Slow responders more likely to have a PD and had higher levels of overall personality pathology.
Reich, 1990 [137]	37 outpatients	PDQ	Within 1 week of intake	Non-PD group had higher GAS scores and more likely to achieve full employment at 6-month follow-up.
Shea et al., 1990 [131]	239 outpatients	PAF	Pretreatment	PD patients less likely to recover following either psychotherapy plus medication or clinical management plus placebo.
Peselow et al., 1992 [124]	68 outpatients	SIDP	Pretreatment	Treatment responders had lower level of overall personality pathology; patients with lower personality pathology fared better at 6-month follow-up.
Diguer et al., 1993 [132]	25 outpatients	PAF	Pretreatment	Co-occurring PD associated with less improvement and greater severity at presentation, post-treatment, and follow-up.

Study	Sample	Instrument	Timing	Findings
Diguer et al., 1993 [132]	239 outpatients	PAF	Within 1 week of intake	PD patients were more depressed at intake, posttreatment, and 6-month follow-up.
Sato et al., 1993 [125]	96 outpatients	SCID-II	After at least 2 months of treatment and HRSD <11	PD patients had significantly worse 4-month outcome; strongest association with failure to remit.
Brophy, 1994 [138]	57 inpatients	PAS	Within 3 days of admission	PD patients more depressed or anxious after 2 weeks.
Fava et al., 1994 [119]	83 outpatients	PDQ-R	Pretreatment	Presence of PD was not associated with worse outcome.
Peselow et al., 1994 [144]	68 outpatients	SIDP	Pretreatment and posttreatment—after 4–5 weeks	Recovered patients were lower in Cluster A and C PDs, whereas there was no difference in Cluster B traits before and after treatment.
Sato et al., 1994 [127]	96 outpatients	SCID-II	After at least 2 months of treatment and HRSD <11	Reanalysis and replication of Sato et al., 1993 [125] (i.e., presence of Cluster A PD worsened outcome).
Sullivan et al., 1994 [143]	103 outpatients	SCID-II	Pretreatment	No significant differences across groups in treatment comparisons, despite trend for BPD group to have worse outcome.
Patience et al., 1995 [134]	113 outpatients	PAS	At end of 16-week treatment phase or earlier if HRSD <7	Fewer patients with PD recovered by end of treatment; no difference in recovery rates at follow-up.
Casey et al., 1996 [136]	40 inpatients	PAS	After discharge from hospital	Patients with PD were more depressed and had more social dysfunction at discharge but not at follow-up.
Sato et al., 1999 [95]	117 outpatients	SCID II	After 2 months of treatment	Greater PD co-occurrence in patients with early-onset MDD than in those with late onset.

[a] Structured Interview for DSM Personality Disorders (SIDP), Personality Diagnostic Questionnaire (PDQ), Structured Clinical Interview for DSM Personality Disorders (SCID-II), Personality Assessment Form (PAF), Personality Assessment Schedule (PAS).
[b] Hamilton Rating Scale for Depression (HRSD).
[c] MDD, major depressive disorder; PD, personality disorder.

TABLE 4 Prognostic Comparison of PD in Responders and Nonresponders

Study [Ref.]	Sample	PD measure[a]	Time of assessment[b]	Results and comment[c]
Tyrer et al., 1983 [122]	48 outpatients 12 inpatients	PAS	Pretreatment	Nonresponders were significantly more likely to have a PD compared with responders.
Sauer et al., 1986 [123]	52 inpatients	Clinical interview	"When patients had improved"	PD, sudden onset of depression, and depressive psychotic features were negatively correlated with 21-day outcome and explained 34% of outcome variance.
Frank et al., 1987 [128]	68 outpatients	PAF	During acute treatment at point that HRSD 7 and RDS 5 for 3 consecutive weeks	Slow responders to psychotherapy and medication had more personality pathology.
Thompson et al., 1988 [130]	79 outpatients	SIDP	Within 12 to 24 months following completion of treatment	Non-PD patients were more likely to not meet criteria for depression following treatment with psychotherapy.
Joffe and Regan, 1989 [118]	42 outpatients	MCMI	After 4 weeks of treatment for nonresponders when HRSD <5	Medication responders had higher mean score on antisocial and paranoid scales of MCMI.

Mazure et al., 1990 [117]	52 inpatients	Not reported	Within 3 days of admission	Absence of PD was associated with lack of response to 1-week hospitalization.
Hoencamp et al., 1994 [120]	119 outpatients	SCID-II	Pretreatment	Dependent, self-defeating, passive-aggressive PD associated with worse outcome; obsessive PD associated with better outcome (medication treatment).
Nelson et al., 1994 [126]	119 outpatients	SCID-II	Pretreatment	Presence of PD associated with worse 4-week outcome.
Orgodniczuk et al., 2001 [145]	144 outpatients	SCID-II	Pretreatment	A greater number of PDs was associated with poor outcome across two forms of short-term psychotherapy.

a Millon Clinical Multiaxial Inventory (MCMI-1), Structured Clinical Interview for DSM Personality Disorders (SCID-II), Personality Assessment Form (PAF), Structured Interview for DSM Personality Disorders (SIDP), Personality Assessment Schedule (PAS).
b Hamilton Rating Scale for Depression (HRSD), Raskin Depression Scale (RDS).
c MDD, major depressive disorder; PD, personality disorder.

and that patients with PDs often misperceive clinician behavior and elicit constrained reactions from clinicians [150]. Clinical wisdom suggests that such difficulties should lead to noncompliance. However, most studies of depressed subjects have not analyzed the association between noncompliance and personality disorder, and of studies that did assess compliance [125,131], there is no systematic evidence suggesting the noncompliant patients are more likely to have personality disorders.

CONCLUSION

The relatively high rates of co-occurrence between MDD and personality disorders are indicative of some positive association between these two disorders. Although co-occurrence affords justification for model building, co-occurrence alone makes little contribution to the search for an explanatory model that is consistent with the available data. However, rates of co-occurrence do prompt the continued expenditure of resources on the difficult project of teasing apart the relationship between depression and personality with the hope that current models may be refined, and that a single parsimonious and pragmatic explanatory model may one day become available.

At present, the taxonomy of psychopathology is itself not fixed, and major depression and personality disorders serve as a reminder of the need to continue conducting taxonomic research. Whether or not it is simply a rite of passage to critique the ICD/DSM, and provide a new system, the common language of the ICD/DSM helps despite any co-occurring constraint [151]. Indeed, the utilization of a common metric is as important as critique of the metric itself. Although, the nosology may be common, current assessment procedures are not.

Despite the advent of multiple explanatory models of illness and little to no methodological consensus in regard to personality disorders, some aggregate findings exist that do inform future research and practice. Such a statement in and of itself is noteworthy given the aforementioned difficulties. Taken together, current epidemiological and clinical data may be brought to bear on pessimistic claims that distinctive patterns are not apparent. In particular, there is a clear association between the co-occurrence of a personality disorder and MDD recurrence. Further, there is an indication that other MDD variables such as those found as subtypes and as a specifier (e.g., chronic) are capable of making specific distinctions.

Although no systematic pattern has emerged, global PD pathology is associated with poor prognosis in the treatment of depression. Although each PD cluster is implicated, there are particular findings that are in need of further study. For example, although BPD is linked to recurrence and chronicity, it is also hypothesized to be a motivating factor in the treatment of depression. On the face of it, these two lines of evidence appear to be incompatible, and suggest that motivation itself is in need of study, as Cluster B PDs may not change after treatment for depression, whereas Cluster A and C PDs do appear to change. It may be that what appears to be extraordinary motivation is in fact another sign of BPD.

It can be concluded that chronic depression and PDs often "go" together. In addition to more taxonomic study and model building, future research might continue study of the relationship of chronicity to PDs by comparison of the chronic specifier to the model of chronicity of double depression with recurrent episodes of MDD that increase in severity over time. In addition, longitudinal study is important in order to determine if and how chronic MDD episodes separate from persistent personality pathology. Yet there is a lack of evidence from such an association from which to conclude if chronic depression leads to PD, is caused by PDs, or is simply associated. Such evidence must be forthcoming if we are to answer the question of whether or not PDs may be considered to be a true risk factor leading to the onset of chronic major depression.

REFERENCES

1. Kraepelin E: Manic-Depressive Insanity and Paranoia. Edinburgh, Scotland: Livingstone, 1921.
2. Schneider K: Clinical Psychopathology. London, Grune & Stratton, 1959.
3. Haslam N, Beck AT: Subtyping major depression: a taxometric analysis. J Abnorm Psychol 1994; 103(4):686–692.
4. Hirschfeld RMA: Commentary. In: Personality and Depression: A Current View. Klein MH, Kupfer DJ, Shea MT, eds. New York: Guilford Press, 1993, pp 127–132.
5. Widiger TA: Personality and depression: assessment issues. In: Personality and Depression: A Current View. Klein MH, Kupfer DJ, Shea MT, eds. New York: Guilford Press, 1993, pp 77–118.
6. Diagnostic and Statistical Manual of Mental Disorders. 4th ed. Washington, DC: American Psychiatric Association, 1994.
7. Diagnostic and Statistical Manual of Mental Disorders. 3rd ed. Washington, DC: American Psychiatric Association, 1980.
8. Kendell RE: The Role of Diagnosis in Psychiatry. Oxford, UK: Blackwell, 1975.
9. Morey L: Classification of mental disorder as a collection of hypothetical constructs. J of Abnorm Psychol 1991; 100:289–293.
10. Livesley WJ: Suggestions for a framework for an empirically based classification of personality disorder. Can J Psychiatry 1998; 43:137–147.

11. Feinstein A: The pre-therapeutic classification of comorbidity in chronic disease. J Chronic Dis 1970; 23:455–462.

12. McGlashan TH, Grilo C, Skodol AE, Gunderson JG, Shea MT, Morey LC, Zanarini MC, Stout RL: The collaborative longitudinal personality disorders study: baseline Axis I/II and II/II diagnostic co-occurrence. Acta Psychiatr Scandi 2000; 102:256–264.

13. Hirschfeld RMA: Personality disorders and depression. Depression Anxiety 1999; 10(4):142–146.

14. Ryder AG, Bagby RM: Diagnostic viability of depressive personality disorder: Theoretical and conceptual issues. J Pers Disord 1999; 13:99–117.

15. Widiger T, Frances A: Towards a dimensional model for the personality disorders. In: Personality Disorders and the Five-Factor Model of Personality. Costa P, Widiger T, eds. Washington, DC: American Psychological Association, 1994, pp 19–39.

16. Lyons MJ, Tyrer P, Gunderson J, Tohen M: Special feature: heuristic models of comorbidity of Axis I and Axis II disorders. J Pers Disord 1997; 11(3):260–269.

17. Tyrer P, Gunderson J, Lyons M, Tohen M: Special Feature: Extent of comorbidity between mental state and personality disorders. J Pers Disord 1997; 11(3):242–259.

18. Dolan-Sewell RT, Krueger RF, Shea MT: Co-occurrence with syndrome disorders. In: Handbook of Personality Disorders: Theory, Research, and Treatment. Livesley WJ, eds. New York: Guilford Press, 2001, pp 84–106.

19. Widiger TA, Clark LA: Toward DSM-V and the classification of psychopathology. Psychol Bull 2000; 126(6):946–963.

20. Klein MH, Wonderlich S, Shea MT. Models of relationships between personality and depression: toward a framework for theory and research. In: Personality and Depression: A Current View. Klein MH, Kupfer DJ, Shea MT, eds. New York: Guilford Press, 1993, pp 1–54.

21. Junker BW, Pilkonis PA: Personality and depression: Modeling and Measurement Issues. In: Personality and Depression: A Current View. Klein MH, Kupfer DJ, Shea MT, eds. New York: Guilford Press, 1993, pp 133–170.

22. Barnett PA: Commentary. In: Personality and Depression: A Current View. Klein MH, Kupfer DJ, Shea MT, eds. New York: Guilford Press, 1993, pp 68–76.

23. Westen D, Shedler J: Revising and assessing axis II, Part: II: Toward an empirically based and clinically useful classification of personality disorders. Am Jo Psychiatry 1999; 156(2):273–285.

24. Nurnberg HG, Woodbury MA, Bogenschutz MP: A mathematical typology analysis of DSM-III-R personality disorder classification: grade of membership technique. Compr Psychiatry 1999; 40(1):61–71.

25. Coyne JC, Whiffen VE: Issues in personality as diathesis for depression: the case of sociotropy–dependency and autonomy–self-criticism. Psychol Bull 1995; 118(3):358–378.

26. Zimmerman M, Coryell WH: DSM-III personality disorders dimensions. J Nerv Ment Dis 1990; 178:686–692.

27. Millon T: The disorders of personality. In: Handbook of Personality: Theory and Research. Pervin LA, ed. New York: Guilford Press, 1990, pp 339–370.

28. Livesley WJ, Jang KL, Vernon PA: Phenotypic and genetic structure of traits delineating personality disorder. Arch Gen Psychiatry 1998; 55:941–948.

29. Cattell RB: The integration of functional and psychometric requirements in a quantitative and computerized diagnostic system. In: New approaches to personality classification. Mahrer AR, ed. New York: Columbia University Press, 1970, pp 9–52.

30. Meehl PE: Bootstrap taxometrics: solving the classification problem in psychopathology. Am Psychol 1995; 50: 266–275.

31. Strube MJ: Evidence for the type in type A behavior: a taxometric analysis. Jo Pers Soc Psycholo 1989; 56:972–987.

32. Trull TJ, Widiger TA, Guthrie P: Categorical versus dimensional status of borderline personality disorder. J of Abnorm Psycholo 1990; 99(1):40–48.

33. Livesley WJ: Conceptual and taxonomic issues. In: Handbook of Personality Disorders: Theory, Research, and Treatment. Livesley WJ, ed. New York: Guilford Press, 2001, pp 3–38.

34. Mahrer AR: So many researchers are sincerely scientific about factitious fictions: Some comments on the DSM classification of personality disorders. J Clin Psychol 2000; 56(12):1623–1627.

35. Eysenck HJ: Personality and experimental psychology: the unification of psychology and the possibility of a paradigm. J of Pers Soc Psychol 1997; 73(6):1224–1237.

36. Zimmerman M: Diagnosing personality disorders: A review of issues and research methods. Arch Gen Psychiatry 1994; 51:225–245.

37. Dowson JH: Assessment of DSM-IIIR personality disorders by self-report questionnaire: The role of informants and a screening test for co-morbid personality disorders (STCPD). Br J Psychiatry 1992; 161:344–352.

38. Zimmerman M, Pfohl B, Coryell W, Stangl D, Corenthal C: Diagnosing personality disorder in depressed patients. Arch Gen Psychiatry 1988; 45:733–737.

39. Zimmerman M, Pfohl BM, Coryell WH, Stangl D, Corenthal C: Personality disorder diagnosis: who should be interviewed? Presented at 143rd Annual Meeting of the American Psychiatric Association, New York, 1990.

40. Rapaport D, Gill MM, Schafer R: Diagnostic Psychological Testing. New York: International Universities Press, 1972.

41. Gunderson JG, Kolb JE, Austin V: The diagnostic interview for borderlines. Am J of Psychiatry 1981; 138:896–903.

42. Kendler KS, Liberman JA, Walsh D: The structured interview for schizotypy (SIS): a preliminary report. Schizophr Bull 1989; 15:559–571.

43. Pfohl B, Blum N, Zimmerman M: Structured Interview for DSM-IV Personality. Washington, DC: American Psychiatric Press, 1997.

44. Loranger AW: Personality Disorder Examination (PDE) Manual. Yonkers, NY: DV Communications, 1988.

45. Millon T: Manual for the Millon Clinical Multiaxial Inventory-III (MCMI-III). Minneapolis, National Computer Systems, 1994.

46. Fossati A, Maffei C, Bagnato M, Donati D, Donini M, Fiorilli M, Novella L, Ansoldi M: Brief communication: criterion validity of the Personality Diagnostic Questionnaire-4+(PDQ-4+) in a mixed psychiatric sample. J Pers Disords 1998; 12(2):172–178.

47. Maffei C, Fossati A, Agostoni I, Barraco A, Bagnato M, Deborah D, Namia C, Novella L, Petrachi M: Interrater reliability and internal consistency of the structured clinical interview for DSM-IV axis II personality disorders (SCID-II), version 2.0. J Pers Disord 1997; 11(3):279–84.

48. Zanarini MC, Skodol AE, Bender D, Dolan R, Sanislow C, Schaefer E, Morey LC, Grilo CM, Shea MT, McGlashan TH, Gunderson JG: The Collaborative Longitudinal Personality Disorders Study: reliability of axis I and II diagnoses. J Pers Disord 2000; 14(4):291–299.

49. Morey LC: An Interpretive Guide to the Personality Assessment Inventory (PAI). Odessa, FL: Psychological Assessment Resources, 1996.

50. Gabbard GO: Finding the "person" in personality disorders. Am J Psychiatry 1997; 154(7):891–893.

51. Westen D, Shedler J: Revising and Assessing Axis II, Part I: Developing a clinically and empirically valid assessment method. Am J of Psychiatry 1999; 156(2):258–272.

52. Pilkonis PA, Hepe CL, Ruddy J, Serrao P: Validity in the diagnosis of personality disorders: The use of the LEAD standard. J Consult Clin Psychol 1991; 3(1):46–54.

53. O'Boyle M, Self D: A comparison of two interviews for DSM-IIIR personality disorders. Psychiatry Res 1990; 32:85–92.

54. Oldham JM, Skodol AE, Kellman HD, Hyler SE, Rosnick L, Davies M: Diagnosis of DSM-IIR personality disorders by two structured interviews: Patterns of comorbidity. Am J Psychiatry 1992; 149(2):213–220.

55. Shectman F: Problems in communicating psychological understanding: why won't they listen to me?! Am Psycholo 1979; 34(9):781–790.

56. Zimmerman M, Coryell W, Black DW: A method to detect intercenter differences in the application of contemporary diagnostic criteria. J Nerv Ment Dis 1993; 181:130–134.

57. Kasch KL, Klein DN: The relationship between age at onset and comorbidity in psychiatric disorders. J Nerv Ment Dis 1996; 184(11):703–707.

58. Schober MF: Does conversational interviewing reduce survey measurement error? Public Opin Q 1998;61(4):576–602.

59. Santor DA, Bagby RM, Joffer RT: Evaluating stability and change in personality and depression. J Pers Soc Psychol 1997; 73(6):1354–1362.

60. Stuart S, Simons AD, Thase ME, Pilkonis P: Are personality assessments valid in acute major depression. J Affect Disord 1992; 24(4):281–289.

61. Ames-Frankel J, Devlin MJ, Walsh BT, Strasser TJ, Sadik C, Oldham JM, Roose SP: Personality disorder diagnosis in patients with bulimia nervosa: clinical correlates and changes with treatment. J Clin Psychiatry 1992; 53(3): 90–96.

62. Ricciardi JN, Baer L, Jenike MA, Fischer SC, Sholtz D, Buttolph ML:

Changes in DSM-III-R axis II diagnoses following treatment of obsessive-compulsive disorder. Am J Psychiatry 1992; 149(6):829–831.

63. McDermut W, Zimmerman M: The effects of personality disorders on outcome in the treatment of depression. In: Mood and Anxiety Disorders. Rush AJ (ed). Philadelphia: Williams & Wilkins, 1998, pp 321–338.

64. Berkson J: Limitations of the application of fourfold table analysis to hospital data. Biometrics Bull 1946; 2(3):47–53.

65. Paris J: Personality disorders in sociocultural perspective. J Pers Disord 1998: 12(4):289–301.

66. Sullivan PF, Kessler RC, Kendler KS: Latent class analysis of lifetime depressive symptoms in the National Comorbidity Survey. Am J Psychiatry 1998; 155:1398–1406.

67. Johnson JG, Cohen P, Skodol AE, Oldham JM, Kasen S, Brook JS: Personality disorders in adolescence and risk of major mental disorders and suicidality during adulthood. Arch Gen Psychiatry 1999; 56:805–811.

68. Lewinsohn PM, Rohde P, Seeley JR, Klein DN: Axis II Psychopathology as a function of axis I disorders in childhood and adolescence. J Am Acad Child Adolesc Psychiatry 1997; 36(12):1752–1759.

69. Lenzenweger MF: Stability and change in personality disorder features: the longitudinal study of personality disorders. Arch of Gen Psychiatry 1999; 56:1009–1015.

70. Kasen S, Cohen P, Skodol AE, Johnson JG, Brook JS: Influence of child and adolescent psychiatric disorders on young adult personality disorder. Am J Psychiatry 1999; 156(10):1529–1535.

71. Zimmerman M, Coryell W: DSM-III personality disorder diagnosis in a nonpatient sample: demographic correlates and comorbidity. Arch Gen Psychiatry 1989; 46:682–689.

72. Daley SE, Hammen C, Burge D, Davila J, Paley B, Linderg N, Herzberg DS: Depression and axis II symptomatology in an adolescent community sample: concurrent and longitudinal associations. J Pers Dis 1999; 13(1):47–59.

73. Daley SE, Hammen C, Davila J, Burge D: Axis II Symptomatology, depression, and life stress during the transition form adolescence to adulthood. J Consult Clin Psychol 1998; 66(4):595–603.

74. Gustafsson L, Jacobsson L: On mental disorder and somatic disease in suicide: a psychological autopsy study of 100 suicides in northern Sweden. Nordic J Psychiatry 2000; 54(6):383–395.

75. Heikkinen ME, Henriksson MM, Isometsa ET, Marttunen MJ, Aro HM, Lonnqvist JK: Recent life events and suicide in personality disorders. J Nerv Ment Dis 1997; 185(6):373–381.

76. Carter JD, Joyce PR, Mulder RT, Sullivan PF, Luty SE: Gender differences in the frequency of personality disorders in depressed outpatients. J Pers Disord 1999; 13(1):67–74.

77. Farmer R, Nelson-Gray RO: Personality disorders and depression: hypothetical relations, empirical findings, and methodological considerations. Clin Psychol Rev 1990; 10:453–476.

78. Kool S, Dekker J, Duijsens IJ, Jonghe Fd: Major depression, double depression, and personality disorders. J Pers Disord 2000; 14(3):274–281.

79. Sato T, Sakado K, Uehara T, Sato S, Nishioka K, Kasahara Y: Personality disorder diagnosis using DSM-IIIR in a Japanese clinical sample with major depression. Acta Psychiatr Scandi 1997; 95:451–453.

80. Dunayevich E, Sax KW, P E Keck J, McElroy SL, Sorter MT, McConville BJ, Strakowski SM: Twelve-month outcome in bipolar patients with and without personality disorders. J Clin Psychiatry 2000; 61(2):134–139.

81. Ferro T, Klein DN, Schwartz JE, Kasch KL, Leader JB: 30-Month stability of personality disorder diagnosis in depressed outpatients. Am J Psychiatry 1998; 155(5):653–659.

82. Rossi A, Marinangeli MG, Butti G, Scinto A, Cicco LD, Kalyvoka A, Petruzzi C: Personality disorders in bipolar and depressive disorders. J Affect Disord 2001; 65:3–8.

83. Oulis P, Lykouras L, Hatzimanolis J, Tomaras V: Comorbidity of DSM-IIR personality disorders in schizophrenic and unipolar mood disorders: a comparative study. Eur Psychiatry 1997; 12(6):316–318.

84. Brooner RK, King VL, Kidorf M, Schmidt CW, Bigelow GE: Psychiatric and substance use comorbidity among treatment-seeking opioid abusers. Archi Gen Psychiatry 1997; 54:1997.

85. Chen C, Tsai S, Su L, Yang T, Tsai C, Hwu H: Psychiatric comorbidity among male heroin addicts: differences between hospital and incarcerated subjects in Taiwan. Addiction 1999; 94(6):825–832.

86. Zanarini MC, Frankenburg FR, Dubo ED, Sickel AE, Trikha A, Levin A, Reynolds V: Axis I comorbidity in borderline personality disorder. Am J Psychiatry 1998; 155(12):1733–1739.

87. Grilo CM, Walker ML, Becker DF, Edell WS, McGlashan TH: Personality disorders in adolescents with major depression, substance use disorders, and coexisting major depression and substance use disorders. J Consult Clin Psychol 1997; 65(2):238–232.

88. Striegel-Moore RH, Garvin V, Dohm FA, Rosenheck RA: Eating disorders in a national sample of hospitalized female and male veterans: detection rates and psychiatric comorbidity. Int J Eating Disord 1999; 25(4):405–414.

89. Skodol AE, Stout RL, McGlashan TH, Grilo CM, Gunderson JG, Shea MT, Morey LC, Zanarini MC, Dyck IR, Oldham JM: Co-occurrence of mood and personality disorders: a report from the collaborative longitudinal personality disorders study (CLPS). Depression Anxiety 1999; 10:175–182.

90. Bunce SC, Coccaro E: Factors differentiating personality disordered individuals with and without a history of unipolar mood disorder. Depression Anxiety 1999; 10(4):147–157.

91. Stormberg D, Rojnningstam E, Gunderson J, Tohen M: Brief Communication: Pathological narcissism in bipolar disorder patients. J Pers Disord 1998; 12(2):179–185.

92. Langs G, Quehenberger F, Fabisch K, Klug G, Fabisch H, Zapotoczky HG: Prevalence, patterns and role of personality disorders in panic disorder

patients with and without comorbid (lifetime) major depression. Acta Psychiatri Scandi 1998; 98:116–123.

93. Gude T, Vaglum P: One-year follow-up of patients with cluster C personality disorders: a prospective study comparing patients with "pure" and comorbid conditions within cluster C, and "pure" C with "pure" cluster A or B conditions. J Pers Dis 2001; 15(3):216–228.

94. Alnaes R, Torgersen S: Personality and personality disorders predict development and relapses of major depression. Acta Psychiatr Scand 1997; 95:336–342.

95. Sato T, Sakado K, Uehara T, Narita T, Hirano S: Personality disorder comorbidity in early-onset versus late-onset major depression in Japan. J Nerv Ment Dis 1999; 187(4):237–242.

96. Vieta E: Personality disorders in bipolar II patients. J Nerv Ment Dis 1999; 187(4):245–248.

97. Fava M, Alpert JE, Borus JS, Nierenberg AA, Pava JA, Rosenbaum JF: Patterns of personality disorder comorbidity in early-onset versus late-onset major depression. Am J Psychiatry 1996; 153(10):1308–1312.

98. Ucok A, Karaveli D, Kundakci T, Yazici O: Comorbidity of personality disorders wiht bipolar mood disorders. Compr Psychiatry 1998; 39(2):72–74.

99. Garyfallos G, Adamopoulou A, Karastergiou A, Voikli M, Sotiropoulou A, Donias S, Giouzepas J, Paraschos A: Personality disorders in dysthymia and major depression. Acta Psychiatr Scand 1999; 99:332–340.

100. Haw C, Hawton K, Houston K, Townsend E: Psychiatric and personality disorders in deliberate self-harm patients. Br J Psychiatry 2001; 178:48–54.

101. Arte-Vaidya N, Hussain SM: Borderline Personality Disorder and bipolar mood disorder: two distinct disorders or a continuum? J Nerv Ment Dis 1999; 187(5):313–315.

102. Akiskal HS, Maser JD, Zeller PJ, Endicott J, Coryell W, Keller M, Warshaw M, Clayton P, Goodwin F: Switching from 'unipolar' to bipolar II: an 11 year prospective study of clinical and temperamental predictors in 559 patients. Arch Gen Psychiatry 1995; 52:114–123.

103. Gunderson JG, Phillips KA: A current view of the interface between borderline personality disorder and depression. Am J Psychiatry 1991; 148:967–975.

104. Westen D, Moses MJ, Silk KR, Lohr NE, Cohen R, Segal H: Quality of depressive experience in borderline personality disorder and major depression: When depression is not just depression. J Pers Disorders 1992; 6:382–393.

105. Westen D: Affect regulation and psychopathology: applications to depression and borderline personality disorder. In: Emotions in Psychopathology: Theory and Research. WF Flack J, Laird JD, ed. New York: Oxford University Press, 1998, pp 394–406.

106. Hartlage S, Arduino K, Alloy LB: Depressive personality characteristics state dependent concomitants of depressive disorder and traits independent of current depression. J Abnorm Psychol 1998; 107(2):349–354.

107. Huprich SK: Depressive personality disorder: theoretical issues, clinical findings, and future research questions. Clini Psychol Rev 1998; 18(5):477–500.

108. Klein DN: Depressive personality in the relatives of outpatients wiht dys-

thymic disorder and episodic major depressive disorder and normal controls. J Affect Disord 1999; 55:19–27.

109. Klein DN, Shih JH: Depressive personality associations with DSM III-R mood and personality disorders and negative and positive affectivity, 30-month stability, and prediction of course of axis I depressive disorders. J of Abnorm Psychol 1998; 107(2):319–327.

110. Kwon JS, Kim YM, Chang CG, Park BJ, Kim L, Yoon DJ, Han WS, Lee HJ, Lyoo IK: Three-year follow-up of women with the sole diagnosis of depressive personality disorder: Subsequent development of dysthymia and major depression. Am J Psychiatry 2000; 157:1966–1972.

111. Lyoo IK, Gunderson JG, Phillips KA: Personality dimensions associated with depressive personality disorder. J Pers Disord 1998; 12(1):46–55.

112. Phillips KA, Gunderson JG, Triebwasser J, Kimble CR, Faedda G, Lyoo K, Renn J: Reliability and validity of depressive personality disorder. Am J Psychiatry 1998; 155:1044–1048.

113. Phillips KA, Gunderson JG: Depressive personality disorder: fact or fiction. J Pers Disord 1999; 13(2):128–134.

114. Frances AJ: The DSM-III personality disorders section: a commentary. Am J Psychiatry 1980; 137:1050–1054.

115. Widiger TA: Depressive personality traits and dysthymia: a commentary on Ryder and Bagby. Jo of Pers Disord 1999; 13(2):135–141.

116. Livesley J: Depressive personality disorder: an introduction. J Pers Disord 1999; 13(2):97–98.

117. Mazure CM, Nelson JC, Jatlow PI: Predictors of hospital outcome without antidepressants in major depression. Psychiatry Res 1990; 33(1):51–58.

118. Joffe RT, Regan JJ: Personality and response to tricyclic antidepressants in depressed patients. J Nerv Ment Disord 1989; 177(12):745–749.

119. Fava M, Bouffides E, Pava JA, McCarthy MK, Steingard RJ, Rosenbaum JF: Personality disorder comorbidity with major depression and response to fluoxetine treatment. Psychother Psychosom 1994; 62:160–167.

120. Hoencamp E, Haffmans PMJ, Duivenvoorden H, Knegtering H, Dijken WA: Predictors of (non-)response in depressed outpatients treated with three-phase sequential medication strategy. J Affect Disord 1994; 31:235–246.

121. Charney DS, Nelson JC, Qunlan DN: Personality traits and disorder in depression. Am J Psychiatry 1981; 138:1601–1604.

122. Tyrer P, Casey P, Gall J: Relationship between neurosis and personality disorder. Br J Psychiatry 1983; 142:404–408.

123. Sauer H, Kick H, Minne HW, al e: Prediction of amitirptyline response: psychopathology vs. neroendocrinology. Int Clin Psychopharmacol 1986(1): 284–295.

124. Peselow ED, Fieve RR, DiFiglia C: Personality traits and response to desipramine. J Affect Disord 1992; 24:209–216.

125. Sato T, Sakado K, Sato S: Is there any specific personality disorder or personality disorder cluster that worsens the short-term treatment outcome of major depression? Acta Psychiatr Scand 1993; 88:342–349.

126. Nelson JC, Mazure CM, Jatlow PI: Characteristics of desipramine-refractory depression. J Clin Psychiatry 1994; 55(1):12–9.

127. Sato T, Sakado K, Sato S, Morikawa T: Cluster A personality disorder: a marker of worse treatment outcome of major depression? Psychiatry Res 1994; 53:153–159.

128. Frank E, Kupfer DJ, Jacob M: Personality features and response to acute treatment in recurrent depression. J Pers Disord 1987; 1:14–26.

129. Pilkonis PA, Frank E: Personality pathology in recurrent depression: nature, prevalence, and relationship to treatment response. Am J Psychiatry 1988; 145:435–441.

130. Thompson L, Gallagher D, Czirr R: Personality disorder and outcome in the treatment of late-life depression. J Geriatr Psychiatry 1988; 21:133–146.

131. Shea MT, Pilkonis PA, Beckham E, Collins JF, Elkin I, Sotsky SM, Docherty JP: Personality disorders and treatment outcome in the NIMH treatment of depression collaborative research program. Am J Psychiatry 1990; 147:711–718.

132. Diguer L, Barber JP, Luborsky L: Three concomitants: personality disorders, psychiatric severity, and outcome of dynamic psychotherapy of major depression. Am J Psychiatry 1993; 150(8):1246–1248.

133. Hardy GE, Barkham M, Shapiro DA, et al.: Impact of cluster C disorder on outcomes of contrasting brief psychotherapies for depression. J Consult Clin Psychol 1995; 63:997–1004.

134. Patience DA, McGuire RJ, Scott AIF, et al. The Edinburgh Primary Care Depression Study: personality disorder and outcome. Br J Psychiatry 1995; 167:324–330.

135. Zimmerman M, Coryell W, Pfohl B, Corenthal C, Stangl D: ECT response in depressed patients with and without a DSM-III personality disorder. Am J Psychiatry 1986; 143:1030–1032.

136. Casey P, Meagher D, Butler E: Personality, functioning, and recovery from major depression. J Nerv Ment Dis 1996; 184:240–245.

137. Reich JH: Effect of DSM-III personality disorders on outcome of tricyclic antidepressant-treated nonpsychotic outpatients with major or minor depressive disorder. Psychiatry Res 1990; 32:175–181.

138. Brophy JJ: Personality disorder, symptoms and dexamethasone suppression in depression. J Affect Disord 1994; 31:19–27.

139. Pfohl B, Stangl D, Zimmerman M: The implications of DSM-III personality disorders for patients with major depression. J Affect Disord 1984; 7:309–318.

140. Black DW, Bell S, Hulbert J, Nasrallah A: The importance of axis II in patients with major depression: a controlled study. J Affect Disord 1988; 14:115–122.

141. Pfohl B, Coryell W, Zimmerman M, et al. Prognostic validity of self-report and interview measures of personality disorder in depressed patients. J Clin Psychiatry 1987; 48:468–472.

142. Shea MT, Widiger TA, Klein MH: Comorbidity of personality disorders and depression: implications for treatment. J Consult Clin Psychol 1992; 60:857–868.

143. Sullivan PF, Joyce PR, Mulder RT: Borderline personality disorder in major depression. J Nerv Ment Dis 1994; 182(9):508–516.
144. Peselow ED, Sanfilipo MP, Fieve RR, Gulbenkian G: Personality traits during depression and after clinical recovery. Bri J Psychiatry 1994; 164:349–354.
145. Ogrodniczuk JS, Piper WE, Joyce AS, McCallum M: Using DSM Axis II information to predict outcome in short-term individual psychotherapy. J Perso Disord 2001; 15(2):110–122.
146. Perry JC, Banon E, Ianni F: Effectiveness of psychotherapy for personality disorders. Am J Psychiatry 1999; 156(9):1312–1321.
147. Wilberg T, Karterud S, Urnes O, Pedersen G, Friis S: Outcomes of poorly functioning patients with personality disorders in a day treatment program. Psychiatr Serv 1998; 49(11):1462–1467.
148. Chiesa M, Fonagy P: Cassel personality disorder study: Methodology and treatment effects. Br J Psychiatry 2000; 176:485–491.
149. Keller MB, Gelenberg AJ, Hirschfeld RMA, Rush AJ, Thase ME, Kocsis JH, Markowitz JC, Fawcett JA, Koran LM, Klein DN, Russell JM, Kornstein SG, McCullough JP, Davis SM, Harrison WM: The treatment of chronic depression, Part 2: A double-blind, randomized trial of Sertraline and Imipramine. J Clin Psychiatry 1998; 59(11):598–607.
150. Wagner CC, Riley WT, Schmidt JA, McCormick MGF, Butler SF: Personality disorder styles and reciprocal interpersonal impacts during outpatient intake interviews. Psychother Res 1999; 9(2):216–231.
151. Widiger TA: Official classification systems. In: Handbook of Personality Disorders: Theory, Research, and Treatment. Livesley WJ, ed. New York: Guilford Press, 2001, pp 60–83.

3

Vulnerability to Chronic Depression: A Review and Preliminary Model

Lawrence P. Riso

Georgia State University
Atlanta, Georgia, U.S.A.

Daniel N. Klein

State University of New York at Stony Brook
Stony Brook, New York, U.S.A.

INTRODUCTION

Although depression has traditionally been conceptualized as an episodic, remitting condition, recent epidemiological studies of community samples and longitudinal studies of depressed patients indicate that a substantial number of individuals suffer from chronic forms of depression. For example, in the National Comorbidity Study, Kessler et al. [1] found that over 6% of a nationally representative community sample had experienced chronic depressions at some point in their lives. In the longitudinal follow-up component of the National Institute of Mental Health (NIMH) Collaborative Depression Study, over 19% of depressed patients experienced a chronic course with episodes lasting at least 2 years, and 7% still had not recovered after 8 years [2,3]. In light of this high prevalence, it is critical to elucidate the vulnerability factors that predispose to chronic depression and the processes that maintain depression after onset.

In the first section of this chapter, we discuss various definitional and conceptual issues in chronic depression. In the following sections, we review the findings for six key risk factors, including familial psychopathology, early adversity, temperament/personality, cognitive factors, interpersonal factors, and chronic stress. Finally, we conclude by offering our own conceptual framework for understanding the origins and development of chronic depression.

DEFINITIONAL AND CONCEPTUAL ISSUES

Chronic depression has been defined in a variety of ways. In this chapter, we will rely on the Diagnostic and Statistical Manual of Mental Disorders DSM-III-R and DSM-IV definitions of chronic depression, which include two major categories: Major Depressive Disorder (MDD), chronic type, and Dysthymic Disorder (DD). Both chronic MDD and DD require a duration of 2 years or longer (although DD can have a duration of only 1 year in children or adolescents) with no more than a 2-month period of remission. The symptom criteria for both diagnoses overlap, but chronic MDD requires a greater number of symptoms than DD. The majority of individuals with DD experience exacerbations meeting criteria for a MDD episode at some point in their lives [4,5]; a pattern that has been referred to as double depression [6]. However, a diagnosis of DD is made only if there were no MDD episodes in the first 2 years of the disturbance. In this way, DD is restricted to individuals with an insidious or gradual onset.

As we discuss below, there is considerable evidence that chronic depressions differ from episodic forms of MDD in many respects. However, at the present time, there is little evidence of significant differences between the various forms of chronic depression. For example, patients with DD and double depression are generally similar with respect to family history of mood and personality disorders [7], childhood adversity [8], Axis I and II comorbidity [9,10], and course and outcome [5,11]. In addition, patients with double depression and chronic MDD are similar with respect to demographics, severity, most indicators of clinical course and psychosocial impairment, comorbidity, family history, and response to antidepressant medication [12]. Hence, in this chapter, we will use the broader rubric of chronic depression rather than emphasizing the finer-grained distinctions between the DSM categories of chronic MDD, DD, and MDD superimposed on DD.

Although there is a large body of literature on predictors of the short-term course and outcome of MDD, there are almost no prospective studies exploring predictors for the development of chronic depression. Thus, we have been forced to rely primarily on cross-sectional studies and longitudinal studies that began after participants had already experienced some degree of chronicity. Most of this research has focused on DD and double depression rather than on chronic MDD. Most studies have compared chronic forms of depression to episodic MDD. However, some have compared DD and double depression to MDD in general without indicating whether patients with chronic MDD were excluded.

There are a variety of variables that distinguish chronic from episodic depression. In this chapter, we will emphasize variables that are likely to play a causal role in the development of chronic depression. We have chosen not to include biological variables in our review. This is not because biological variables are unlikely to contribute to the development of chronic depression, but because the literature on biological risk factors in chronic depression is still quite limited and permits few firm conclusions [13,14]. In addition, we will attempt to distinguish between variables that play a qualitative versus quantitative role in the development of chronic, as opposed to episodic, depressions. Variables that play a qualitative role are specific to chronic depression; that is, they distinguish individuals with chronic depressions from those with episodic depressions, but do not differentiate persons with episodic depression from nondepressed individuals. Variables that play a quantitative role also distinguish individuals with chronic depression from those with episodic depression; however, persons with episodic depression differ significantly from nondepressed individuals. Thus, quantitative risk variables play a role in episodic depression but an even stronger role in chronic depression.

POTENTIAL VULNERABILITY FACTORS

Familial Aggregation

There is some evidence that a family history of mood disorders is associated with a poorer course and outcome in follow-up studies of MDD [15–18]. Consistent with this notion, the relatives of patients with chronic depression have higher rates of depressive disorders than the relatives of patients with episodic depressions [19,20]. The elevated rate of mood disorders in the relatives of patients with chronic depression appears to be largely attributable to an increased rate of DD in relatives of patients with chronic compared to episodic depression [20]. Interestingly, the rates of chronic depression in the relatives of episodic depressives and normal controls are similar [20], suggesting that there is specificity of familial aggregation of chronic depression. The evidence for specificity of aggregation of chronic depression is supported by two other studies reporting an increased rate of chronic depression in the relatives of individuals with chronic compared to episodic depressions [21,22].

Finally, familial loading of DD, but not MDD, predicted a poorer course in a 5-year follow-up of outpatients with chronic depression [11]. Taken together, these findings suggest that family history of chronic depression may be a qualitative risk factor for chronic depression.

Family history of personality disorders may also increase the risk for chronic depression. Klein et al. [20] found that outpatients with chronic depression had a significantly higher rate of personality disorders in their relatives compared to patients with episodic MDD. However, probands with episodic MDD had a significantly higher rate of personality disorders in relatives than normal controls, indicating that this is a quantitative rather than qualitative risk factor.

Few twin and adoption data on chronic depression are available. Thus, at this point, it is impossible to disentangle genetic from environmental influences on the familial transmission of chronic depression.

Early Adversity

A number of studies have reported that childhood adversity, including experiences such as sexual and physical abuse and parental neglect, indifference, and rejection, is associated with a poorer course and outcome in MDD [23–30]. It is of note that several studies have reported greater childhood adversity in patients with chronic than episodic depressions [8,31,32]. Importantly, this finding does not appear to be due to the effects of comorbid personality disorders [8]. Finally, among outpatients with chronic depression, early adversity predicted a poorer course and outcome in a 5-year follow-up [11]. Since patients with episodic MDD also report having experienced greater childhood adversity than normal controls [8], early adversity may be a quantitative rather than a qualitative risk factor for chronic depression. Indeed, early adversity appears to influence a broad spectrum of psychopathology, and is associated with an increased risk for a number of non–mood disorders [33,34].

Several methodological issues warrant consideration in evaluating these data. First, all of these studies assessed childhood adversity retrospectively while patients were experiencing significant depressive symptomatology [13]. Although long-term prospective studies are needed, there is substantial evidence that retrospective reports of early adversity are at least moderately accurate, and are not influenced by clinical state at the time of the assessment [35,36].

Second, numerous studies have documented that parents with mood disorders and other forms of psychopathology exhibit significant deficits in their parenting behavior [37,38]. Thus, it is conceivable that the relationship between chronic depression and early adversity is attributable to the greater familial loading of mood and personality disorders in the families of chronic depressives. However, a recent study found that the differences in childhood adversity between patients with chronic and episodic depressions persisted even after controlling for parental psychopathology [39]. Similarly, Hayden and Klein [11] reported that childhood adversity continued to predict the course of chronic depression after controlling for parental psychopathology.

Given that the association between childhood adversity and chronic depression is not explained by parental psychopathology, it is also conceivable that it mediates or moderates the effects of psychopathology in parents. For example, parental psychopathology may increase the risk to offspring by increasing maladaptive parenting behavior and family conflict (mediation), or parental psychopathology may interact with childhood adversity by increasing the risk to offspring (moderation). However, Lizardi and Klein [39] did not find evidence of mediation or moderation, and they concluded that familial liability and early adversity represented independent influences on chronic depression.

Childhood adversity often antedates chronic depression by many years. This makes it less likely that childhood adversity has direct effects on chronicity. Rather the influence of childhood adversity is likely to be mediated by more proximal processes. For example, childhood adversity may influence personality and personality disorders [40,41], interpersonal styles [25], and styles of information processing [42,43], which in turn increase the risk for chronic depression. There is also evidence that childhood adversity can have long-term effects on neurobiological functioning that may increase the risk for depression [44].

Another potential effect of early adversity is its impact on attachment representations. Patients with DD and no comorbid borderline personality disorder exhibit high rates of insecure attachment that are similar to patients with borderline personality disorder (and no DD) [45]. Moreover, there are higher rates of insecure attachment in DD than MDD [46]. Unfortunately, studies of attachment in chronic depression have tended to assess subjects while they are acutely ill. Moreover, the extent to which attachment representations reflect current relationship functioning versus internal working models of relationships remains unclear [47].

Temperament, Personality, and Personality Disorders

During the past century, a number of prominent clinical investigators have argued that particular types of temperament, including the depressive, hypomanic, cyclothymic, and irritable (i.e., mixed depressive and hypomanic) temperaments, are precursors of the major mood disorders [48–50].

Of these, the depressive temperament has been the focus of the greatest empirical research. The depressive temperament (also referred to as the depressive personality) includes such characteristics as a usual mood of dejection, gloominess, and joylessness; feelings of inadequacy and low-self-esteem; proneness to being self-critical and self-derogatory; brooding and being given to worry; negativism and being judgmental of others; pessimism; and proneness to feelings of guilt and remorse [48,51,52]. Although the depressive temperament overlaps considerably with milder forms of chronic depression such as DD, the two constructs are conceptually and empirically distinguishable [53,54].

Although many studies have documented an association between depressive temperament and depressive disorders in general [53], several studies have indicated that the relationship may be specific to chronic forms of depression. Thus, Klein et al. [21] found that depressive personality traits in the offspring of depressed individuals were related to chronic forms of depression in parents. More recently, Klein [55] reported that there was a significantly higher level of depressive personality traits in the relatives of patients with chronic depression than in the relatives of patients with episodic MDD and the relatives of normal controls, who did not differ from each other. Finally, a prospective study [56] found that depressive personality traits predicted the first lifetime onset of DD but not MDD. Taken together, these findings suggest that depressive personality traits may be a qualitative risk factor for chronic forms of depression.

Although depressive personality has typically been conceptualized as a temperamental substrate for mood disorders, it likely represents a socially and cognitively mediated elaboration of more fundamental temperamental processes [57]. In order to delineate these more fundamental processes, it may be helpful to draw on concepts and measures of temperament from the literature on child development.

Contemporary models of child temperament tend to emphasize individual differences in emotionality [58,59]. The two temperament traits that have received the most attention with regard to risk for mood disorders in the developmental literature are low positive emotionality (PE) and behavioral inhibition. There is some overlap between these constructs. Low PE refers to low levels of positive affects including diminished enthusiasm and joy, energy, affiliation, and dominance [60]. Behavioral inhibition refers to wariness/fear, diminished activity, and a lack of approach in novel situations [61]. Several studies have reported that the infants and young children of parents with depressive disorders exhibit lower PE and greater behavioral inhibition than offspring of nondepressed parents [62–64]. Moreover, Neff and Klein [65] found that among the toddlers of mothers with a history of MDD, low child PE was significantly correlated with chronicity of maternal depression even after controlling for the mother's style of interacting with their child.

Several prospective studies have also reported data suggesting that low PE and behavioral inhibition predict the subsequent development of depressive disorders, particularly chronic depression. Caspi et al. [66] reported that children rated as socially reticent, inhibited, and easily upset at age 3 had elevated rates of depressive (but not anxiety or substance use) disorders at age 21. Similarly, van Os et al. [67] found that physicians' ratings of behavioral apathy at ages 6, 7, and 11 years predicted chronic depression in middle adulthood. Finally, Gjerde [68] found that experts' Q-sort ratings of shyness and withdrawal in 3 to 4 year-old children predicted self-reported chronic depressive symptoms at age 23 years in women, although not in men.

These data are consistent with recent work on adult personality and depression. Most models of adult personality structure include the higher order dimensions of PE and negative emotionality (NE). Negative emotionality overlaps with, but is broader than, the construct of behavioral inhibition. It reflects sensitivity to negative stimuli, resulting in a range of negative moods, including sadness, fear, anxiety, guilt, and anger [60].

Watson and Clark [69] have hypothesized that low PE and high NE form the core of the depressive temperament and predispose to depressive disorders. This model has received some support in the literature. Thus, persons with MDD tend to report diminished levels of PE even after they have recovered, and NE appears to predict the subsequent onset of a first lifetime depressive episode (see Ref. 57 for a review).

PE and NE may play a particularly important role in chronic forms of depression. A number of studies have reported that increased levels of NE predict a poorer course and outcome of depression over periods ranging up to 18 years [27,70,71]. In addition, several studies have reported that individuals with chronic depression report lower levels of PE and higher levels of NE than persons with episodic MDD both while in episode [72] and after recovery [73]. Finally, Hayden and Klein [11] found that higher NE was associated with a poorer 5-year outcome in DD.

There is also strong evidence for a link between chronic depression and Axis II personality disorders. Thus, personality disorders predict a poorer course of depression [74], as well as a poorer outcome in chronic depression [11]. In addition, a number of studies have reported increased rates of personality disorders in patients with chronic compared to episodic depression [75–77]. The most common personality disorders in chronic depression are from DSM-IV Cluster B, particularly borderline and histrionic, and Cluster C, especially avoidant and dependent. Importantly, similar findings have been obtained with both patients' and informants' reports [75]. However, the rate of personality disorders also appears to be elevated in episodic depressions [78], suggesting that this is probably a quantitative rather than qualitative risk factor.

The mechanisms linking temperament and personality disorders to chronicity of depression are unclear. Akiskal [4] has suggested that there are at least two distinct pathways to chronic depression—one associated with the depressive temperament and the other associated with unstable, or Cluster B, personality disorders. However, this typology has not been confirmed in recent studies [79,80]. Another possibility is that both depressive temperament and personality disorders have a shared genetic or family environmental liability. For example, there is evidence for shared familial etiological influences for DD and Cluster B personality disorders [81]. Alternatively, temperament/personality may have a direct influence on depression [82]. Finally, temperamental and personality factors may influence other variables, such as social functioning and stress [83–85], that contribute to the persistence of depression.

Interpersonal Factors

Coyne has long argued that interpersonal difficulties play an important role in prolonging depressive episodes [86,87]. According to Coyne's theory, the depressed individual has a negative impact on others, particularly family members and friends, by excessively seeking assurances of love and support. These excessive demands often become aversive and begin to erode important relationships. The depressed individual perceives that the support he or she is receiving is diminishing and escalates his or her demands on others, resulting in an increasingly vicious cycle.

Research examining interactions with depressed individuals provides some support for Coyne's theory [87]. However, most of these studies have focused on relationships with strangers or recent acquaintances rather than family members and close friends, and few studies have examined these processes longitudinally over periods of longer than a few weeks [88]. As a result, there are no studies specifically testing the importance of Coyne's theory in the development or maintenance of chronic forms of depression.

Joiner [89] has further elaborated on the interpersonal processes described by Coyne [86]. Joiner distinguishes between erosive and self-propagating processes. Erosive processes involve the passive loss of personal and social resources, whereas self-propagatory processes are more active and involve the loss of resources through behaviors initiated by the depressed individual. Both processes are hypothesized to be involved in the development of chronic depression. As the literature has tended to focus on erosive processes, Joiner emphasizes the potential role of self-propagatory processes that include stress generation, negative feedback seeking, excessive reassurance seeking, conflict avoidance, and blame maintenance (i.e., persistent negative schemata of others).

Although there are few data explicitly testing these theories in chronic depression, numerous studies have reported that low social support, conflicted familial and marital relationships, and interpersonal difficulties are associated with a poorer course and outcome of depression [25,27,90]. In addition, there are data indicating that chronic depressives have poorer interpersonal relationships than episodic depressives [19,91,92]. Persons with chronic depression continue to experience interpersonal difficulties even after recovery [93], indicating that these deficits are not simply epiphenomena of the depressed state. As noted earlier, interpersonal problems may play an important role in mediating the relationship between some of the more distal risk factors (e.g., early adversity, temperament/personality) and chronic depressive outcomes [25].

Cognitive Factors

Personality and temperament may be expressed, in part, in the form of biases in attributions and information processing, particularly concerning emotionally valenced information that is self-relevant. Thus, Teasdale [94,95] and Nolen-Hoeksema [96] have proposed cognitive theories of chronicity of depression. Teasdale's differential activation hypothesis suggests that depression activates certain negative constructs, which in turn create a negative interpretation of new events. Nolen-Hoeksema's response style theory suggests that rumination in response to depressed mood (as opposed to active problem solving) prolongs depression.

A number of recent studies have tested Nolen-Hoeksema's hypothesis that rumination leads to more prolonged depressive episodes with mixed results [28,97–100]. Unfortunately, none of these studies has tested the theory in a carefully defined group of participants with chronic depression or followed participants for long enough periods to examine the development of chronicity.

There is some indication that other cognitive variables such as dysfunctional attitudes [19], attributional style [101], and global autobiographical recall [102] are associated with a poor course of depression. However, research into these factors has either been cross sectional [19] or involved relatively short follow-up periods [101,102]. Moreover, the state versus traitlike nature of these variables continues to be debated [103].

Chronic Stress

In a number of studies, stressful life events do not appear to distinguish chronic from episodic forms of depression [104–106]. However, it is important to distinguish between acute and chronic stressors, as the latter would be expected to play a greater role in chronic depression [13,107]. Indeed, Klein et al. [19] reported that outpatients with chronic depression reported a significantly higher level of chronic stress than patients with episodic MDD, but the two groups did not differ on acute life events. Moreover, in a 5-year follow-up of a different sample of chronically depressed outpatients, Hayden and Klein [11] found that chronic stress predicted outcome over and above the effects of familial psychopathology, early adversity, personality, and comorbidity.

Although acute life events do not appear to play a major role in the development of chronic depression, they may be influential in triggering exacerbations such as superimposed MDD episodes in DD. Thus, Moerk and Klein [108] reported that an acute life stressor in the context of an ongoing chronic stressor predicted the onset of a MDD episode in outpatients with DD.

Like interpersonal factors, chronic stress may play an important mediating role between some of the more distal risk factors (e.g., early adversity, temperament/personality) and chronic depressive outcomes [84]. In addition, chronic stressors may interact with some of these vulnerabilities to increase the duration of depression.

In some cases, severe and enduring stressors may initiate and maintain chronic depression even in the absence of marked preexisting vulnerabilities, particularly in the context of limited environmental and psychosocial resources. For example, chronic depression can develop in the face of a chronic and incapacitating illness or the chronic illness or death of a significant other [109]. Unfortunately, it is often difficult to date the onsets of chronic stressors and chronic depression precisely enough to establish a clear temporal relationship. Moreover, it can be difficult to distinguish between stressors that are independent and those that are produced by the chronically depressed state itself. In order to address these problems, Dura et al. [110] examined the onset of chronic depression in the spouses of individuals with progressive dementia. Despite being comparable on demographic characteristics, prior history of depression, and family history of mood disorders, a significantly greater proportion of caregivers than controls developed DD.

HETEROGENEITY IN CHRONIC DEPRESSION: THE EARLY-LATE ONSET DISTINCTION

There are likely to be important sources of heterogeneity in chronic depression apart from the distinctions between DD, double depression, and chronic MDD. The subtyping approach that has received the greatest empirical support to date is the early- versus late-onset distinction.

First proposed by Akiskal [4,111], the early-late onset distinction was incorporated into the DSM-III-R and DSM-IV categories for DD. The early-onset subtype of DD begins before age 21 years, whereas the late-onset subtype begins at age 21 years or older. Recent work suggests that this distinction may also apply to chronic MDD [112], and may in fact be relevant for depressive disorders in general [113–115]. Several studies have reported that in patients with DD, those with the early-onset subtype are more likely than those with the late-onset subtype to experience major depressive episodes and comorbid anxiety, substance use, eating, and personality disorders [77,116, 117]. Patients with early-onset DD also have a significantly greater level of childhood adversity [118], higher rates of mood disorders in relatives [116,117], and a more severe short-term course [116] than patients with late-onset DD. Finally, the early-onset subtype may exhibit increased rates of nonsuppression on the dexamethasone suppression test [119]. As noted above, similar results have been reported in a sample of outpatients with chronic MDD [112]. Thus, although several smaller studies have reported negative [120,121] and equivocal [122] findings, the available data suggest that the early-late onset distinction captures important variance in chronic depression and may be relevant to understanding vulnerability factors.

A SCHEMATIC MODEL

Figure 1 presents a preliminary model of the development of chronic depression based on the work reviewed above (also see Ref. 123) for a model that overlaps in important respects. It is offered as a means of organizing the work that has been done so far and as a heuristic for further research in this area. The model includes the following variables and hypothesized causal linkages.

Family History of Chronic Depression

As discussed earlier, a familial predisposition for chronic depression may be one of the few specific, or qualitative, risk factors for chronic depression. Family history of depression in general may also contribute to the risk for chronic depression, but probably only in so far as it confers a general vulnerability for depression, and by definition depression has to precede the development of chronicity.

Family History of Personality Disorders

As reviewed above, there is some evidence suggesting that family history of personality disorders may be a quantitative risk factor for chronic depression in that it is associated with risk for depression in general, but an even greater familial loading is associated with chronic depression. The curved arrow

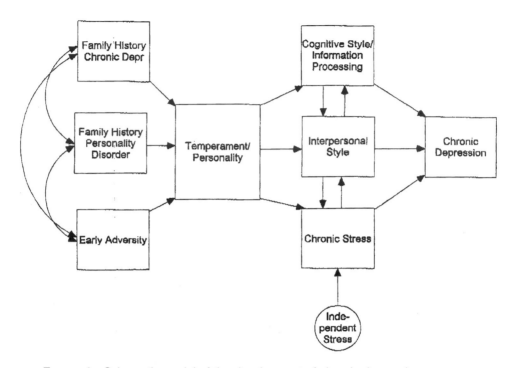

FIGURE 1   Schematic model of the development of chronic depression.

linking family history of chronic depression and family history of personality disorders in Figure 1 reflects evidence for common familial etiological influences between DD and at least some Axis II conditions [81].

Early Adversity

There is strong evidence that childhood adversity contributes to chronicity of depression, although it probably serves as a quantitative rather than a qualitative risk factor. The curved arrows linking early adversity to family history of chronic depression and family history of personality disorder in Figure 1 reflect the fact that offspring of parents with depression and personality disorders are at increased risk for adverse childhood environmental experiences. However, as discussed above, parental psychopathology does not appear fully to account for the association between early adversity and chronicity of depression. Rather the limited evidence available suggest that early adversity is a distinct vulnerability factor with an additive effect [39].

Temperament/Personality

There is some evidence that low PA, behavioral inhibition, and NA may be part of an underlying temperamental substrate for chronic forms of depression. However, further work is necessary to delineate the boundaries and overlap between these constructs and to determine whether their effects are additive or interactive.

There is also preliminary evidence suggesting that depressive personality is a qualitative risk factor for chronic depression. Depressive personality is correlated with low PA and high NA, but appears to have predictive power over and above these two temperament dimensions [124], which is consistent with the possibility that depressive personality develops somewhat later in the causal chain.

Finally, comorbid personality disorders may contribute to the development of chronic depression. Some of the DSM-IV personality disorders are also likely to derive from temperamental processes such as NA and behavioral inhibition [60]. In addition, there is some overlap between depressive personality and the DSM Axis II disorders (particularly avoidant personality disorder [53]).

Further work is also needed to understand the contributions of genetic and early environmental influences on these temperament and personality traits. There is evidence that family history of chronic depression is related to depressive personality [55], although the role of genetic versus environmental factors is unclear. There is strong evidence of genetic determinants in PA and NA [125] and possibly in behavioral inhibition [126]. A number of the DSM personality disorders aggregate in families, although twin and adoption data are limited [127]. Finally, there is evidence that early environmental adversity has an important influence on a number of personality disorders [40,41], although few studies have used genetically informative designs.

Cognitive Style/Information Processing

There is growing interest in the role of cognitive and information processing styles in the maintenance of depression, and this promises to be an active area of research in the near future. There is some evidence that certain cognitive variables that are associated with a poorer course of depression (attributional style, autobiographical memory) are influenced by childhood adversity [42, 43] and by family history of depression [128]. Work is clearly needed on the relationship between temperament and personality variables and cognitive and information processing variables in depression, although there is some interesting evidence of links between personality disorders and attributional style [42]. The direction of causality between these domains will be very difficult to establish, however, and may require longitudinal studies of young children [129].

Interpersonal Style

As discussed earlier, it appears likely that interpersonal variables contribute to the persistence and maintenance of depression. There is also evidence that parental depression and personality disorders influence their offspring's interpersonal functioning [130], and that early adversity influences adult interpersonal functioning [131]. In addition, there is a substantial literature documenting associations between personality and interpersonal functioning [132], although establishing the direction of causality between these often overlapping constructs is challenging. There is also emerging evidence of links between interpersonal processes and cognitive variables such as ruminative response style [133]. Fewer studies have determined whether the impact of familial psychopathology and early adversity on interpersonal functioning is direct or mediated by temperament/personality variables. However, there is some evidence that the effects of personality on the course of depression are at least partially mediated by interpersonal processes [134].

Chronic Stress

As reviewed above, there is some evidence indicating that chronic, but not acute, stress plays a role in the chronicity of depression. As these chronic stressors are often interpersonal in nature, it may be difficult to separate interpersonal and other chronic stress domains in Figure 1. There is also evidence suggesting that stress influences depressive cognitive style [128], although more work in this area is needed.

In many cases, depressed individuals may actively contribute to generating stressful events that are dependent on their own behavior. Indeed, there is evidence indicating that depressed persons continue to generate stress even after recovery, suggesting that this phenomenon is due to traitlike personality features or stable interpersonal or cognitive styles rather than the presence of depressive symptoms [135]. Importantly, the rate of dependent life events appears to be particularly high in patients with chronic forms of depression [136].

However, chronic stressors can also be partially or completely independent of the depressed individual's behavior (e.g., a chronic, impairing medical condition in the patient or a significant other). This may be particularly common in late-onset chronic depressions [109]. Hence, Figure 1 includes a residual influence on chronic stress that reflects independent stressors (i.e., not influenced by other variables in the model such as personality and interpersonal style).

Chronic Depression

Although chronic depression is presented as the dependent variable in this model, it is likely that there are reciprocal links between depression and the three proximal factors: information processing [95,96], interpersonal factors [86], and psychosocial stress [107]. Thus, it is likely that depression contributes to perpetuating itself via a number of indirect processes.

Finally, it is important to consider the heterogeneity of chronic depression [4]. It is likely that all factors will not be equally important in all cases. The early-late onset distinction may be particularly important in this regard [123]. Thus, familial psychopathology, early adversity, and temperament/personality may play a greater role in early-onset chronic depression [112,116], whereas independent sources of chronic stress play a greater role in late-onset chronic depression [110].

CONCLUSION

In this chapter, we have focused on factors and processes that appear to contribute to the development of chronicity in depression, including familial psychopathology, early adversity, temperament/personality, cognitive styles and information processing, interpersonal styles, and chronic stress. We attempted to integrate these domains and presented a preliminary framework that we hope will be informative and have heuristic value. Many of the causal links contain a degree of speculation, and some of the domains overlap. Thus, the model will undoubtedly require revision in light of further research.

Most of the research on chronic depression to date has focused on DD and double depression. In this chapter, we chose to focus on chronic depression in general rather than incorporating the finer-grained distinctions between DD, chronic MDD, and double depression. Although recent research has failed to uncover many differences between these conditions [12], further work on this issue is needed.

Our model does not attempt to account for sex differences in chronic depression. As with acute depression, chronic depression appears to be more common in women [1]. This sex difference may, in part, result from the moderating effects of sex on the temperament–chronic depression relationship [53].

Research into the mechanisms of chronic depression is difficult. Although longitudinal studies are of critical importance, it is extremely difficult to assess the hypothesized vulnerability factors prior to the onset of chronic depression, particularly in early-onset cases. However, in light of the prevalence of chronic depression and the significant impairment associated with it, further work in this area should be accorded high priority.

REFERENCES

1. Kessler RC, McGonagle KA, Zhao S, Nelson CB, Hughes M, Eshleman S, Wittchen H-U, Kendler, KS. Lifetime and 12-month prevalence of DSM-III-R psychiatric disorders in the United States: results from the National Comorbidity Survey. Arch Gen Psychiatry 51:8–19, 1994.

2. Keller MB, Hanks DL. Course and natural history of chronic depression. In: JH Kocsis and DN Klein, eds. Diagnosis and Treatment of Chronic Depression. New York: Guilford Press, 1995, pp 58–72.

3. Keller MB, Lavori PW, Mueller TI, Endicott J, Coryell W, Hirschfeld RMA, Shea T. Time to recovery, chronicity, and levels of psychopathology in major depression. Arch Gen Psychiatry 49:809–816, 1992.

3a. Diagnostic and Statistical Manual of Mental Disorders. 3rd ed., rev. Washington, DC: American Psychiatric Association, 1980.

3b. Diagnostic and Statistical Manual of Mental Disorders. 4th ed. Washington, DC: American Psychiatric Association, 1994.

4. Akiskal HS. Dysthymic disorder: psychopathology of proposed chronic depressive subtypes. Am J Psychiatry 140:11–20, 1983.

5. Klein DN, Schwartz JE, Rose S, Leader JB. Five-year course and outcome of dysthymic disorder: a prospective, naturalistic follow-up study. Am J Psychiatry 157:931–939, 2000.

6. Keller MB, Shapiro RW. Double depression: superimposition of acute depressive episodes on chronic depressive disorders. Am J Psychiatry 139:438–442, 1982.

7. Donaldson SK, Klein DN, Riso LP, Schwartz JE. Comorbidity between dysthymic and major depressive disorders: a family study. J Affect Disord 42:103–111, 1997.

8. Lizardi H, Klein DN, Ouimette PC, Riso LP, Anderson RL, Donaldson SK. Reports of the childhood home environment in early-onset dysthymia and major depression. J Abnorm Psychol 140:132–139, 1995.

9. Klein DN, Riso LP, Anderson RL. DSM-III-R dysthymia: antecedents and underlying assumptions. In: Experimental Personality and Psychopathology Research. New York: Springer, 1993, pp 222–253.

10. Pepper CM, Klein DN, Anderson RL, Riso LP, Ouimette PC, Lizardi H. DSM-III-R axis I comorbidity in dysthymia and major depression. Am J Psychiatry 152:239–247, 1995.

11. Hayden EP, Klein DN. Outcome of dysthymic disorder at 5-year follow-up: the effect of familial psychopathology, early adversity, personality, comorbidity, and chronic stress. Am J Psychiatry 158:1864–1870, 2001.

12. McCullough JP, Klein DN, Keller MB, Holzer CE, Davis SM, Kornstein SG, Howland RH, Thase ME, Harrison WM. Comparison of DSM-III-R chronic major depression and major depression superimposed on dysthymia (double depression): validity of the distinction. J Abnorm Psychol 109:419–427, 2000.

13. Riso LP, Miyatake R, Thase ME. The search for determinants of chronic depression: a review of six factors. J Affect Disord. In press.

14. Thase ME, Howland RH. Biological processes in depression: an updated review and integration. In: EE Beckham, WR Leber, eds. Handbook of Depression. 2nd ed. New York: Guilford Press, 1995, pp 213–279.
15. Gonzales LR, Lewinsohn PM, Clarke GN. Longitudinal follow-up of unipolar depressives: an investigation of predictors of relapse. J Consult Clin Psychol 53:461–469, 1985.
16. Duggan C, Sham P, Minne C, Lee A, Murray R. Family history as a predictor of poor long-term outcome in depression. Br J Psychiatry 173:527–530, 1998.
17. Lewinsohn PM, Rhode P, Seeley JR, Klein DN, Gotlib IH. Natural course of adolescent major depressive disorder in a community sample: predictors of recurrence in young adults. Am J Psychiatry 157:1584–1591, 2000.
18. Scott J. Chronic depression. Br J Psychiatry 153:287–297, 1988.
19. Klein DN, Taylor ET, Dickstein S, Harding K. Primary early-onset dysthymia: comparison with primary nonbipolar nonchronic major depression on demographic, clinical, familial, personality, and socioenvironmental characteristics and short-term outcome. J Abnorm Psychol 97:387–398, 1988.
20. Klein DN, Riso LP, Donaldson SK, Schwartz JE, Anderson RL, Ouimette PC, Lizardi H, Aronson TA. Family study of early-onset dysthymia: mood and personality disorders in relatives of outpatients with dysthymia and episodic major depression and normal controls. Arch Gen Psychiatry 52:487–496.
21. Klein DN, Clark DC, Dansky L, Margolis ET. Dysthymia in the offspring of parents with primary unipolar affective disorder. J Abnorm Psychol 97:265–274, 1988.
22. Goodman DW, Goldstein RB, Adams PB, Horwath E, Sobin C, Wickramaratne P, Weissman MM. Relationship between dysthymia and major depression: an analysis of family study data. Depression 2:252–258, 1994/1995.
23. Andrews B. Bodily shame as a mediator between abusive experiences and depression. J Abnorm Psychol 104:277–285, 1995.
24. Andrews B, Hunter E. Shame, early abuse, and course of depression in a clinical sample: preliminary study. Cognition d Emotion 11:373–381, 1997.
25. Brown GW, Moran P. Clinical and psychosocial origins of chronic depressive episodes: I. A community survey. Br J Psychiatry 165:447–456, 1994.
26. Brown GW, Harris TO, Hepworth C, Robinson R. Clinical and psychosocial origins of chronic depressive episodes: II. A patient inquiry. Br J Psychiatry 165:457–465, 1994.
27. Kendler KS, Walters EE, Kessler RC. The prediction of length of major depressive episodes: results from an epidemiolocal study of female twins. Psychol Med 27:107–117, 1997.
28. Lara ME, Klein DN, Kasch KL. Psychosocial predictors of the short-term course and outcome of major depression: a longitudinal study of a nonclinical sample with recent-onset episodes. J Abnorm Psychol 109:644–650, 2000.
29. Zlotnick C, Ryan CE, Miller IW, Keitner GI. Childhood abuse and recovery from major depression. Child Abuse Neglect 19:1513–1516, 1995.
30. Zlotnick C, Warshaw M, Meredith S, Shea MT, Keller MB. Trauma and

chronic depression among patients with anxiety disorders. J Consult Clin Psychology 65:333–336, 1997.

31. Alnaes R, Torgersen S. Characteristics of patients with major depression in combination with dysthymic or cyclothymic disorders: childhood and precipitating events. Acta Psychiatr Scand 79:11–18, 1989.

32. Rosenthal TR, Akiskal HS, Scott-Strauss A, Rosenthal RH, David M. Familial and developmental factors in characterological depressions. J Affect Disord 3:183–192, 1981.

33. Dinwiddie SH, Heath AC, Dunne MP, Bucholz KK, Madden PAF, Slutske WS, Bierut LJ, Statham DB, Martin NG. Early sexual abuse and lifetime psychopathology: a co-twin–control study. Psychol Med 30:41–52, 2000.

34. Kessler RC, Davis CG, Kendler KS. Childhood adversity and adult psychiatric disorder in the US National Comorbidity Survey. Psychol Med 27:1101–1119, 1997.

35. Brewin CR, Andrews B, Gotlib IH. Psychopathology and early experience: a reappraisal of retrospective reports. Psychol Bull 113:82–98, 1993.

36. Maughan B, Rutter M. Retrospective reporting of childhood adversity: assessing long-term recall. J Pers Disord 11:19–33, 1997.

37. Goodman SH, Gotlib IH. Risk for psychopathology in the children of depressed mothers: a developmental model for understanding mechanisms of transmission. Psychol Rev 106:458–490, 1999.

38. Lovejoy MC, Graczyk PA, O'Hare E, Neuman G. Maternal depression and parenting behavior: a meta-analytic review. Clin Psychol Rev 20:561–592, 2000.

39. Lizardi H, Klein DN. Parental psychopathology and reports of the childhood home environment in adults with early-onset dysthymic disorder. J Nerv Ment Dis 188:63–70, 2000.

40. Johnson JG, Cohen P, Kasen S, Smailes E, Brook JS. Association of maladaptive parental behavior with psychiatric disorder among parents and their offspring. Arch Gen Psychiatry 58:453–460, 2001.

41. Zanarini MC, Williams AA, Lewis RE, Reich RB, Vera SC, Marino MF, Levin A, Yong, L, Frankenburg FR. Reported pathological childhood experiences associated with the development of borderline personality disorder. Am J Psychiatry 154:1101–1106, 1997.

42. Rose DT, Abramson LY. Developmental predictors of depressive cognitive style: research and therapy. In: D Cicchetti, S Toth, eds. Rochester Symposium on Developmental Psychopathology, 1992, pp 323–349.

43. Kuyken W, Brewin CR. Autobiographical memory functioning in depression and reports of early abuse. J Abnorm Psychol 104:585–591, 1995

44. Heim C, Nemeroff CB. The role of childhood trauma in the neurobiology of mood and anxiety disorders: preclinical and clinical studies. Biol Psychiatry 49:1023–1039, 2001.

45. Patrick M, Hobson P, Castle D, Howard R, Maughan B. Personality disorder and the mental representation of early social experience. Dev Psychopathol 6:375–388, 1994.

46. Fonagy P, Leigh T, Steel M, Steele H, Kennedy R, Mattoon G, Target M, Gerber A. The relation of attachment status, psychiatric classification, and response to psychotherapy. J Consult Psychol 64:22–31, 1996.

47. van Ijzendorn M. Adult attachment representations, parental responsiveness, and infant attachment: a meta-analysis on the predictive validity of the Adult Attachment Interview. Psychol Bull 117:387–403, 1995.

48. Akiskal HS. Validating affective personality types. In: Robins L, Barrett J, eds. The Validity of Psychiatric Diagnosis. New York: Raven Press, 1988, pp 217–227.

49. Kraepelin E. Manic depressive insanity and paranoia. Edinburgh: Livingstone, 1921.

50. Kretschmer E. Physique and Character. New York: Harcourt, Brace, 1925.

51. Gunderson JG, Phillips KA, Triebwasser JT, Hirschfeld RMA. The diagnostic interview for depressive personality. Am J Psychiatry 151:1300–1304.

52. Schneider K. Psychopathic Personalities. London: Cassell, 1958.

53. Klein DN, Vocisano C. Depressive and self-defeating (masochistic) personality disorders. In: Millon T, Blaney PH, Davis RD, eds. Oxford Textbook of Psychopathology. New York: Oxford University Press, 1999, pp 653–673.

54. Phillips KA, Gunderson JG, Hirschfeld RM, Smith LE. A review of the depressive personality. Am J Psychiatry 147:830–837, 1990.

55. Klein DN. Depressive personality in the relatives of outpatients with dysthymic disorder and episodic major depressive disorder and normal controls. J Affect Disord 55:19–27, 1999.

56. Kwon JS, Kim Y-M, Chang C-G, Park B-J, Kim L, Yoon DJ, Han W-S, Lee H-J, Lyoo IK. Three-year follow-up of women with the sole diagnosis of depressive personality disorder: subsequent development of dysthymia and major depression. Am J Psychiatry 157:1966–1972, 2000.

57. Klein DN, Durbin CE, Shankman SA, Santiago NJ. Depression and personality. In: Gotlib IH, Hammen CL, eds. Handbook of Depression and Its Treatment. New York: Guilford Press, 2002, pp 115–140.

58. Goldsmith HH, Campos JJ. Toward a theory of infant temperament. In: Emde RN, Harmon RJ, eds. The Development of Attachment and Affiliative Systems. New York: Plenum, 1982, pp 161–193.

59. Rothbart MK, Bates JE. Temperament. In Eisenberg N, ed. Handbook of Child Psychology. Vol. 3. Social, Emotional, and Personality Development. 5th ed. New York: Wiley, 1998, pp 105–176.

60. Clark LA, Watson D. Temperament: a new paradigm for trait psychology. In: Pervin LA, John OP, eds. Handbook of Personality: Theory and Research. 2nd ed. New York: Guilford Press, 1999, pp 399–423.

61. Kagan J, Reznick JS, Snidman N. The physiology and psychology of behavioral inhibition in children. Child Dev 55:1459–1473, 1987.

62. Field T. Infants of depressed mothers. Dev Psychopathol 4:9–66, 1992.

63. Kochanska G. Patterns of inhibition to the unfamiliar in children of normal and affectively ill mothers. Child Devl 62:250–263, 1991.

64. Rosenbaum JF, Biederman J, Hirshfeld-Becker DR, Kagan J, Snidman N,

Friedman D, Nineberg A, Gallery DJ, Faraone SV. A controlled study of behavioral inhibition in children of parents with panic disorder and depression. Am J Psychiatry 157:2002–2010, 2000.

65. Neff C, Klein DN. The relationships between maternal behavior and psychopathology and offspring adjustment in depressed mothers of toddlers. Presented at the Annual Meeting of the Society for Research in Psychopathology, Palm Springs, CA, 1992.

66. Caspi A, Moffitt TE, Newman DL, Silva PA. Behavioral observations at age 3 years predict adult psychiatric disorders. Arch Gen Psychiatry 53:1033–1039, 1996.

67. van Os J, Jones P, Lewis G, Wadsworth M, Murray R. Developmental precursors of affective illness in a general population birth cohort. Arch Gen Psychiatry 54:625–631, 1997.

68. Gjerde PF. Alternative pathways to chronic depressive symptoms in young adults: gender differences in developmental trajectories. Child Dev 66:1277–3000, 1995.

69. Watson D, Clark LA. Depression and the melancholic temperament. Eur J Pers 9:351–366, 1995.

70. Duggan CG, Lee AS, Murray RM. Does personality predict long-term outcome in depression? Br J Psychiatry 157:19–24, 1990.

71. Surtees PG, Barkley C. Future imperfect: the long-term outcome of depression. Br J Psychiatry 164:327–341, 1994.

72. Klein DN, Taylor EB, Harding K, Dickstein S. Double depression and episodic major depression: demographic, clinical, familial, personality, and socioenvironmental characteristics and short-term outcome. Am J Psychiatry 145:1226–1231, 1988.

73. Hirschfeld RMA. Personality and dysthymia. In SW Burton and HS Akiskal, eds. Dysthymic Disorder. London: Gaskell, 1990, pp 69–77.

74. Shea MT, Widiger TA, Klein MH. Comorbidity of personality disorders and depression: implications for treatment. J Consult Clin Psychol 60:857–868, 1992.

75. Pepper CM, Klein DN, Anderson RL, Riso LP, Ouimette PC, Lizardi H. DSM-III-R axis II comorbidity in dysthymia and major depression. Am J Psychiatry 152:239–247, 1995.

76. Markowitz JC. Comorbidity of dysthymic disorder. In: JH Kocsis, DN Klein, eds. Diagnosis and Treatment of Chronic Depression. New York: Guilford Press, 1995, pp 41–57.

77. Garyfallos G, Adamopoulou A, Karastergiou A, Voikli M, Sotiropoulou A, Donias S, Giouzepas J, Paraschos A. Personality disorders in dysthymia and major depression. Acta Psychiatr Scand 99:332–340, 1999.

78. Corruble E, Ginestet D, Guelfi JD. Comorbidity of personality disorders and unipolar major depression: a review. J Affect Disord 37:157–170, 1996.

79. Anderson RL, Klein DN, Riso LP, Ouimette PC, Lizardi H, Schwartz JE. The subaffective-character spectrum subtyping distinction in primary early-onset dysthymia: a clinical and family study. J Affect Disord 38:13–22, 1996.

80. Schrader GD. An attempt to validate Akiskal's classification of chronic depression using cluster analysis. Compr Psychiatry 36:344–352, 1995.
81. Riso LP, Klein DN, Ferro T, Kasch KL, Pepper CM, Schwartz JE, Aronson TA. Understanding the comorbidity between early-onset dysthymia and cluster B personality disorders: a family study. Am J Psychiatry 153:900–906, 1996.
82. Daley SE, Hammen C, Burge D, Davila J, Paley B, Lindberg N, Herzberg DS. Depression and Axis II symptomatology in an adolescent community sample: concurrent and longitudinal associations. J Pers Disord 13:47–59, 1999.
83. Daley SE, Burge D, Hammen C. Borderline personality disorder symptoms as predictors of 4-year romantic relationship dysfunction in young women: addressing issues of specificity. J Abnorm Psychol 109:451–460, 2000.
84. Daley SE, Hammen C, Davila J, Burge D. Axis II symptomatology, depression, and life stress during the transition from adolescence to adulthood. J Consult Clin Psychol 66:595–603, 1998.
85. Nelson DR, Hammen C, Daley SE, Burge D, Davila J. Sociotropic and autonomous personality styles: contributions to chronic life stress. Cog Ther Res 25: 61–76, 2001.
86. Coyne JC. Depression and the response of others. J Abnorm Psychol 43:43–48, 1976.
87. T Joiner and JC Coyne, eds. The Interactional Nature of Depression: Advances in Interpersonal Approaches. Washington, DC: American Psychological Association, 1999.
88. Lara ME, Klein DN. Psychosocial processes underlying the maintenance and persistence of depression: implications for understanding chronic depression. Clin Psychol Rev 5:553–570, 1999.
89. Joiner TE. Depression's vicious scree: self-propagating and erosive processes in depression chronicity. Clin Psychol Sci Pract 7:203–218, 2000.
90. Keitner GI, Ryan CE, Miller IW, Norman WH. Recovery and major depression: factors associated with twelve-month outcome. Am J Psychiatry 149:93–99, 1992.
91. Hays JC, Krishnan K, Ranga R, George LK, Pieper CF, Flint EP, Blazer DG. Psychosocial and physical correlates of chronic depression. Psychiatry Res 72: 149–159, 1997.
92. Swindle RW, Cronkite RC, Moos RH. Risk factors for sustained nonremission of depressive symptoms: a 4-year follow-up. J Nerv Ment Dis 186:462–469, 1998.
93. Klein DN, Lewinsohn PM, Seeley JR. Psychosocial characteristics of adolescents with a past history of dysthymic disorder: comparison with adolescents with past histories of major depressive and non-affective disorders, and never mentally ill controls. J Affect Disord 42:127–135, 1997.
94. Teasdale JD. Negative thinking in depression: cause effect or reciprocal relationship? Adv Behav Res Ther 5:3–26, 1983.
95. Teadale JD. Cognitive vulnerability to persistent depression. Cognition Emotion 2:247–274, 1988.

96. Nolen-Hoeksema S. Responses to depression and their effects on duration of depressive episodes. J Abnorm Psychol 100:569–582, 1991.
97. Just N, Alloy CB. The response styles theory of depression: tests and an extension of the theory. J Abnorm Psychol 106:221–229, 1997.
98. Nolen-Hoeksema S. The role of rumination in depressive disorders and mixed anxiety/depressive symptoms. J Abnorm Psychol 109:504–511, 2000.
99. Nolen-Hoeksema S, McBride A, Larson J. Rumination and psychological distress among bereaved partners. J Pers Soc Psychol 72:855–862, 1997.
100. Nolen-Hoeksema S, Morrow J, Fredrickson BL. Response styles and the duration of episodes of depressed mood. J Abnorm Psychol 102:20–28, 1993.
101. McCullough JP, Kasnetz MD, Braith JA, Carr KF, Cones JH, Fielo J, Martelli MF. A longitudinal study of an untreated sample of predominately late onset characterological dysthymia. J Nerv Ment Dis 176:658–667, 1988.
102. Brewin CR, Reynolds M, Philip T. Autobiographical memory precesses and the course of depression. J Abnorm Psychol 108:511–517, 1999.
103. Ingram RE, Christian H. Cognitive science of depression. In: DJ Stein, JE Young, eds. Cognitive Science and Clinical Disorders. San Diego: Academic Press, 1992, pp 187–209.
104. Billings AG, Moos RH. Life stressors, social resources affect post-treatment outcomes among depressed patients. J Abnorm Psychol 94:140–153, 1985.
105. Cronkite RC, Moos RH, Twohey J, Cohen C, Swindle Jr R. Life circumstances and personal resources as predictors of the ten-year course of depression. Am J Commun Psychol 26:255–280, 1998.
106. Ravindran AV, Griffiths J, Waddell C, Anisman H. Stressful life events and coping styles in relation to dysthymia and major depressive disorder: variations associated with alleviation of symptoms following pharmacotherapy. Prog Neuropsychopharmacol Biol Psychiatry 19:637–653, 1995.
107. Ravindran AV, Merali Z, Anisman H. Dysthymia: a biological perspective. In: J Licinio, CL Bolis, P Gold, eds. Dysthymia: From Clinical Neuroscience to Treatment. Geneva, World Health Organization, 1997, pp 21–44.
108. Moerk KM, Klein DN. The development of major depressive episodes during the course of dysthymic and episodic major depressive disorders: a retrospective examination of life events. J Affect Disord 58:117–123.
109. Akiskal H. Factors associated with incomplete recovery in primary depressive illness. J Clin Psychiatry 43:266–271. 1982.
110. Dura JR, Stukenberg KW, Kiecolt-Glaser JK. Chronic stress and depressive disorders in older adults. J Abnorm Psychol 99:284–290, 1990.
111. Akiskal HS, King D, Rosenthal TL, Robinson D, Scott-Strauss A. Chronic depressions: part I: clinical and familial characteristics in 137 probands. J Affect Disord 3:297–315, 1981.
112. Klein DN, Schatzberg AF, McCullough JP, Dowling F, Goodman D, Howland RH, Markowitz JC, Smith C, Thase ME, Rush AJ, LaVange L, Harrison WM, Keller MB. Age of onset in chronic major depression: Relation to demographic and clinical variables, family history, and treatment response. J Affect Disord 55:149–157, 1999.

113. Fava M, Alpert JE, Borus JS, Nierenburg AA, Pava JA, Rosenbaum JF. Patterns of personality disorder comorbidity in early-onset versus late-onset major depression. Am J Psychiatry 153:1308–1312, 1996.
114. Kasch KL, Klein DN. The relationship between age at onset and psychiatric disorders. J Nerv Ment Dis 184:703–707.
115. Weissman MM, Wickramaratne P, Merikangas KR, Leckman JF, Prusoff BA, Caruso KA, Kidd KK, Gammon GD. Onset of major depression in early adulthood: increased familial loading and specificity. Arch Gen Psychiatry 41:1136–1143, 1984.
116. Klein DN, Taylor EB, Dickstein S, Harding K. The early-late onset distinction in DSM-III-R dysthymia. J Affect Disord 14:25–33, 1988.
117. Klein DN, Schatzberg AF, McCullough JP, Keller MB, Dowling F, Goodman D, Howland RH, Markowitz JC, Smith C, Miceli R, Harrison WM. Early-versus late-onset dysthymic disorder: comparison in outpatients with super-imposed major depressive episodes. J Affect Disord 52:187–196, 1999.
118. Horwitz JA. Early-onset versus late-onset chronic depressive disorders: comparison of retrospective reports of coping with adversity in the childhood home environment. MA thesis, Virginia Commonwealth University, Richmond, VA, 2001.
119. Szadoczky E, Fazekas I, Rihmer Z, Arato M. The role of psychosocial and biological variables in separating chronic and non-chronic major depression and early-late onset dysthymia. J Affect Disord 32:1–11, 1994.
120. Miller IW, Norman WH, Dow MG. Psychosocial characteristics of "double depression." Am J Psychiatry 143:1032–1044, 1986.
121. McCullough JP, Braith JA, Chapman RC, Kasnetz MD, Carr KF, Cones JH, Fielo J, Shoemaker OS, Roberts WC. Comparison of early and late onset dysthymia. J Nerv Ment Dis 178:577–581, 1990.
122. Shores MM, Glubin T, Cowley DS, Dager SR, Roy-Burne PP, Dunner DL. The relationship between anxiety and depression: a clinical comparison of generalized anxiety disorder, dysthymic disorder, panic disorder, and major depressive disorder. Compr Psychiatry 33:237–244, 1992.
123. McCullough JP. Treatment for Chronic Depression: Cognitive Behavioral Analysis System of Psychotherapy. New York: Guilford Press, 2000.
124. Klein DN, Shih JH. Depressive personality: associations with DSM-III-R mood and personality disorders and negative and positive affectivity, 30-month stability, and prediction of course of Axis I depressive disorders. J Abnorm Psychol 107:319–327, 1998.
125. Plomin R, Caspi A. Behavioral genetics and personality. In: LA Pervin, OP John, eds. Handbook of Personality: Theory and Research. 2nd ed. New York: Guilford Press, 1999, pp 251–276.
126. DiLalla LF, Falligant EL. An environmental and behavioral genetic perspective on behavioral inhibition in toddlers. In: LF DiLalla, SMC Dollinger, eds. Assessment of Biological Mechanisms Across the Life Span. Hillsdale, NJ: Lawrence Erlbaum, 1995, pp 91–119.
127. Nigg JT, Goldsmith HH. Genetics of personality disorders: prspectives from personality and psychopathology research. Psychiatry Bull 115:346–380, 1994.

128. Garber J. Predictors of depressive cognitions in young adolescents. Cog Ther Res 25:353–376, 2001.
129. Hamburg SR. Inherited hypohedonia leads to learned helplessness: a conjecture updated. Rev Gen Psychol 24: 384–403, 1998.
130. Hammen C, Brennan PA. Depressed adolescents of depressed and nondepressed mothers: Tests of an interpersonal impairment hypothesis. J Consult Clin Psychol 69:284–294, 2001.
131. DiLillo D. Interpersonal functioning among women reporting a history of childhood sexual abuse: empirical findings and methodological issues. Clin Psychol Rev 21:553–576, 2001.
132. Benjamin LS. An interpersonal theory of personality disorders. In: JF Clarkin, MF Lenzenweger, eds. Major Theories of Personality Disorder. New York: Guilford Press, 1996, pp 141–220.
133. Nolen-Hoeksema S, Davis CG. "Thanks for sharing that": ruminators and their social support networks. J Pers Soc Psychol 77:801–814, 1999.
134. Lara ME, Leader J, Klein DN. The association between social support and course of depression: is it confounded with personality? J of Abnorm Psychol 106:478–482, 1997.
135. Hammen CL. The generation of stress in the course of unipolar depression. J Abnorm Psychol 100:555–561, 1991.
136. Harkness KL, Luther J. Clinical risk factors for the generation of life events in major depression. J Abnorm Psychol 110:564–572, 2001.

4

Biological Factors in Chronic Depression

David Mischoulon, Darin D. Dougherty, and Maurizio Fava

Massachusetts General Hospital
and Harvard Medical School
Boston, Massachusetts, U.S.A.

INTRODUCTION

No one really knows why some people get depressed—or fail to respond to antidepressant or psychotherapeutic treatment—but it is probably the result of a combination of factors. Historically, several nonbiological, psychoanalytically and cognitively based theories—such as aggression turned inward, object loss, loss of self-esteem, cognitive, learned helplessness, and negative reinforcement, among others [1,2]—have been widely used to explain major depression as well as most other mood disorders.

With the growing development of biology and neuroscience, however, our understanding of major depression is now broader and more sophisticated. Although psychodynamic factors, along with psychosocial and environmental stressors, may account, at least in part, for many cases of depression, certain individuals are likely born with a *biological* predisposition and vulnerability to depression. This vulnerability may be based on a variety of genetic and physiological factors, and the current belief is that biological factors are at least necessary, if not sufficient, for the development of depression [3,4].

The goal of this chapter will be (1) to review what is known about the biological basis for major depression and (2) to review how this increased understanding of the pathophysiology of major depression may impact diagnosis and treatment of depression. We will review the genetics of depressive disorders, biological correlates of depressive states, and some established biological models of depression including the monoamine hypotheses, as well as endocrine and physiological models. These ever-developing models reflect our increased understanding of the pathophysiology of depression and may serve in the development of a more accurate diagnosis of major depression, and may elucidate the therapeutic mechanisms of action of antidepressant therapies.

GENETICS OF DEPRESSION

Genetics have been demonstrated to play a prominent role in the expression of many medical disorders, such as Huntington's disease, sickle cell anemia, and Tay-Sachs disease. However, our understanding of genetics in psychiatric disorders is relatively limited. Heritability is thought to be involved in a broad spectrum of psychiatric disorders, although the extent of this involvement is unclear. For example, there appears to be a fairly strong genetic component in schizophrenia, bipolar disorder, and alcoholism, but the source and nature of the vulnerability is a mystery.

Morbidity risk among first-degree relatives of individuals with different psychiatric disorders has been examined in numerous studies with varying results. For example, the risk of developing bipolar disorder for individuals with a first-degree relative who has the disorder is between 4 and 9% [5], and the risk for schizophrenia is between 3 and 7% [6]. Thus, the risk of developing these psychiatric disorders in these individuals is markedly higher than what is reflected in the general population. Concordance for illness among twins has also been studied. In schizophrenia, for example, there is a 30–80% concordance among monozygotic twins [6]; in bipolar and other mood disorders, the concordance is 30–90% among monozygotic twins [5], and 34% among dizygotic twins [5].

The pattern for transmission of risk for unipolar depression is not as well characterized as for some other psychiatric disorders. There are several mechanisms of heredity or gene transfer [5], but those thought to be involved in the transmission of mental illness are likely multifactorial with varying degrees of penetrance [1]. Family studies suggest that transmission risk is greater in women [7], and is greatest with early-onset, recurrent forms of depression [8]. The risk for depression in first-degree relatives of depressed individuals is estimated to be two to six times the average [9]. Twin studies suggest a higher concordance in monozygotic versus dizygotic twins [10], and adoption studies suggest a significant genetic contribution to unipolar depression [10]. Current research has focused on linkage studies and candidate genes, but results so far have not yielded a specific "depression gene."

To conclude, although the genetic diathesis of depression is not well understood, depressive syndromes and disorders have well-demonstrated familial patterns of transmission. It is therefore reasonable to suppose that a significant genetic contribution underlies the transmission of depressive vulnerability [11], particularly in the case of bipolar depression. With regard to chronic depressive illness, a stronger genetic load may contribute to more refractory depressive states, but this remains to be clarified.

CELLULAR AND NEUROCHEMICAL CORRELATES OF DEPRESSIVE STATES

There are several lines of evidence which suggest that depression can arise in the context of exogenous and endogenous biological manipulation. Examples include depression secondary to administration of medications such as reserpine and the interferons [12,13], medical disorders such as stroke, pancreatic cancer, and Parkinson's disease [14–17], as well as induced neurochemical imbalances, as seen with tryptophan depletion [18] and deep brain stimulation [19].

By the same reasoning, biological therapies have been widely demonstrated to relieve depression, often without a need for concomitant "talking" psychotherapies or other psychosocial interventions. Examples of biological treatments include antidepressant medications, electroconvulsive therapy (ECT) [20], psychosurgery [21], repetitive transcranial magnetic stimulation (RTMS) [22], and vagus nerve stimulation [23].

Finally, several studies have found common biochemical characteristics in many depressed individuals [24]. These include decreased 5-hydroxyindoleacetic acid (5-HIAA), a serotonin metabolite, in the cerebrospinal fluid (CSF) of unmedicated depressed patients, decreased serotonin and 5-HIAA in brain tissue, decreased plasma tryptophan, and increased density of 5HT2-binding sites in the brain tissue of suicide victims [24]. Many depressed patients also have decreased homovanillic acid (HVA), a metabolite of dopamine, in their CSF, although this finding is not consistent [25,26]. Likewise, variations in urine, CSF, and plasma levels of cortisol, norepinephrine, and norepinephrine metabolites such as 3-methoxy-4-hydroxyphenylglycol (MHPG) (which may best reflect brain norepinephrine) have been demonstrated in depressed states, and have varied with response and nonresponse to antidepressant treatment, but again without a truly consistent pattern [27–34].

With regard to more chronic depressive states, studies have attempted to characterize differences and similarities between dysthymia—a milder, chronic depressive disorder—and major depression. Studies have focused on rapid eye movement (REM) latency, electrodermal activity, and thyroid function, but findings have been mixed. Investigations using the dexamethasone suppression test (DST), catecholamine measurements, and other electroencephalogram (EEG) sleep variables have shown more consistent differences between dysthymia and major depression [35–37]. For example, patients with major depressive disorder have a shorter duration of total sleep time, a longer sleep latency, and a lower sleep efficiency than dysthymics, although similar sleep architecture and REM sleep characteristics are found in both [38]. Early-onset dysthymics, compared to late-onset dysthymics and chronic depressives, have been shown to have a higher rate of DST nonsuppression and blunted thyroid-stimulating hormone (TSH) responses after thyrotropin-releasing hormone (TRH) administration during a period of double depression [38]. DST may differentiate severe melancholic depression, mania, or acute psychosis from chronic psychosis (87% specificity) or dysthymia (77% specificity) [36]. Dysthymia, as opposed to other depressive types, has also been associated with increased circulation of natural killer (NK) cells [39] and interleukin-1β (IL-1β) [40].

Likewise, treatment studies of dysthymic patients have shown that fluoxetine responders, when compared to nonresponders, have higher pretreatment plasma cortisol levels following dexamethasone administration, higher pretreatment 6-sulfatoxymelatonin levels, lower pretreatment monoamine oxidase (MAO) activity, and lower pretreatment urinary 5-HIAA and metanephrine levels. Following treatment, urinary 5-HIAA tended to be decreased in nonresponders and increased in responders [39,41].

Taken together, these findings strongly suggest that there is a biological basis for at least some dysthymias and other chronic depressive states, and that it may involve the hypothalamic-pituitary-adrenal (HPA) axis and the serotonergic, noradrenergic, and dopaminergic systems.

BIOLOGICAL MODELS OF DEPRESSION

Although the data reviewed support the idea of a biological substrate for depression, the actual mechanisms that ultimately result in depression and its alleviation are not clear. Several biological models have been put forth since the 1960s to attempt to explain the nature of depression. The first of these was the *biogenic amine imbalance theory*, which suggested that depression was the result of dysregulation of aminergic transmission. The *neurophysiological theory* developed concurrently with the biogenic amine theory, and proposed that electrophysiological disturbance, particularly neuronal hyperexcitability and the kindling phenomenon, contributed to depression. Later in the 1960s, *neuroendocrine models* emphasized the interplay between neurotransmitters and endocrine axes as potential explanations for depression. And in the 1970s, we saw the emergence of the *final common pathway model*, which proposed that a stress diathesis interaction converging on the midbrain was responsible for depression and affected mechanisms of rewards and biorhythms [42]. These models and the evidence for and against them will be reviewed.

Biogenic Amine Imbalance

The biogenic amine hypothesis was based on two sets of observations. First, it was known that reserpine caused a decrease in blood pressure by depletion of biogenic amines, and also caused depression in some individuals. Second, tricyclic antidepressants were known to increase the functional capacity of biogenic amines—particularly norepinephrine—in the brain, suggesting the correction of a noradrenergic imbalance present in these depressed patients. Indeed, norepinephrine-containing neurons are involved in many functions that are disturbed in major depression including mood, arousal, appetite, reward, and drives [1,42]. The connection between depletion and imbalance of norepinephrine and major depression was proposed by several investigators [43–46]. Janowsky [46] suggested that depression resulted specifically from *noradrenergic dysregulation*, a state of oscillation from one output mode to another at different phases of depressive illness. In this model, bipolar depression was thought to involve decreased noradrenergic output, and unipolar depression was thought to involve increased noradrenergic output (a process similar to anxiety). In addition, the observation that cholinergic neurons are generally antagonistic to catecholaminergic neurons led to the *cholinergic-noradrenergic imbalance hypothesis* [46,47], which suggested that an imbalance between these systems resulted in depression.

These early investigations led to the birth of a "pharmacological bridge" between these phenomena [1], and to this day, the development of novel antidepressants that work primarily by increasing the availability of neurotransmitters in the neuronal synapse has been driven largely by the biogenic amine hypothesis.

The serotonergic model followed the noradrenergic model and was based on similar principles [45,48]. Serotonergic neurons are important in the regulation of mood, sleep, and inhibitory control [1], all of which may be disturbed in depressed states. The *permissive biogenic amine hypothesis* suggested that a decrease in serotonin caused an increase in catecholamine-mediated depressive or manic states. Evidence for this included the fact that an intact serotonergic system is needed for optimal function of noradrenergic neurons, and that depletion of the serotonin precursor tryptophan annuled the efficacy of antidepressants. However, 1-tryptophan supplementation, also referred to as "precursor loading," was never a clear success in the treatment of depression, so this mechanism is still controversial [1]. Likewise, catecholamine precursor loading has been even less successful in reversing depression [1]. ECT studies have also shed doubt on the classic biogenic amine model, as ECT treatment may *decrease* plasma norepinephrine in melancholic/psychotic depressive illness, and this decrease seems to correlate with clinical improvement [49].

With regard to dopaminergic mechanisms of depression, it has been shown that some depressed patients have decreased homovanillic acid (HVA), a metabolite of dopamine, in their CSF, but this finding is not consistent [25,26]. Dopaminergic neurons are important in regulation of psychomotor activity [1], which is often disturbed in depression. Neuroendocrine studies that have assessed dopaminergic status by measuring prolactin and growth hormone levels following administration of dopamine agonists have not convincingly demonstrated dopaminergic dysfunction in depression. However, dopaminergic psychostimulant augmentation strategies have been shown to be effective in the treatment of major depression [50], and overall the evidence suggests a role for dopaminergic dysfunction in depression.

There are, however, many inconsistencies in the biogenic amine hypothesis of depression. For example, the time lag of the antidepressant effect (usually 3–6 weeks) suggests that the antidepressant mechanism is not purely dependent on neurotransmitter imbalances, as these imbalances are generally corrected within hours of the first dose of antidepressant administered [51]. Recently, the monoamine theory has been further challenged by the purported mechanisms of some of the newer antidepressant agents, as they suggest that depression may develop by pathways different from those mediated by the biogenic amines [52,53]. Examples of such medications include the substance P (SP) antagonists and hypericum (St. John's wort).

Substance P is a peptide that transmits in pain endings of the spinal cord. Synthetic SP antagonists have not demonstrated substantial analgesic properties, but they may possess antidepressant effects [53–56]. SP antagonists are believed to be active in areas of the brain involved in emotion and stress [56]. SP antagonists given after a stressful event may decrease the effects of stress, so they may have a potential role in posttraumatic stress disorder (PTSD) treatment as well [57]. It is possible that antidepressants may decrease production of endogenous SP, and SP may be a component of the final common pathway in depression. Because there is no known interconnection between SP and the monoamine systems, the biogenic amine model of depression must be called into question.

Another challenge to the biogenic amine model of depression is the use of hypericum (St. John's wort) as an antidepressant. The mechanism of action of hypericum probably involves multiple components, some similar to those of conventional antidepressants. These include monoamine reuptake inhibition, postsynaptic receptor downregulation, and monoamine oxidase inhibitor (MAOI) activity [58]. But hypericin, believed to be one of the key active components, does not cross the blood-brain barrier [58]. It may therefore contribute to hypericum's effect by inhibiting monocyte production of interleukins, resulting in a decrease of corticotropin-releasing hormone (CRH), hence of cortisol, and thus may regulate the hypothalamic-pituitary-adrenal (HPA) axis (Fig. 1) [58].

It is sobering to note that after three decades of research, we have not proved that either a deficiency or an excess of biogenic amines in specific brain structures is necessary or sufficient for the occurrence of mood disorders [1]. The data reviewed suggest that the picture is much more complicated. Other areas that require investigation, for example, include dopamine's role in atypical and bipolar depression or mania [25,26], as well as the role of

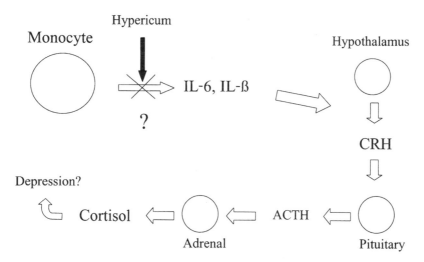

FIGURE 1 Hypericum mechanism? This model proposes that hypericum (St. John's wort) may function by inhibiting production of interleukins, resulting in a decrease in production of cortisol, which has been implicated in the development of depression. However, given the various chemicals in hypericum, it is likely that its mechanism of action may involve various different pathways. (Adapted from Nierenberg AA, Mischoulon D, DeCecco L. St. John's wort: A critique of antidepressant efficacy and possible mechanisms of action. In: Mischoulon D, Rosenbaum J, eds. Natural Medications for Psychiatric Disorders: Considering the Alternatives. Philadelphia: Lippincott Williams & Wilkins, 2002, p. 7. Used with kind permission from the publishers.)

serotonin in suicidality (especially impulsive suicidality) rather than specifically in the pathophysiology of depression [59]. Although we are far from a complete understanding of depressogenic pathways, it is clear that dimensional neurochemical disturbance is present in depression, as well as in most psychiatric disorders such as obsessive compulsive disorder (OCD), bulimia nervosa, panic disorder, and schizophrenia. Although environment may affect neurochemistry, it is likely that genetics play a prominent role in the neurochemical disturbances seen in major depression as well.

Neuroendocrine Models

The neuroendocrine model of depression suggests that the imbalances in neurotransmitters noted in many psychiatric disorders may result from endocrine dysfunction [1]. Specifically, neurotransmitter deficits may result from disinhibition of the HPA axis, which may be due to perturbation of limbic-diencephalic neurotransmission balance, leading to depression. In this regard, steroid overproduction is the most widely studied process thought to be involved in the pathophysiology of depression. Lines of evidence for this include increased CRF in the CSF of depressed patients as well as in the CSF of rats and primates exposed to early-life stress [60]. These increases in CRF are likely due to hyperactivity of the HPA axis, which normalizes with antidepressant treatment [60]. Additional evidence supporting the HPA axis dysregulation model includes the finding of decreased CRF receptor binding sites in the prefrontal cortex of depressed suicide victims [61].

Given the proposed relationship between hormone dysregulation and depression, *neuroendocrine indices* have been studied as potential tools for the diagnosis and characterization of depression. The best-known index is the DST [62]. The theory behind the DST suggests that the altered HPA axis in depression is resistant to normal suppression by dexamethasone administration. The DST has revealed abnormal HPA axis suppression in many, but not all, studies of depressed patients. Other examples of neuroendocrine indices include the blunted growth hormone (GH) response usually seen with administration of clonidine (an alpha$_2$ agonist and antimanic agent) [62], and the blunted TSH response with administration of TRH [62]. Unfortunately, as with the DST, these indices lack *specificity* (similar abnormalities are found in other psychiatric disorders) and *sensitivity* (many depressed individuals exhibit patterns similarly to nondepressed controls). Although often used in research settings, these indices have never gained widespread use in diagnosis and characterization of depressive disorders.

Neurophysiological models have also been proposed as explanations for the pathophysiology of depression. For instance, the model of *electrolyte metabolism and neuronal hyperexcitability* [1,45] suggests that excess residual sodium ions move into neurons and cause neurophysiological disturbances that may lead to depression. However, research suggests that this phenomenon would be more likely to explain mania rather than depression [1]. This model may, therefore, account for mixed mood states and provide a rationale for the antidepressant role of the antimanic agent lithium.

The *rhythmopathology model* [1] is based in part on the ancient Greek theory of geophysical influences. These influences were thought to contribute to abnormalities of circadian regulation of temperature, activity, and sleep. Depressed patients have been shown to be phase advanced in many rhythms, particularly decreased latency to REM sleep. Therefore, shortened REM latency has been proposed as a biological test for depression, but its lack of specificity has limited its acceptability as a diagnostic tool. Sleep deprivation and exposure to bright light have been shown, in some instances, to correct phase disturbances and alleviate depression, particularly in cases of periodic/seasonal illness. These phenomena, although supported by limited evidence, suggest that midbrain dysregulation may be a common neurophysiological pathway for major depression.

In summary, although these neuroendocrine-based models are of limited specificity individually, the majority of depressed patients demonstrate at least some neuroendocrine abnormalities. These disparate neuroendocrine abnormalities likely represent a shared pathophysiological mechanism for depression. Finally, it is possible that endocrine dysregulation may account for more refractory or chronic illness, as it is known that patients with complicated medical illnesses such as fibromyalgia may be more prone to depression and may be more difficult to treat [63].

Final Common Pathway

The final common pathway model developed with the growth of molecular biology in the 1970s and 1980s [1,64,65]. Monoamines are known to interact with neuronal receptors, G-proteins, and second messengers, leading to interactions with the cell's gene transcription machinery. These receptor-to-gene pathways are likely involved in the pathophysiology of depression (Fig. 2), and antidepressant treatments may exert their effects by impacting these pathways. Monoamine and neuroendocrine imbalances result in intracellular and intranuclear changes that may account for the kindling phenomenon in recurrent and/or chronic illness [65]. Investigation into molecular abnormalities associated with major depression have demonstrated that imbalances of neurotrophic factors such as brain-derived neurotrophic factor (BDNF) (Fig. 3) are present during the depressed state. BDNF is thought to be involved in the production of neurons in the hippocampus and other brain areas [66]. Studies have shown that immobilization stress in rats causes

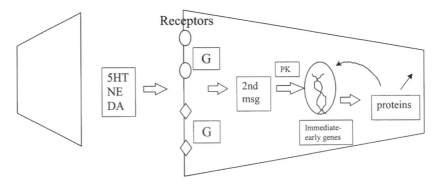

FIGURE 2 Intracellular pathways. Neurotransmitters (5HT, NE, DA) may interact with specific postsynaptic receptors, which in turn set off a second-messenger cascade, ultimately resulting in the transcription and synthesis of cellular proteins, in part through immediate-early gene activation. These proteins, after undergoing various modifications, act within the nucleus of the cell, leading to the synthesis of other proteins, and may also act within the cell to carry out specific functions which eventually translate into the clinical antidepressant effect.

decreased BDNF in the hippocampus. Chronic stress or glucocorticoid administration to rats and primates also causes neuron atrophy/death in the hippocampus, perhaps secondary to BDNF underproduction [64]. Finally, antidepressants have been shown to reverse some of the brain alterations and BDNF imbalances found in these models [64,67,68].

Although there are limited human data in this regard, the final common pathway model is attractive in that it proposes a "funnel" for the varying

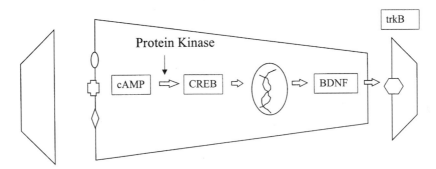

FIGURE 3 Neurotrophic factors. It has been suggested that CREB's intranuclear action leads to the production of BDNF, which in turn interacts with trkB and may somehow result in alleviation of depression.

neurotransmitter and hormone imbalances thought to be involved in depression. In addition, the involvement of the gene transcription and translation machinery followed by protein synthesis and modification serves to explain the time lag of antidepressant response, as these mechanisms can require several weeks until the final protein products have been rendered biochemically active [65,51].

In summary, molecular mechanisms are understood primarily in the context of antidepressant *treatment* rather than in the development of depressive symptoms. In recent years, research on antidepressant action has focused largely on molecular and intracellular mechanisms. This focus will likely yield new insights into the understanding of the causes of acute and chronic depression and may result in the development of more effective pharmacological treatments.

FUNCTIONAL NEUROANATOMY OF MAJOR DEPRESSION

Although cellular level and neurochemical studies of major depression have yielded useful information regarding the pathophysiology of major depression, these abnormalities must be understood in the context of the brain as a whole. With the advent of powerful techniques such as electroencephalography and functional neuroimaging that allow investigators to measure whole brain function, the role of specific brain regions and neural systems in the pathophysiology of major depression can be explored.

Electroencephalography

Electroencephalography (EEG) utilizes electrodes placed on the scalp to measure cortical surface electrical activity. Many studies have attempted to characterize EEG sleep patterns in major depression and other disorders, and some EEG changes have been well-documented in patients with major depression. These EEG changes include decreased sleep efficiency, increased nighttime awakenings, decreased stage 2 sleep, decreased REM latency, increased REM density, increased sleep-onset REM, decreased delta amplitude, and decreased slow wave sleep (SWS) [69–74], although other studies have presented contradictory data [75–77] (Table 1).

Some studies have shown that EEG changes correlate with scores on depression scales such as the Hamilton-D (HAM-D) scale [78,79] and the Beck Depression Inventory (BDI) [79]. Other significant findings include a higher mean REM factor among nonresponders to antidepressants [80], suggesting a unique substrate to more refractory and chronic depressive states. Another study examining patients with dysthymia versus recurrent nonmelancholic major depression revealed similar sleep architectures in both

TABLE 1 Sleep Cycle

NREM (slow wave sleep)	Characteristics
Stage 1	Drowsiness (theta)
Stage 2	Light sleep (sleep spindles, K-complex)
Stage 3	Deep sleep (delta/slow wave sleep)
Stage 4	Deep sleep (delta/slow wave sleep)
REM (fast, alpha)	Very still, loss of tone, variable eye movements, dreams

groups [37], suggesting a biological overlap between these two chronic forms of depression.

Slow wave sleep inversely correlates with age and the presence of personality disorder symptoms in depressed individuals [80], which may contribute to greater chronicity and refractoriness [81–83]. DST abnormalities correlate with stage 2, slow wave, and REM sleep [78], suggesting that depression may be an overarroused state. Cognitive-behavioral therapy (CBT) has been shown to normalize REM latency, sleep efficiency, and REM density [84]; and interpersonal therapy (IPT) has been shown to increase sleep latency and REM latency [85], supporting the proposal that psychotherapies, like medications, also have the potential to alter brain structure and function.

Quantitative EEG (QEEG) measures coherence (synchronized activity between brain regions) and cordance (associated with cerebral perfusion) in the brain [86]. Depression may result in decreased cordance in QEEG measures [87], particularly a decrease in prefrontal activity in responders to antidepressants, and may therefore predict treatment response or refractoriness in some individuals [88,89].

Clearly, there is no consistent evidence of REM or non-REM (NREM) sleep involvement in clinical mechanisms of acute or chronic depression. As with the other diagnostic tests reviewed, EEG lacks diagnostic utility, sensitivity, and specificity [90,91], and published studies are generally hampered by small patient samples and limited reproducibility. Some of the EEG abnormalities observed in depression may represent an epiphenomenon, may be a reflection of depressive states secondary to different underlying mechanisms, or may simply represent markers of vulnerability to depression [92]. Treatment studies with psychotherapy, antidepressants, and ECT have also failed to demonstrate a consistent trend of EEG pattern normalization [93–99]. More studies comparing different therapies for depression are needed in order to clarify the relationship between EEG changes and depression.

Neuroimaging

A large number of both structural and functional neuroimaging studies have been conducted in patients with major depression. Structural neuroimaging studies utilize either computed tomography (CT) or magnetic resonance imaging (MRI), whereas functional neuroimaging studies utilize positron emission tomography (PET), single photon CT (SPECT), or functional MRI (fMRI). Data collected in studies of depressed patients using these different modalities have converged to reveal structures and neural networks that are consistently implicated in the pathophysiology of MDD [100,101].

Structural Neuroimaging Studies

Early structural neuroimaging studies of MDD involved collecting standard clinical CT or MRI studies in depressed patients and healthy volunteers. Analyses typically involved having radiologists interpret the studies or using basic measurements (e.g., venticular-brain ratios) to compare the two groups. These early investigations demonstrated that white matter hyperintensities, likely secondary to vascular disease, are more prevalent in patients with late-onset MDD. Additionally, these rudimentary studies suggested that there are nonspecific brain volumetric differences in depressed patients when compared to healthy volunteers. However, it was the introduction of morphometric MRI (mMRI) techniques that allowed investigators to compare volumes of specific brain structures or regions. mMRI involves collecting images at a higher resolution than is typically utilized in standard clinical situations and then using computer-aided techniques to parcellate brain structures or regions on a slice-by-slice basis in order to determine their volumes. mMRI studies have reported decreased volume in the frontal cortex, hippocampus, amygdala, and basal ganglia (including caudate nucleus and putamen) in depressed patients [102].

Functional Neuroimaging Studies

Functional imaging technologies such as PET, SPECT, and fMRI provide in vivo measurements of changes in indices (e.g., cerebral blood flow and cerebral metabolic rate) that are associated with neuronal activity. These technologies may be used in conjunction with countless study designs including comparisons of resting regional cerebral metabolic rate (rCMR) in separate populations and measurements of changes in regional cerebral blood flow (rCBF) during cognitive or affective tasks [103].

Early functional neuroimaging studies of MDD used PET and SPECT to measure rCMR or rCBF while the subjects did little except lie still in the PET or SPECT camera. Dozens of these resting, or *neutral-state*, studies of MDD have been completed to date. Comparing neutral-state rCMR or rCBF in groups of depressed patients and healthy volunteers provides a measure of gross functional differences in the brain at rest much like a standard resting electrocardiogram (ECG) measures electrical activity in the heart at rest. The most consistent findings in these neutral-state neuroimaging studies of depressed patients have been *decreased* rCMR or rCBF in dorsolateral prefrontal cortex (DLPFC) and basal ganglia, *increased* rCMR or rCBF in the ventromedial prefrontal cortex (VMPFC) and amygdala, and *both* increases and decreases in different regions of the cingulate cortex [104]. As described above, volumetric abnormalities in many of these same brain regions have been demonstrated in mMRI studies of patients with MDD.

Activation studies involve measuring rCBF during an experimental task and during a control task or resting state. Differences in rCBF between the experimental task and control task are assumed to be related to performing the experimental task. If neutral state studies are analogous to a standard resting ECG, then activation studies are analogous to a cardiac stress test. Activation studies should be able to detect more subtle differences between populations than neutral-state studies. Standard activation designs involve cognitive tasks (e.g., various memory tests, the Stroop Test and the Wisconsin Card Sorting Test) or affective tasks which typically involve inducing different emotions using autobiographical scripts or during the viewing of emotionally laden films or pictures. Although many cognitive and affective activation studies have been conducted with healthy volunteers using functional neuro-imaging techniques, few to date have included patients with MDD. The activation studies that have included patients with MDD have demonstrated blunted activation of anterior paralimbic regions such as the prefrontal cortex and ACC during both cognitive and affective tasks in depressed patients when compared to healthy volunteers [105]. Future studies of patients with MDD using functional neuroimaging and activation paradigms should further elucidate the pathophysiology of MDD.

Synthesis of Neuroimaging Data

The brain regions implicated in the pathophysiology of MDD by functional neuroimaging studies are intricately interconnected with one another. In addition, these brain regions play important roles in domains of brain function that are often abnormal during major depressive episodes (MDEs). For example, activation of the DLPFC has been demonstrated during cognitive tasks in healthy volunteers. Thus, the decreased rCMR or rCBF in the DLPFC of depressed patients may be associated with the cognitive disturbances that are common during MDEs. Both the VMPFC and amygdala play vital roles in emotional and autonomic responses to stimuli. Thus, the increased rCMR or rCBF in these brain regions during MDEs may be associated with many of the neurovegetative symptoms of MDD.

attention-cognition

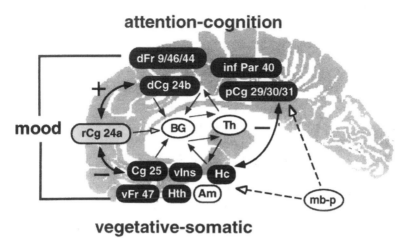

mood

vegetative-somatic

FIGURE 4 Compartmental model of depression. Brain regions consistently identified in neuroimaging studies of major depression and represented in this schematic model. Regions with known anatomical interconnections are grouped into three main compartments: dorsal (*shaded regions under the heading "attention-cognition"*), ventral (*shaded regions above the heading "vegetative-somatic"*), and rostral anterior cingulate cortex (*rCg 24a*). Depressive illness is associated with decreases in dorsal limbic and neocortical regions and relative increases in ventral paralimbic areas; with successful treatment there is a reversal of these findings. The model proposes that illness remission occurs when there is inhibition of the overactive ventral regions and activation of the previously hypofunctioning dorsal areas (*arrows connecting compartments to rCg 24a*). Integrity of the rostral cingulate (*rCg 24*), with its direct anatomical connections to both the dorsal and ventral compartments, is postulated to be additionally required for the ocurrence of these adapative changes, since pretreatment metabolism in this region uniquely predicts antidepressant response. *White regions* delineate brain regions potentially critical to the evolution of the model but where changes have not been consistently identified across neuroimaging studies. *Arrows*: 1) identify segregated ventral and dorsal compartment afferents and efferents to and from the striatum (caudate, putamen, nucleus accumbens) and thalamus (predominantly mediodorsal and anterior thalamus), although individual cortical-striatal-thalamic pathways are not delineated; 2) indicate reciprocal connections through the anterior and posterior cingulate linking the dorsal and ventral compartments. *Dotted lines* indicate serotonergic projections to limbic, paralimbic, subcortical, and cortical regions in both compartments. *Dorsal*: dFr=dorsolateral prefrontal; inf Par= inferior parietal; dCg=dorsal anterior cingulate; pCg=posterior cingulate. *Ventral*: Cg25=subgenual (infralimbic) cingulate; vIns=ventral anterior insula; Hc=hippocampus; vFr=ventral frontal; Hth=hypothalamus. rCg=rostral anterior cingulate. White: mb-p=midbrain-pons; BG=basal ganglia; Th=thalamus; Am=amygdala. Numbers are Brodmann designations. (Reprinted from J Neuropsychiatry 1997; 9:471, Fig 1. Used with kind permission from American Psychiatric Press, Inc.)

Contemporary functional models of MDD account for the fact that many of the brain regions that demonstrate decreased activity are dorsal to the brain regions that demonstrate increased activity in depressed patients. Mayberg [106] has proposed a three-compartment model of MDD (Fig. 4) that includes dorsal and ventral compartments. The dorsal compartment, which demonstrates decreased activity during MDEs, includes brain regions involved in normal attention and cognition such as the DLPFC and dorsal divisions of the cingulate cortex. The ventral compartment, which demonstrates increased activity during MDEs, includes brain regions involved in vegetative and somatic functions such as the VMPFC, ventral divisions of the cingulate cortex, and the amygdala. Following successful treatment, the activity in both of these compartments normalizes (i.e., dorsal compartment activity increases and ventral compartment activity decreases). The third compartment simply includes the rostral cingulate cortex (RCC). The RCC has extensive connections with both the dorsal and ventral compartments. In addition, there is some evidence that increased metabolism in the RCC in patients with MDD predicts response to antidepressant treatment, whereas decreased metabolism in the RCC predicts nonresponse to antidepressant treatment. Therefore, the RCC is purported to play a significant regulatory role in the network of brain regions included in this contemporary three-compartment model for the pathophysiology of MDD.

CONCLUSION

There are multiple lines of evidence to support a biological basis for depression. It is likely that there is an interaction between genetic endowment and environmental factors that alter brain structure and function, thus contributing to depressed states. However, the precise mechanisms by which this genetic/biological vulnerability is linked to environmental stress is still unclear. Despite the many technologies and biochemical modalities available, contradictory and inconsistent data suggest that none of these is sophisticated enough yet to provide a clear diagnosis or characterization of acute or chronic depressive states, or any significant leads as to optimal approaches to treatment. The future looks promising, however, and in that spirit, we offer the following speculations about the roles of these technologies in the years to come.

Genetic studies will likely gain a prominent role in predictive and/or preventive function, and may one day provide the framework for gene therapy of depression and other psychiatric disorders. Genetic markers may be found to identify individuals at risk for chronicity and treatment resistance, and genetic tests for enzymes involved in the metabolism of antidepressants (e.g., CYP-2D6 and CYP-2C19) may help identify individuals who may be slow or fast metabolizers, hence allowing for more effective dosing strategies and choice of medication [107].

Molecular and biochemical studies will provide further clarification of the current postulated mechanisms of depression, and will likely elucidate novel mechanisms of acute and chronic depression. In addition, we may gain a more precise understanding of specific loci in the brain where antidepressants exert their effect, and this may lead to the development of a faster-acting and more uniformly effective antidepressant with a more benign side effect profile.

Imaging studies will utilize increasingly sophisticated experimental designs that will reveal which brain regions are involved in emotion regulation in healthy volunteers and how these brain regions are functioning abnormally during major depressive episodes. Neuroimaging may also be useful for predicting treatment response or nonresponse to different therapeutic interventions and may help elucidate the mechanisms of action of these therapies.

Finally, we hope that these lines of investigation will also help to develop a more sophisticated understanding of the interface between medical and psychiatric illnesses, and that this may help to "legitimize" depression as a *medical* illness, hence bridging the ever-wide gap between psychiatry and medicine.

REFERENCES

1. Akiskal H. Mood Disorders: introduction and overview. In: Kaplan HI, Saddock BJ, eds. Comprehensive Texbook of Psychiatry. 6th ed. Baltimore: Williams & Wilkins, 1995, pp 1067–1079.
2. Gabbard GO. Mood disorders: psychodynamic etiology. In: Kaplan HI, Saddock BJ, Eds. Comprehensive Texbook of Psychiatry. 6th ed. Baltimore: Williams & Wilkins, 1995, pp. 1116–1123.
3. Rowe DC. Do people make environments or do environments make people? Ann NY Acad Sci 2001; 935:62–74.
4. Wong ML, Licinio J. Research and treatment approaches to depression. Nat Rev Neurosci 2001; 2(5):343–351.
5. Merikangas KR, Kupfer DJ. Mood disorders: genetic aspects. In: Kaplan HI, Saddock BJ, eds. Comprehensive Texbook of Psychiatry. 6th ed. Baltimore: Williams & Wilkins, pp. 1102–1116.
6. Kendler KS, Diehl SD. Schizophrenia: Genetics. In: Kaplan HI, Saddock BJ, eds. Comprehensive Texbook of Psychiatry. 6th ed. Baltimore: Williams & Wilkins, 1995, pp. 942–957.
7. Kendler KS, Gardner CO, Neale MC, Prescott CA. Genetic risk factors for major depression in men and women: similar or different heritabilities and same or partly distinct genes? Psychol Med 2001; 31(4):605–616.

8. Warner V, Weissman MM, Mufson L, Wickramaratne PJ. Grandparents, parents, and grandchildren at high risk for depression: a three-generation study. J Am Acad Child Adolesc Psychiatry 1999; 38:289–296.

9. Kendler KS, Gardner CO Jr. Twin studies of adult psychiatric and substance dependence disorders: are they biased by differences in the environmental experiences of monozygotic and dizygotic twins in childhood and adolescence? Psychol Med 1998; 28:625–633.

10. Wender PH, Kety SS, Rosenthal D, Schulsinger F, Ortmann J, Lunde I. Psychiatric disorders in the biological and adoptive families of adopted individuals with affective disorders. Arch Gen Psychiatry 1986; 43:923–929.

11. Kendler KS, Thornton LM, Gardner CO. Genetic risk, number of previous depressive episodes, and stressful life events in predicting onset of major depression. Am J Psychiatry 2001 Apr; 158(4):582–586.

12. Patten SB, Love EJ. Drug-induced depression. Incidence, avoidance and management. Drug Saf 1994; 10:203–219.

13. Valentine AD Meyers CA, Kling MA, Richelson E, Hauser P. Mood and cognitive side effects of interferon-alpha therapy. Semin Oncol 1998; 25(1, Suppl 1):39–47.

14. Cunningham LA. Depression in the medically ill: choosing an antidepressant. J Clin Psychiatry 1994; 55(9, Suppl A):90–97.

15. Joffe RT, Rubinow DR, Denicoff KD, Maher M, Sindelar WF. Depression and carcinoma of the pancreas. Gen Hosp Psychiatry 1986; 8:241–245.

16. Robinson RG, Kubos KL, Starr LB, Rao K, Price TR. Mood disorders in stroke patients. Importance of location of lesion. Brain 1984; 107:81–93.

17. Cummings JL, Masterman DL. Depression in patients with Parkinson's disease. Int J Geriatr Psychiatry 1999; 14:711–718.

18. Delgado PL, Miller HL, Salomon RM, Licinio J, Krystal JH, Moreno FA, Heninger GR, Charney DS. Tryptophan-depletion challenge in depressed patients treated with desipramine or fluoxetine: implications for the role of serotonin in the mechanism of antidepressant action. Biol Psychiatry 1999; 46:212–220.

19. Bejjani BP, Damier P, Arnulf I, Thivard L, Bonnet AM, Dormont D, Cornu P, Pidoux B, Samson Y, Agid Y. Transient acute depression induced by high-frequency deep-brain stimulation. N Engl J Med. 1999 May 13; 340(19):1476–1480.

20. Bailine SH, Rifkin A, Kayne E, Selzer JA, Vital-Herne J, Blieka M, Pollack S. Comparison of bifrontal and bitemporal ECT for major depression. Am J Psychiatry 2000;157:121–123.

21. Bridges P. Psychosurgery for resistant depression: progress and problems. Int Clin Psychopharmacol. 1991; 6(Suppl 1):73–80.

22. Loo C, Mitchell P, Sachdev P, McDarmont B, Parker G, Gandevia S. Double-blind controlled investigation of transcranial magnetic stimulation for the treatment of resistant major depression. Am J Psychiatry 1999; 156: 946–948.

23. Rush AJ, George MS, Sackeim HA, Marangell LB, Husain MM, Giller C,

Nahas Z, Haines S, Simpson RK Jr, Goodman R. Vagus nerve stimulation (VNS) for treatment-resistant depressions: a multicenter study. Biol Psychiatry 2000; 47:276–286.

24. Owens MJ, Nemeroff CB. Role of serotonin in the pathophysiology of depression: focus on the serotonin transporter. Clin Chem 1994; 40:288–295.

25. Kapur S, Mann JJ. Role of the dopaminergic system in depression. Biol Psychiatry 1992; 32:1–17.

26. Willner P. Dopamine and depression: a review of recent evidence. II. Theoretical approaches. Brain Res Review 1983; 6:225–236.

27. Loo H, Scatton B, Dennis T, Benkelfat C, Gay C, Poirier-Littre MF, Garreau M, Vanelle JM, Olie JP, Deniker P. (Study of noradrenaline metabolism in depressed patients by the determination of plasma dihydroxyphenylethylene glycol.) Encephale 1983; 9(4):297–316.

28. Roy A, Pickar D, Linnoila M, Doran AR, Ninan P, Paul SM. Cerebrospinal fluid monoamine and monoamine metabolite concentrations in melancholia. Psychiatry Res 1985; 15(4):281–92.

29. Roy A, Linnoila M, Karoum F, Pickar D. Relative activity of metabolic pathways for norepinephrine in endogenous depression. Acta Psychiatr Scand 1986; 73(6):624–628.

30. Roy A, Pickar D, De Jong J, Karoum F, Linnoila M. Norepinephrine and its metabolites in cerebrospinal fluid, plasma, and urine. Relationship to hypothalamic-pituitary-adrenal axis function in depression. Arch Gen Psychiatry 1988; 45(9):849–857.

31. Roy A, Linnoila M, Karoum F, Pickar D. Urinary-free cortisol in depressed patients and controls: relationship to urinary indices of noradrenergic function. Psychol Med 1988; 18(1):93–98.

32. Beckmann H, Goodwin FK. Antidepressant response to tricyclics and urinary MHPG in unipolar patients. Clinical response to imipramine or amitriptyline. Arch Gen Psychiatry 1975; 32(1):17–21.

33. Scatton B, Loo H, Dennis T, Benkelfat C, Gay C, Poirier-Littre MF. Decrease in plasma levels of 3,4-dihydroxyphenylethyleneglycol in major depression. Psychopharmacology (Berl) 1986; 88(2):220–225.

34. Siever LJ, Uhde TW, Jimerson DC, Lake CR, Kopin IJ, Murphy DL. Indices of noradrenergic output in depression. Psychiatry Res 1986; 19(1):59–73.

35. Howland RH, Thase ME. Biological studies of dysthymia. Biol Psychiatry 1991; 30(3):283–304.

36. Arana GW, Baldessarini RJ, Ornsteen M. The dexamethasone suppression test for diagnosis and prognosis in psychiatry. Commentary and review. Arch Gen Psychiatry 1985; 42(12):1193–1204.

37. Arriaga F, Cavaglia F, Matos-Pires A, Lara E, Paiva T. EEG sleep characteristics in dysthymia and major depressive disorder. Neuropsychobiology 1995; 32(3):128–131.

38. Szadoczky E, Fazekas I, Rihmer Z, Arato M. The role of psychosocial and biological variables in separating chronic and non-chronic major depression and early-late-onset dysthymia. J Affect Disord 1994; 32(1):1–11.

39. Ravindran AV, Griffiths J, Merali Z, Anisman H. Primary dysthymia: a study of several psychosocial, endocrine and immune correlates. J Affect Disord 1996; 40(1–2):73–84.

40. Anisman H, Ravindran AV, Griffiths J, Merali Z. Endocrine and cytokine correlates of major depression and dysthymia with typical or atypical features. Mol Psychiatry 1999; 4(2):182–188.

41. Ravindran AV, Bialik RJ, Lapierre YD. Primary early onset dysthymia, biochemical correlates of the therapeutic response to fluoxetine: I. Platelet monoamine oxidase and the dexamethasone suppression tests. J Affect Disord 1994; 31(2):111–117.

42. Akiskal H, McKinney W. Overview of recent research in depression: integration of 10 conceptual models into a comprehensive clinical frame. Arch Gen Psychiatry 1975; 32: 285–305.

43. Schildkraut JJ. The catecholamine hypothesis of affective disorders: a review of supporting evidence. Am J Psychiatry 1965; 122(5):509–522.

44. Bunney WE Jr, Davis JM. Norepinephrine in depressive reactions. A review. Arch Gen Psychiatry. 1965; 13(6):483–494.

45. Coppen A. The biochemistry of affective disorders. Br J Psychiatry 1967; 113:1237–1264.

46. Janowsky DS, el-Yousef MK, Davis JM, Sekerke HJ. A cholinergic-adrenergic hypothesis of mania and depression. Lancet 1972 S3; 2(7778): 632–635.

47. Janowsky DS. Is cholinergic sensitivity a genetic marker for the affective disorders? Am J Med Gen 1994; 54:335–344.

48. Lapin IP, Oxenkrug GF. Intensification of the central serotoninergic processes as a possible determinant of the thymoleptic effect. Lancet 1969; 1(7586): 132–6.

49. Kelly CB, Cooper SJ. Plasma noradrenaline response to electroconvulsive therapy in depressive illness. Br J Psychiatry 1997; 171:182–186.

50. Nierenberg AA, Dougherty DD, Rosenbaum JF. Dopaminergic agents and stimulants as antidepressant augmentation strategies. J Clin Psychiatry 1998; 59(Suppl 5):60–63.

51. Mischoulon D. Why do antidepressants take so long to work? Am Soc Clin Psychopharmacol Prog Notes 1997; 8:9–11.

52. Nutt D. Substance P antagonists: a new treatment for depression? Lancet 1998; 352:1644–1646.

53. Kramer MS, Cutler N, Feighner J, Shrivastava R, Carman J, Sramek JJ, Reines SA, Liu G, Snavely D, Wyatt-Knowles E, Hale JJ, Mills SG, MacCoss M, Swain CJ, Harrison T, Hill RG, Hefti F, Scolnick EM, Cascieri MA, Chicchi GG, Sadowski S, Williams AR, Hewson L, Smith D, Carlson EJ, Hargreaves RJ, Rupniak NM. Distinct mechanism for antidepressant activity by blockade of central substance P receptors. Science 1998; 281:1640–1645.

54. Argyropoulos SV, Nutt DJ. Substance P antagonists: novel agents in the treatment of depression. Expert Opin Invest Drugs 2000; 9(8):1871–1875.

55. Baby S, Nguyen M, Tran D, Raffa RB. Substance P antagonists: the next

breakthrough in treating depression? J Clin Pharm Ther. 1999 Dec; 24(6):461–469.

56. Lieb K, Fiebich BL, Berger M. (Substance P receptor antagonists—a new antidepressive and anxiolytic mechanism?) Nervenarzt. 2000; 71(9):758–761.

57. Friedman MJ. What might the psychobiology of posttraumatic stress disorder teach us about future approaches to pharmacotherapy? J Clin Psychiatry 2000; 61(Suppl)7:44–51.

58. Mischoulon D. Herbal remedies for mental illness. Psychiatr Clin North Am Ann Drug Ther 1999; 6:1–20.

59. Mann JJ, Brent DA, Arango V. The neurobiology and genetics of suicide and attempted suicide: a focus on the serotonergic system. Neuropsychopharmacology 2001; 24(5):467–477.

60. Arborelius L, Owens MJ, Plotsky PM, Nemeroff CB. The role of corticotropin-releasing factor in depression and anxiety disorders. J Endocrinol 1999; 160:1–12.

61. Nemeroff CB, Owens MJ, Bissette G, Andorn AC, Stanley M. Reduced corticotropin releasing factor binding sites in the frontal cortex of suicide victims. Arch Gen Psychiatry 1988; 45(6):577–579.

62. Green AI, Mooney JJ, Posener, JA, Schildkraut JJ. Mood disorders: biochemical aspects. In: Kaplan HI, Saddock BJ, Eds. Comprehensive Texbook of Psychiatry. 6th ed. Baltimore: Williams & Wilkins, 1995, pp 1089–1102.

63. McBeth J, Silman AJ. The role of psychiatric disorders in fibromyalgia. Curr Rheumatol Rep 2001; 3(2):157–164.

64. Duman RS, Heninger GR, Nestler EJ. A molecular and cellular theory of depression. Arch Gen Psychiatry 1997; 54:597–606.

65. Post RM. Transduction of psychosocial stress into the neurobiology of recurrent affective disorder. Am J Psychiatry 1998; 149:999–1010.

66. Gould E. Serotonin and hippocampal neurogenesis. Neuropsychopharmacology 1999; 21:46S–51S.

67. Nibuya M, Morinobu S, Duman RS. Regulation of BDNF and trkB mRNA in rat brain by chronic electroconvulsive seizure and antidepressant drug treatments. J Neurosci 1995; 15(11):7539–47.

68. Nibuya M, Nestler EJ, Duman RS. Chronic antidepressant administration increases the expression of cAMP response element binding protein (CREB) in rat hippocampus. J Neurosci 1996; 16(7):2365–72.

69. Armitage R, Hoffmann R, Trivedi M, Rush AJ. Slow-wave activity in NREM sleep: sex and age effects in depressed outpatients and healthy controls. Psychiatry Res 2000; 95(3):201–213.

70. Dykierek P, Stadtmulter G, Schramm P, Bahro M, van Calker D, Braus DF, Steigleider P, Low H, Hohagen F, Gattaz WF, Berger M, Riemann D. The value of REM sleep parameters in differentiating Alzheimer's disease from old-age depression and normal aging. J Psychiatry Res 1998; 32(1):1–9.

71. Thase ME. Depression, sleep, and antidepressants. J Clin Psychiatry 1998; 59(Suppl)4:55–56.

72. Lauer CJ, Krieg JC. Slow-wave sleep and ventricular size: a comparative

study in schizophrenia and major depression. Biol Psychiatry 1998; 44(2):121–128.

73. Hoffmann R, Hendrickse W, Rush AJ, Armitage R. Slow-wave activity during non-REM sleep in men with schizophrenia and major depressive disorders. Psychiatry Res 2000 ;95(3):215–225.

74. Armitage R. Microarchitectural findings in sleep EEG in depression: diagnostic implications. Biol Psychiatry 1995; 37:72–84.

75. Armitage R, Emslie GJ, Hoffmann RF, Rintelmann, J, Rush AJ. Delta sleep EEG in depressed adolescent females and healthy controls. J Affect Disord 2001; 63 (1–3):139–148.

76. Dahabra S, Ashton CH, Bahrainian M, Britton PG, Ferrier IN, McAllister VA, Marsh VR, Moore PB. Structural and functional abnormalities in elderly patients clinically recovered from early and late-onset depression. Biol Psychiatry 1998; 44:34–46.

77. Debener S, Beauducel A, Nessler D, Brocke B, Heilemann H, Kayser J. Is resting anterior EEG alpha asymmetry a trait marker for depression? Findings for healthy adults and clinically depressed patients. Neuropsychobiology. 2000; 41(1):31–37.

78. Hubain PP, Staner L, Dramaix M, Kerkhofs M, Papadimitriou G, Mendlewicz J, Linkowski P. The dexamethasone suppression test and sleep electro-encephalogram in nonbipolar major depressed inpatients: a multivariate analysis. Biol Psychiatry 1998; 43:220–229.

79. Perlis ML, Giles DE, Buysse DJ, Thase ME, Tu X, Kupfer DJ. Which depressive symptoms are related to which sleep electroencephalographic variables? Biol Psychiatry 1997; 42:904–913.

80. Buysse DJ, Hall M, Tu XM, Land S, Houck PR, Cherry CR, Kupfer DJ, Frank E. Latent structure of EEG sleep variables in depressed and control subjects: descriptions and clinical correlates. Psychiatry Res 1998; 79(2):105–122.

81. Reynolds CF 3rd, Alexopoulos GS, Katz IR, Lebowitz BD. Chronic depression in the elderly: approaches for prevention. Drugs Aging 2001; 18(7): 507–514.

82. Hirschfeld RM. Personality disorders and depression: comorbidity. Depression Anxiety 1999; 10(4):142–146.

83. DeBattista C, Mueller K. Is electroconvulsive therapy effective for the depressed patient with comorbid borderline personality disorder? J ECT 2001; 17(2):91–98.

84. Thase ME, Fasiczka AL, Berman SR, Simons AD, Reynolds CF 3rd. Electroencephalographic sleep profiles before and after cognitive behavior therapy of depression. Arch Gen Psychiatry 1998; 55:138–144.

85. Buysse DJ, Frank E, Lowe KK, Cherry CR, Kupfer DJ. Electroencephalographic sleep correlates of episode and vulnerability to recurrence in depression. Biol Psychiatry 1997; 41(4):406–418.

86. Leuchter AF, Cook IA, Uijtdehaage SH, Dunkin J, Lufkin RB, Anderson-Hanley C, Abrams M, Rosenberg-Thompson S, O'Hara R, Simon SL, Osato

S, Babaie A. Brain structure and function and the outcomes of treatment for depression. J Clin Psychiatry 1997; 58(Suppl)16:22–31.

87. Leuchter AF, Cook IA, Uijtdehaage SH, Dunkin J, Lufkin RB, Anderson-Hanley C, Abrams M, Rosenberg-Thompson S, O'Hara R, Simon SL, Osato S, Babaie A. Brain structure and function and the outcomes of treatment for depression. J Clin Psychiatry 1997; 58(Suppl)16:22–31.

88. Cook IA, Leuchter AF. Prefrontal changes and treatment response prediction in depression. Semin Clin Neuropsychiatry 2001; 6(2):113–120.

89. Cook IA, Leuchter AF, Witte E, Abrams M, Uijtdehaage SH, Stubbeman W, Rosenberg-Thompson S, Anderson-Hanley C, Dunkin JJ. Neurophysiologic predictors of treatment response to fluoxetine in major depression. Psychiatry Res 1999; 85(3):263–73.

90. Buysse DJ, Kupfer DJ. Diagnostic and research applications of electroencephalographic sleep studies in depression. Conceptual and methodological issues. J Nerv Ment Dis 1990; 178:405–414.

91. Eiber R, Escande M. (Sleep electroencephalography in depression and mental disorders with depressive comorbidity.) Encephale 1999; 25(5):381–390.

92. Fulton MK, Armitage R, Rush AJ. Sleep electroencephalographic coherence abnormalities in individuals at high risk for depression: a pilot study. Biol Psychiatry 2000; 47(7):618–625.

93. Van Bemmel AL. The link between sleep and depression: the effects of antidepressants on EEG sleep. J Psychosom Res 1997; 42:555–564.

94. Nofzinger EA, Berman S, Fasiczka A, Miewald JM, Meltzer CC, Price JC, Sembrat RC, Wood A, Thase ME. Effects of bupropion SR on anterior paralimbic function during waking and REM sleep in depression: preliminary finding using. Psychiatry Res 2001 Apr 10; 106(2):95–111.

95. Landolt HP, Raimo EB, Schnierow BJ, Kelsoe JR, Rapaport MH, Gillin JC. Sleep and sleep electroencephalogram in depressed patients treated with phenelzine. Arch Gen Psychiatry 2001; 58(3):268–276.

96. Pizzagalli D, Pascual-Marqui RD, Nitschke JB, Oakes TR, Larson CL, Abercrombie HC, Schaefer SM, Koger JV, Benca RM, Davidson RJ. Anterior cingulate activity as a predictor of degree of treatment response in major depression: evidence from brain electrical tomography analysis. Am J Psychiatry 2001; 158(3):405–415.

97. Hese RT, Jedrzejewska B. (Multiple EEG examinations in patients with refractory endogenous depression after unilateral ECT). Psychiatr Pol 1999; 33(6):897–907.

98. Buysse DJ, Kupfer DJ, Cherry C, Stapf D, Frank E. Effects of prior fluoxetine treatment on EEG sleep in women with recurrent depression. Neuropsychopharmacology 1999; 21(2):258–267.

99. Buysse DJ, Tu XM, Cherry CR, Begley AE, Kowalski J, Kupfer DJ, Frank E. Pretreatment REM sleep and subjective sleep quality distinguish depressed psychotherapy remitters and nonremitters. Biol Psychiatry 1999; 45(2):205–213.

100. Dougherty D, Rauch SR. Neuroimaging and neurobiological models of depression. Harv Rev Psychiatr 1997; 5:138–159.
101. Drevets WC. Integration of structural and functional imaging: examples in depression research. In: Dougherty DD, Rauch SR, eds. Psychiatric Neuroimaging Research: Contemporary Stratagies. Washington, DC: American Psychiatric Press, 2001, pp 249–290.
102. Sheline YI. 3D MRI studies of neuroanatomic changes in unipolar major depression: the role of stress and medical comorbidity. Biol Psychiatry 2000; 48:791–800.
103. Dougherty DD, Rauch SR, eds. Psychiatric Neuroimaging Research: Contemporary Stratagies.Washington DC: American Psychiatric Press, 2001.
104. Drevets WC. Neuroimaging studies of mood disorders. Biol Psychiatry 2000;48:813–829.
105. Dougherty DD, Mayberg HS. Neuroimaging studies of treatment response: the example of major depression. In: Dougherty DD, Rauch SR, eds. Psychiatric Neuroimaging Research: Contemporary Stratagies. Washington, DC: American Psychiatric Press, 2001, pp 179–192.
106. Mayberg HS. Limbic-cortical dysregulation: a proposed model of depression. J Neuropsychiatry Clin Neurosci 1997;9:471–481.
107. Steimer W, Muller B, Leucht S, Kissling W. Pharmacogenetics: a new diagnostic tool in the management of antidepressive drug therapy. Clin Chim Acta 2001; 308(1–2):33–41.

5

Family and Genetic Studies of Depression

Jordan W. Smoller and Roy H. Perlis
Massachusetts General Hospital
and Harvard Medical School
Boston, Massachusetts, U.S.A.

INTRODUCTION

Major depressive disorder (MDD) is a common and often disabling disorder, with an estimated lifetime prevalence of 17% [1]. In 1999, unipolar depression ranked fifth among the leading causes of disease burden worldwide [2]. Given its high prevalence and associated morbidity, efforts to improve our understanding and treatment of depression have urgent public health significance. Over the past two decades, the genetic basis of depression has been studied with increasingly sophisticated epidemiological and molecular genetic methods. Despite variation in the populations studied and methods of assessment, family and twin studies have provided compelling evidence that major depression is familial and that genes account for a substantial proportion of this familiality. Molecular genetic studies of depression are now appearing with increasing frequency and offer the promise of identifying specific susceptibility genes. In the sections that follow, we will review this work, highlighting both established findings and unresolved questions about the genetic basis of depression. In particular, we will see that the heterogeneity and complexity of the phenotype of depression represent significant challenges to the progress of molecular genetic studies. To date, no specific susceptibility genes have been established, but with advances in phenotypic character-ization, molecular genetic technologies, and statistical methods, the pros-pect of identifying such genes has become a foreseeable goal.

PSYCHIATRIC GENETIC RESEARCH: A FRAMEWORK

We will review the genetics of depression using a framework that Faraone and Tsuang have called the "chain of psychiatric genetic research" [3], a series of study designs used to answer questions about the genetic epidemiology and molecular genetics of psychiatric disorders. The initial question is whether a disorder or trait "runs in families." Family studies address this question by comparing the prevalence of the disorder in relatives of affected individuals (cases) to that in relatives of unaffected individuals (controls). A higher prevalence (recurrence risk) among relatives of affected probands indicates that the disorder can be familial, but it does not necessarily mean that genes are involved; a disorder may run in families for nongenetic (environmental) reasons. The second question of interest is whether familial transmission of a disorder is attributable to genetic factors. Here, twin and adoption studies can be used to estimate the relative contributions of genetic and environmental influences. Estimates of heritability (the proportion of phenotypic variance in a population that is attributable to genetic factors) can be derived from these studies and provide an indication of the magnitude of genetic influences. Having established that genes may play a role in the disorder, segregation analyses and other statistical techniques are sometimes used to answer the third question: What is the mode of inheritance of the genetic liability (e.g., dominant, polygenic)? Ultimately, however, molecular genetic methods are required to address the question of what specific genes are involved. Two general approaches are used to identify such genes. Genome scan linkage studies involve testing whether any of a large number of DNA markers, placed at intervals along all the chromosomes, is coinherited with (linked to) the phenotype of interest. If a chromosomal region is linked to the disorder, this supports the possibility that a susceptibility gene lies in that region; additional methods can then be used to "fine map" and isolate the gene. The advantage of this approach is that it does not require any a priori knowledge about what genes may be involved. The other approach involves testing genes that are plausible "candidate" genes by virtue of prior knowledge about their function or chromosomal location. Candidate gene testing is often done using association methods which examine whether a particular allele (or variant) of the gene is associated with the disorder among affected individuals. This can be done either by comparing the frequency of an allele in the affected cases to that in unrelated controls or by examining whether a particular allele is transmitted within a family to affected individuals more often than chance expectation. Candidate gene association studies have the advantage that they can be more powerful than linkage analyses under certain circumstances [4].

GENETIC EPIDEMIOLOGY OF MAJOR DEPRESSION

Family Studies

A substantial body of evidence has established that MDD is a familial phenotype. This finding has been replicated in family studies using a range of methods (e.g., family history reports vs. direct-interview assessments), proband groups (e.g., parents, children, siblings), and diagnostic criteria [5–21]. In case-control family studies, the risk of depression to relatives of depressed probands has been significantly higher than the risk to relatives of unaffected controls, with relative risks ranging from approximately twofold to ninefold [5,7,8,16,17,21,22].

Although the consistency of findings is persuasive, a number of the available studies may be difficult to interpret in light of methodological limitations. For example, some studies have used the family history method, which can be less sensitive than direct-interview methods for detecting psychopathology in relatives [23]. In other studies, assignment of diagnoses has not been blind with respect to diagnostic status of other family members.

Sullivan and colleagues (2000) [24] performed a meta-analysis of family, twin, and adoption studies of depression. The studies they selected met five a priori inclusion criteria: (1) explicit distinction between unipolar and bipolar disorder; (2) systematic proband recruitment and ascertainment of relatives; (3) direct collection of diagnostic data (e.g., rather than relying on family history reports); (4) use of operationalized diagnostic criteria; and (5) diagnostic determination blind to ascertainment source and diagnoses of other relatives. They identified five family studies that met these criteria [5,7,17,25,26]. All five studies provided evidence in support of the familiality of depression, with morbidity risks ranging from 15.2 to 21.6% for relatives of affected probands and 5.5 to 10.6% for relatives of control probands. The summary odds ratio across the studies was 2.84 (95% CI: 2.31–3.49), indicating that the prevalence of depression was nearly threefold higher in the relatives of affected probands compared to the relatives of unaffected controls.

Again, although family studies can support the possibility that genes influence the development of depression, they cannot prove it. How much of the familial aggregation of depression is attributable to genetic factors? Adoption and twin studies can address this question by examining the relative contributions of genetic and environmental influences on a phenotype.

Adoption Studies

Adoption studies can help distinguish genetic and environmental influences on family resemblance by comparing rates of a disorder in biological family members to those in adoptive family members. If genes influence the risk of a disorder, biological (genetically related) family members should resemble each other more than do adoptive (environmentally related) family members. Unfortunately, adoption studies are logistically difficult to conduct and are subject to a number of potential confounds [27]. For example, adoptive parents and biological parents of adoptees may not be representative of the general population on variables relevant to the study question (e.g., family and personal history of psychopathology). In addition, the social and ethnic background of biological and adoptive families may be correlated due to "selective placement" of adoptees. The availability and interpretability of adoption studies of mood disorders have therefore been somewhat limited.

Von Knorring and colleagues [28] studied biological and adoptive families of 115 adoptees with mood disorders (51 had primary unipolar depressive disorders) or histories of substance abuse and compared them to 115 matched control families. They did not find evidence of excessive transmission of depression among biological relatives, although diagnoses were made based on records rather than direct interviews. Cadoret and colleagues [29] also did not find significant evidence for a genetic basis of depression in their study of 443 adoptees. Although structured psychiatric interviews were performed for the adoptees and their adoptive parents, the study has methodological limitations, because diagnoses were made indirectly for biological relatives from available records and because most of the biological parents had not passed through the age of risk for mood disorders. In a reanalysis of data from this study, Sullivan and colleagues [24] note that the association between depression in adoptees and their biological parents is nominally significant when data for both genders are combined. Wender and colleagues [30] used Danish adoption records to ascertain 71 adoptee probands affected with mood disorders and 71 unaffected control adoptees. These investigators observed a significantly higher rate of unipolar depression in biological relatives of affected probands than in adoptive relatives, although, again, psychiatric diagnoses of biological and adoptive relatives were derived from available psychiatric and death records rather than direct interviews.

In general, adoption studies of depression have found only modest support for genetic influences, but their interpretability has been limited by the use of indirect assessments, older diagnostic criteria, and modest sample sizes.

Twin Studies

Twin studies typically compare the concordance rates of a disorder between monozygotic twins (who are essentially genetically identical) and dizygotic twins (who share on average half of their genes). Assuming that shared environmental influences on monozygotic (MZ) twins are not different from environmental influences on dizygotic (DZ) twins (the "equal environments assumption"), then significantly higher concordance rates in MZ twins reflect the action of genes. Nevertheless, an MZ concordance rate that is less than 100% means that environmental factors influence the phenotype. Twin studies can also be used to estimate the contribution of genetic and environmental factors to the variance in liability to the disorder [27]. These are often partitioned into three components: additive genetic influences, shared familial environment (e.g., social class during childhood, parents' rearing style), and individual-specific environment (e.g., stressful life events). The *heritability* of the disorder is an estimate of the proportion of phenotypic variance that can be attributed to genetic influences. Heritability refers to the strength of genetic influences in a population—not a particular individual— and heritability estimates may differ depending on the population studied.

Overall, twin studies of major depression have provided consistent evidence that genes account for at least a moderate proportion of the familial aggregation of major depression. In almost all recent twin studies, concordance rates for MZ twins have exceeded those for DZ twins [24,31]. For studies published since 1985, the MZ concordance rates have typically fallen in the range of 30–50%, whereas DZ concordance rates have typically ranged from 12 to 40%, with somewhat higher rates seen in female compared with male twin pairs [24,31].

Sullivan and colleagues [24] found five twin studies that met their meta-analysis inclusion criteria (described above). Three involved community samples of twin pairs [32–35], one examined a clinical sample [36], and one included both a community and clinical sample [37]. The estimates of heritability in these studies ranged from 17 to 78%. Applying model fitting techniques to data from all of the studies, Sullivan and colleagues computed summary estimates of the components of variance in the liability to major depression. In their best-fitting model, only genetic and individual-specific environmental effects contributed. The summary heritability was 37% (95% CI: 33–42%), with a larger share of the variance explained by individual-specific environment (63%, 95% CI: 58–67%). The absence of a significant effect of shared family environment suggests that the familial aggregation of major depression is due mostly or entirely to genetic influences.

Segregation Analysis

In light of evidence that genes contribute substantially to the familial aggregation of MDD, segregation analysis can be useful in defining the mode of inheritance of the genetic liability. In general terms, such analyses involve fitting various statistical models of inheritance (e.g., dominant, recessive, multifactorial polygenic) to the observed pattern of disease in pedigrees and determining which modes of inheritance are consistent or inconsistent with the observed data. This information, in turn, can be used to motivate and guide linkage studies. In particular, linkage analysis is more likely to be successful if the mode of inheritance reflects the action of a single or small number of major genes rather than many genes of small effect. Several early segregation analyses of depression were unable to distinguish clearly between single major locus (SML) inheritance and non-genetic transmission [38–40] or between SML and polygenic or multifactorial inheritance in affected pedigrees [41,42]. More recently, Marazita and colleagues [43] performed a segregation analysis on 50 multigenerational pedigrees ascertained through a proband with early-onset (≤age 25 years), recurrent (two or more episodes) depression. When the affected phenotype of relatives was defined narrowly (as recurrent depression), their best-fitting model was a recessive SML. For the broader phenotype of any major affective illness in relatives, the best-fitting model was a codominant major locus transmitted in mendelian fashion. Another segregation analysis of recurrent, early-onset depression in a larger sample of 81 families (4 of which were included in the previous report of Marazita and colleagues) also supported single major locus effects, with a sex-independent mendelian codominant model of transmission for recurrent MDD and a sex-independent mendelian dominant model for transmission of the broader phenotype of major mood disorder (43a). These studies support the possibility that major genes for subtypes of unipolar depression may exist and may be detectable if probands are selected for a severe, early-onset phenotype. Nevertheless, this and other such studies have not resolved the precise mode of inheritance of the genetic liability to major depression. Given the fact that MDD is relatively common and phenotypically complex, it seems unlikely that one or a few major genes will explain the genetic basis of most cases of the disorder. Even if major loci do contribute to the disorder within some families, it is possible that different major genes are segregating in different families (genetic heterogeneity), a circumstance which can complicate linkage analyses [43].

Dissecting the Genetic Epidemiology of MDD

Taken together, the family, adoption, and twin studies reviewed above suggest that genes influence the risk of major depression. These studies can also address a number of secondary questions of interest about the genetic epidemiology of depression. We examine these in the sections below.

What Is the Relationship Between Genetic Risk and Stressful Life Events in Determining Risk for Depression?

As reviewed above, twin studies have demonstrated that the heritability of MDD is moderate (approximately 40%), implying that environmental factors also play a substantial role in risk for the disorder. In fact, most of the residual variance appears to be accounted for by environmental influences that are specific to the individual [24]. This is consistent with the substantial body of evidence implicating stressful life events as triggers of depressive episodes [44,45]. However, defining the contributions and interactions of genetic and environmental influences on MDD has proved to be a complex endeavor. Interestingly, data from family and twin studies indicate that the liability to experience adverse life events can itself be familial/ genetic [46–48], and that genetic risk factors for depression increase the probability of experiencing or reporting stressful life events [49,50], although the latter phenomenon has not been seen in all studies [21]. In a large sample of female twin pairs from the Virginia Twin Registry, Kendler and colleagues [51] observed a gene-environment interaction in which genes influencing depression acted in part by increasing the susceptibility of individuals to the depressogenic effects of stressful life events. In a subsequent analysis [49], they estimated that roughly 10–15% of the impact of genes on risk for MDD is mediated through increasing the probability of experiencing stressful life events. Other twin analyses have substantiated the existence of gene-environment interactions whereby genes influence susceptibility to adverse effects of life events [52].

Finding that the relationship between stressful life events and onset of MDD weakened as the number of recurrent episodes increases (suggesting a "kindling" effect), Kendler and colleagues [53] recently examined patterns of recurrence and genetic risk among their female twin pair cohort. They observed evidence for distinct pathways to recurrent MDD, depending on genetic risk. Higher genetic risk (indexed here by having a cotwin with MDD) appeared to produce a "prekindling" effect whereby recurrent episodes are likely to occur in the absence of environmental triggers. Among those at low genetic risk, however, stressful life events may initially precipitate depressive episodes, and these episodes may then reduce the threshold for spontaneous recurrent episodes.

Are There Gender Differences in the Genetic Liability to Depression?

Epidemiological studies have shown that the lifetime prevalence of major depression is approximately two to three times higher among women compared to men [1,54]. This disparity raises the question of whether there are etiological differences in the liability to depression in women versus men. In general, family studies have not indicated that relatives of depressed women are at higher risk than relatives of depressed men [5,9,12,55]. The heritability of depression in studies of female twin pairs [56] has been similar to that reported for male twin pairs [33]. In their population-based sample of 3790 twin pairs from the Virginia Twin Registry, Kendler and Prescott [34,35] reported a heritability of 34% for the liability to depression in both men and women. The genetic correlation in the liability to major depression in the two sexes was 0.52, suggesting substantial but not complete overlap of the genetic factors affecting depression in women and men. In their meta-analysis, Sullivan et al. [24] found no consistent gender differences in heritability across the five studies they examined. However, in one of those studies, using a large community-based sample (of 2662 Australian twin pairs), Bierut et al. [32] found significantly different estimates of heritability of major depression in women (36–44%) compared to men (18–24%). Most recently, Kendler and colleagues [57] reported similar results in a follow-up study of nearly 3000 twin pairs who underwent diagnostic assessments on two occasions. In their best-fitting model, the heritability of liability to depression was 57% for women and 43% for men, and the correlation of genetic factors between the sexes was 0.55. These results suggest that genes influence risk of depression in both men and women, although the magnitude of the effect may be somewhat stronger in women, and that the genes involved are not entirely the same for the two sexes. The existence of sex-specific susceptibility loci has recently received some support in molecular genetic studies of recurrent, early-onset depression (57a,b).

Are There Features or Subtypes of Depression that Are More Familial?

Depression is a complex and heterogeneous disorder. The identification of phenotypic features that reflect a stronger familial or genetic loading could have important implications for both clinicians and researchers. Clinically, evidence of higher genetic loading might signal greater vulnerability to recurrent depression [53] or the need for increased vigilance for signs of disorder in offspring. For researchers seeking to identify the genes involved in MDD, features which indicate increased genetic loading may facilitate genetic linkage and association studies by defining phenotypes with a stronger genetic "signal to noise ratio."

Does the strength of genetic influences vary with how broadly or narrowly one defines a case of depression? Kendler and colleagues [58] examined the heritability of nine commonly used research definitions of major depression in their population-based female twin sample (N = 1033 pairs). They found that the heritability of broadly and narrowly defined depression was consistently in the range of 33–45%; however, definitions that excluded cases of secondary depression demonstrated lower heritability (21–24%). A more recent study of 2662 Australian twin pairs similarly found no difference in the heritability of narrowly or broadly defined depression [32]. Subsyndromal forms of depression also appear to be familial [59]. In their twin sample, Kendler et al. [60] applied latent class analysis to the DSM-III-R symptoms of depression and identified three depressive syndromes which differed by symptom constellations, associated comorbidity, and severity. These were labeled "mild typical" depression, "severe typical" depression, and "atypical" depression. They found that concordance rates for the atypical and severe typical subtypes were high in MZ twin pairs but not DZ twin pairs, suggesting a genetic component to the expression of these depressive syndromes.

A number of clinical features of depression have been reported to predict greater familial risk of the disorder in relatives of affected probands. For example, recurrent depression has been associated with greater familial loading in several family and twin studies [8,9,22,36,61,62]. In the large Virginia Twin Registry sample, Kendler and colleagues found that recurrence in an index twin predicted MDD in the cotwin. In fact, the familial risk of MDD was highest for intermediate levels of recurrence (7 to 9 lifetime episodes), decreasing again if the index twin had 10 or more episodes.

Some family studies have supported the hypothesis that familial risk of depression is related to the severity and impairment associated with depression among affected probands [61], although others have not [14,55]. In their study of male twin pairs (N = 3372), Lyons and colleagues [33] found evidence of moderate heritability (39%) for severe/psychotic major depression but not for mild or moderate major depression or for dysthymia. Severe/psychotic depression was defined in terms of excess symptoms beyond the diagnostic threshold, greater impairment, and/or delusions or hallucinations. In their female twin sample, Kendler and Gardner [59] found that risk of depression in a cotwin was a monotonic function of severity, impairment, or number of depressive symptoms in the index twin, although the degree of impairment and number of symptoms were not significant predictors in their larger sample of both male and female twins [35,62].

Numerous family and twin studies have examined whether early age at onset of depression is associated with stronger familial transmission. Sullivan and colleagues (2000) have pointed out that two features of these studies complicate their interpretation. First, the age cut-off used to define "early-onset" has varied across studies from < 20 years to < 52 years; and second, apparent effects of age at onset may be confounded if age cohort effects on the incidence of depression are not accounted for. Nevertheless, a number of studies have observed an association between age at onset and familiality of depression.

In an analysis of more than 200 families, Weissman et al. [63] found an inverse relationship between proband age of onset and familial risk of depression. Relatives of probands with onset before age 20 years had the highest risk of depression, whereas relatives of probands with onset after age 40 years had rates that only slightly exceeded those of relatives of unaffected probands. In addition, early-onset depression itself appeared to be a familial phenotype in that probands with age of onset < 20 years were the group most likely to have relatives with onset < 20 years and were nearly eight times more likely to have relatives with this age of onset compared to unaffected probands. In another analysis [64], this group found that parents with early-onset MDD (< age 20 years) were more likely to have children with early-onset MDD, particularly prepubertal-onset depression. In an independent family study sample, Weissman and colleagues [17] again provided evidence for the specificity of early-onset depression. They found that relatives of early-onset (< 30 years) probands had a more than fivefold increased risk of early-onset MDD but did not have an excess risk of later onset. Other family history and direct-interview family studies have supported an inverse relationship between familial risk of depression and age of onset [8,9,12,22,65]. In particular, recurrent early-onset depression has been associated with higher rates of MDD in first-degree relatives [8,22,65a] Weissman and colleagues [55] applied multivariate modeling techniques to family data from the large Yale–National Institute of Mental Health (NIMH) collaborative family study to identify subtypes which confer greatest familial risk of depression. They examined several stratifying factors including proband age at onset, recurrence, suicidality, symptom patterns, and comorbidity. Of these, only three subgroupings independently predicted increased risks of MDD in relatives: early age at onset (< 30 years), a history of anxiety disorder, or a history of secondary alcoholism.

On the other hand, it is not clear that the inverse relationship between age of onset and familial risk holds at younger ages of onset. For example, in a longitudinal family study, Harrington and colleagues [20] found that familial risk of depression was nonsignificantly *lower* in relatives of probands with prepubertal onset compared to those with postpubertal onset. Twin studies provide mixed evidence for early age of onset as an index of genetic loading for MDD. In their large study of male twin pairs, Lyons et al. [33] found that early-onset (< 30 years) MDD was significantly more heritable (47%) than later-onset depression (10%). However, Kendler and colleagues [62] did not find evidence supporting age of onset as a familial risk factor for MDD in another large sample of twins. In an analysis of data from their large population-based sample of 3786 twin pairs, they found only three features in a depressed twin that strongly predicted MDD in the cotwin: intermediate levels of recurrence, long duration of episodes, and recurrent thoughts of death or suicide [35,62].

In sum, both narrowly and broadly defined MDD appear to be moderately heritable, although certain features of depression may reflect stronger genetic influence. Although not uniformly observed, there is evidence that early age of onset, recurrence, and greater severity are associated with stronger familial transmission.

What Is the Genetic Relationship Between Unipolar Depression and Other Disorders?

Studies of the familial and genetic relationship between MDD and other disorders can help clarify the etiological relationships among disorders and the boundaries between them. Early genetic epidemiological studies often combined cases of unipolar and bipolar disorder in examining the familial basis of mood disorders. A substantial body of clinical, biological, and treatment studies support a distinction between these disorders, although the boundary between them may not be easily defined [66]. For the most part, family and genetic studies have suggested that relatives of unipolar probands have an elevated risk of unipolar disorder but not a substantially elevated risk of bipolar disorder; however, some studies have found an excess of bipolar disorder in relatives of unipolar probands [31,66]. On the other hand, the risk of unipolar disorder is elevated among relatives of bipolar probands, particularly if relatives without recurrent depression are included [31,66]. One difficulty faced in family studies of the unipolar-bipolar distinction is the fact that some proportion of individuals with apparent unipolar disorder may go on to have hypomanic or manic episodes, and indicators of "potential bipolarity" have been difficult to identify [67,68]. Overall, it has been difficult to establish the extent to which unipolar and bipolar disorders coaggregate in families. Interestingly, some genetic linkage studies of bipolar disorder have found stronger evidence of linkage when unipolar disorder is included in the affected phenotype definition [69,70].

Other psychiatric disorders commonly co-occur with unipolar disorder in probands and their relatives. Do these disorders share genetic determinants with depression? The relationship between depression and alcoholism has been addressed in several family, twin, and adoption studies with mixed results. Based in part on family history data, Winokur and colleagues [71] distinguished depressed individuals with familial pure depressive disease (only depressions in the family) from those with depression spectrum disease (in which there is also a family history of alcoholism). Differences in clinical features, course, treatment response, and laboratory findings suggested that these may represent distinct subtypes [72]. There has been a large number of studies examining whether alcoholism and depression may be alternate expressions of a shared genetic diathesis, but conflicting results have been reported. Several family studies have been consistent with independent transmission of the disorders [7,73], whereas others have provided evidence of cotransmission [74,75]. In a large population-based sample, Grant and colleagues [76] found elevated rates of alcoholism among relatives of probands with MDD alone, which is consistent with the hypothesis that these disorders share genetic determinants. Similarly, in another population-based sample, Kendler and colleagues [77] observed increased risk of alcoholism in relatives of depressed probands and increased risk of depression in relatives of alcoholic probands. Twin and adoption studies have also supported the possibility of shared genetic influences on depression and alcoholism [30,78–80]. In a recent genetic linkage study, Nurnberger and colleagues [81] found evidence of linkage to chromosome 1 for the phenotype of "alcoholism or depression," providing further support for the hypothesis some of the genetic liability to both disorders is overlapping.

The frequent lifetime comorbidity of anxiety and depressive disorders and the fact that antidepressant medications are effective treatments for both groups of disorders have raised the possibility that they reflect a shared diathesis [82]. Although there have been exceptions [26,83,84], for the most part, family history and family studies of anxiety neurosis [85,86] or panic disorder probands [17,87–92] have not found evidence of increased familial rates of MDD in the absence of comorbid MDD in the proband. Family studies of depressed probands suggest that panic occurring secondary to depression is associated with familial risk of MDD but not panic disorder [41,93–96]. Studies of children at risk for anxiety or depressive disorders have yielded somewhat conflicting results, with some studies suggesting that children of depressed parents are at increased risk for anxiety disorders [97] and others finding an increased risk of depression but not anxiety disorders [94,98]. In a recent high risk study of offspring of parents with panic disorder, major depression, or their combination, Biederman and colleagues [99] found that parental major depression was associated with increased risk of major depression, social phobia, separation anxiety disorder, and multiple anxiety disorders in offspring; parental panic disorder alone, however, did not increase offspring risk of major depression. Family studies have also produced conflicting results with regard to familial coaggregation of MDD with phobic disorders or generalized anxiety disorder, with some studies supporting [74,100] and others not a familial relationship [91,101–103]. However, data from population-based twin studies have indicated that there are varying degrees of overlap between the genetic determinants of MDD and the anxiety disorders. In a sample of female twins from the Virginia Twin Register, Kendler and colleagues found modest shared genetic influences for MDD and phobias and substantial overlap between MDD and generalized anxiety disorder (GAD) [104–106]. In multivariate modeling of data for six disorders [106], they observed two common genetic factors, with MDD and GAD loading most highly on one factor and panic disorder, phobic disorders, and bulimia loading most highly on the other. In another sample that included both male and female twin pairs and both clinical and population-based samples, Roy and colleagues [107] again observed essentially complete overlap between the genetic determinants of MDD and GAD. To the extent that depression and anxiety disorders share genetic determinants, some of this may reflect heritable personality traits that predispose to both kinds of disorders. For example, family and twin studies have demonstrated that temperamental traits such as neuroticism and behavioral inhibition are heritable and have a familial/genetic link to both depression and anxiety disorders [108–111].

MOLECULAR GENETICS OF DEPRESSION

Molecular Genetic Approaches

Taken together, the genetic epidemiological data reviewed above have established that genes play some role in the development of MDD. In light of this, there is an increasingly intensive effort to identify the specific genes that are involved using molecular genetic techniques. The recent completion of a draft sequence of the human genome [112,113] has provided an important tool for such studies and should facilitate the localization of susceptibility genes. Nevertheless, molecular studies face significant obstacles because, as we have seen, unipolar depression is likely to be genetically and phenotypically complex. That is, it is possible that multiple genes of relatively small effect contribute to the disorder and different genes may be operating in different families. In addition, the optimal definition of the heritable phenotype is not clear; the DSM-IV diagnosis of MDD may be a heterogeneous category, and its genetic basis may overlap to varying degrees with other psychiatric disorders, with dysthymia, and with nonsyndromal psychological traits and symptoms [59,78,106,114,115].

Two general approaches are widely used to identify susceptibility genes for complex disorders. The first, linkage analysis, examines whether polymorphisms in DNA markers of known chromosomal location are coinherited with ("linked to") the disorder within families. Evidence of linkage indicates that a susceptibility gene may reside in the chromosomal region containing the linked marker. Linkage analysis can be conducted using markers spread across the entire genome (a whole genome scan), allowing investigators to look for susceptibility loci without requiring prior knowledge of the function or location of the genes involved. Statistical evidence of linkage is often determined by calculating a LOD score (logarithm of the odds in favor of linkage) and/or a P value. The LOD score compares the likelihood of obtaining the observed genotypes and phenotypes when linkage is present to the likelihood assuming no linkage. Traditionally, a LOD score of 3 (corresponding to odds of 1000:1 in favor of linkage) has been the threshold for declaring linkage, but for complex disorders such as psychiatric illnesses, higher thresholds (3.3–3.6) have been recommended [116]. Traditional LOD score linkage analysis has been most successfully applied when a single major gene is involved and the mode of inheritance (e.g., dominant, recessive) is known. Because these assumptions can rarely be used with psychiatric phenotypes, other (non-parametric) methods which do not require knowledge of mode of inheritance are routinely utilized. Typically, these approaches rely on statistical analysis of allele sharing within a family. If alleles at a locus tend to be shared by affected family members, this implies that the locus is linked to a disease gene.

The second widely used approach, association analysis, examines whether particular alleles of genes or markers are statistically associated with the presence of the phenotype of interest across families. For example, case-control association studies examine whether an allele is significantly more common among affected individuals (cases) than among unaffected controls. These methods can be more powerful than linkage analysis for detecting genes of modest effect [4], making them an attractive approach for the study of complex phenotypes like unipolar depression in which the genetic liability may reflect multiple genes of relatively small effect. Three circumstances may produce an apparent association between a given allele and the phenotype. First, the allele may, in fact, be a susceptibility allele for the disorder (a true positive). Second, the allele may be in "linkage disequilibrium" with a true susceptibility allele; that is, the tested allele may so physically close to the susceptibility allele that recombination events between the two have not substantially reduced their coinheritance in a population. Finally, the association may be spurious if the genetic backgrounds of the case and control groups are not well matched (population stratification). If an ethnic group that happens to have a high frequency of the candidate allele is overrepresented in the case group, the allele will be statistically associated with the phenotype even though it may play no causal role. Family-based association methods such as the transmission/disequilibrium test (TDT) avoid this problem by testing the transmission of alleles within families [117].

A third method for identifying the location of a disease gene involves cytogenetic studies which can examine whether a disorder is associated with chromosomal abnormalities (e.g., deletions, translocations). The co-occurrence of such an abnormality with a psychiatric disorder provides evidence that a gene influencing the disorders resides in the region of the abnormality.

Linkage Studies of Depression

Prior to the 1990s, linkage analysis of depression was impeded in part by the limited availability of polymorphic genetic markers. Several early linkage reports focused on phenotypic subtypes which had been suggested by Winokur [118]. Pure depressive disease (PDD) was contrasted with depressive spectrum disease (DSD) by having a later age of onset (typically > 40 years), absence of familial alcoholism and antisocial personality, less familial loading for affective disorder and other comorbidity, and an equal sex distribution of affective disorder in the family (as opposed to a female predominance in DSD). Tanna and colleagues [119] examined 29 polymorphic loci in 13 families ascertained for PDD. Using sibling pair methods of analysis and combining their results with those of two of their earlier studies, they found modest evidence of linkage (nominal $P < .05$) to the ABO and MNS blood group markers (on chromosomes 9q and 4q, respectively) and the immunoglobulin κ locus on chromosome 2p. This group examined the same markers in 27 families ascertained for DSD and found some evidence for linkage ($P = .006$) to the orosomucoid (ORM) locus on chromosome 9q. However, the same result was obtained when the affected phenotype was defined as "any psychiatric illness."

More recently, Balciuniene and colleagues [120] conducted a linkage analysis of recurrent major depression in five large Swedish families. They examined markers on chromosomes (4p, 16, 18, and 21) which had previously been claimed to harbor susceptibility loci for bipolar disorder, but no evidence of significant linkage was detected. In another study of 34 pedigrees ascertained through probands with early-onset (< 25 years) recurrent depression, no evidence of linkage or association was found between the core phenotype (or broader affective disorder phenotypes) and any of 38 polymorphisms in 12 genes related to neuroendocrine or serotonergic systems [121].

A linkage analysis of depression and alcoholism was recently reported by investigators in the Collaborative Study of the Genetics of Alcoholism (COGA), a multicenter linkage study focusing on identification of genes influencing alcoholism. Numberger and colleagues [81] performed a genomic scan on a sample of 105 families, a replication sample of 157 families, and a combined dataset of all of these families. Ascertainment was based on the family's having three alcoholic members (including the proband). Depression was defined as the presence of either DSM-III-R major depression or "depressive syndrome" (meeting all criteria for major depression except for the exclusion of organic factors in initiating or maintaining the disorder). Analyses were performed using nonparametric methods. When the affected phenotype was defined as "alcoholism or depression," a LOD score of 5.12 in the initial sample was found on chromosome 1p, with a lower LOD score in the replication sample (1.52) but still significant (LOD score = 4.66) in the combined sample. This linkage peak appeared to be broad, covering 60 cM, so further fine mapping is needed to clarify the location of a susceptibility locus on chromosome 1 if one exists. A locus on chromosome 2 also showed evidence of linkage in the combined dataset (LOD = 3.26) for this phenotype. Loci on chromosomes 6 and 16 also achieved LOD scores > 3.0 in the initial sample but not in the replication or combined samples. For the phenotype of "comorbid alcoholism and depression," the peak LOD score (0.00 in the initial sample, 4.12 in the replication sample, and 2.16 in the combined sample) was seen at a locus on chromosome 2 nearly 150 cM distal to the chromosome 2 locus linked to the "alcoholism or depression" phenotype. When the phenotype was defined as "depression with or without alcoholism," peak evidence of linkage was seen when only independent sibling pairs were analyzed on chromosome 7 (LOD = 3.97 in the initial dataset, 2.87 in the combined dataset) and chromosome 12 (LOD = 3.05 in the replication dataset, 1.41 in the combined). The observation of a chromosome 1 locus that may influence alcoholism or depression raises the possibility that there are susceptibility genes which may be variably expressed as one or the other phenotype. The fact that most of those affected with alcoholism were men, whereas most of those affected with depression were women suggests that gender may be involved in the variable expression. Nurnberger et al. note that this pattern of familial affection is reminiscent of Winokur and colleagues' description of depressive spectrum disease [118]. It should be noted that this sample was ascertained for alcoholism and that the depression phenotype included depression secondary to substance use; thus, it is not clear that similar results would be expected in a linkage study that specifically examined primary unipolar depression.

A combination of linkage and cytogenetic methods implicated another area of chromosome 1 in a study of a large Scottish extended pedigree in which a balanced translocation involving chromosome 11 (1;11)(q42;q14.3) appeared to segregate with a phenotype that included schizophrenia and mood disorders [122]. Under a dominant model of inheritance, highly significant linkage (maximum LOD = 7.1) was observed between the translocation and a phenotype that included schizophrenia, recurrent major depression, and bipolar disorder. When the affected phenotype was restricted to those with mood disorders (11 with recurrent major depression and 1 with bipolar disorder), the maximum LOD score remained highly significant at 4.5. Two genes on chromosome 1, labeled "disrupted in schizophrenia 1" (*DISC1*) and "disrupted in schizophrenia 2" (*DISC2*), are disrupted by the translocation [123]. These genes, whose precise function is unclear, can thus be considered to be candidate genes for psychotic and mood disorders, although initial linkage and association analyses in schizophrenia and bipolar disorder have been negative [124].

Recent studies of recurrent (two or more episodes), early-onset (first episode before age 25) MDD have implicated other chromosomal regions. Zubenko and colleagues (57a) performed a case-control analysis of polymorphic markers spaced at approximately 10 cM intervals across the genome in 100 cases and 100 unaffected controls and found nominally significant evidence of association with recurrent, early-onset MDD (RE-MDD) for 19 of the 387 markers. Sixteen of these were associated in only one sex (7 in men only and 9 in women only). One of these markers, on chromosome 2, was associated with RE-MDD in women but not men in both the case-control analysis and a TDT analysis of 81 families (124a). It is not clear to what extent the affected probands in the family sample are independent of those in the case-control sample. However, the marker is relatively close to the region on chromosome 2 that showed some evidence of linkage to comorbid alcoholism and depression in the COGA sample described above. Nonparametric linkage analysis showed evidence of linkage to other markers in this region of chromosome 2q33-q35 in the same set of 81 families, again only in female affected relative pairs (57b). LOD scores greater than 3.0 were observed for a pair of adjacent markers using the RE-MDD phenotype and increased as the phenotype definition broadened, exceeding 6.0 for the phenotype of "major or minor mood disorder." The *CREB1* gene, located in the 451 kb interval between these markers, has been suggested as a candidate locus because it encodes a transcription factor whose expression may mediate some effects of antidepressants. The TDT and nonparametric affected relative analysis are both tests of linkage and their application in the same set of families would not represent strictly independent replications. In any case, the simple sequence repeat markers tested are unlikely to be causally associated with MDD but might be in linkage disequilibrium with a susceptibility allele. Additional studies will be needed to determine whether a genetic variant in this region of chromosome 2 is in fact associated with MDD, but these analyses provide intriguing evidence for the existence of sex-specific susceptibility loci.

Overall, linkage analyses have not yet established any chromosomal regions as harboring susceptibility genes for MDD. However, a large NIMH-funded collaborative linkage study of early-onset, recurrent major depression is currently underway and may soon yield important information about the location of such genes. The preliminary evidence of linkage to regions of chromosomes 1 and 2 merits further study.

Candidate Gene Association Studies of Depression

As noted above, association methods may be more powerful than linkage for detecting genes of modest effect. However, a relative disadvantage of association methods is that (thus far) they have been feasible only for "candidate" loci–that is, loci suspected of being involved in the disorder based on prior knowledge about their function or chromosomal location. This presents a dilemma for psychiatric genetics: Given our limited understanding of the pathophysiology of disorders like unipolar depression, almost all brain-expressed genes may be plausible candidates but few are compelling. To date, most candidate gene–association studies of depression have focused on genes involved in neurotransmitter and neuropeptide pathways that have been previously implicated in the biology and treatment of depression. The most widely investigated neurobiological pathways have been those involved in serotonergic neurotransmission and other monoamine systems. As with many association studies, substantial heterogeneity exists among the reported results, with subsequent studies often showing only modest correlation with initial results [125]. Publication bias against negative studies and true population diversity have been suggested as reasons for discrepant results. Thus, although we discuss some preliminary findings below, larger meta-analyses may be required to confirm or dismiss the hypotheses they raise.

Serotonin-Related Genes

A number of lines of evidence implicate serotonin in the neurobiology of depression (see Chap. 4), particularly the observed efficacy of serotonin reuptake inhibitors (SSRIs) in the treatment of major depression. The SSRIs block reuptake by acting on the serotonin transporter (5HTT), and the gene encoding this transporter has been one of the most extensively studied candidate genes for mood and anxiety disorders. This gene, located on the long arm of chromosome 17, has at two relatively common polymorphisms which have been investigated in MDD. The first is located in the second intron, and consists of a variable number of tandem repeats (VNTR) [126,127]. The functional significance of the polymorphism is unclear, although studies in mouse embryonic cells and human platelets suggest that certain alleles may enhance 5HTT gene expression [128,129]. Several initial studies indicated an association between the 9-repeat allele and risk of MDD [130,131]. However, in a meta-analysis that included European-Caucasian samples of 299 patients with MDD and 772 controls, Furlong and colleagues [132] found no significant association between any VNTR allele and MDD.

The other well-characterized polymorphism lies in the promoter region of the 5HTT gene, the so-called 5HTT gene-linked polymorphic region (5HTTLPR). Two common alleles exist and are distinguishable by the insertion("long"allele) or deletion ("short" allele) of a 44–base pair sequence [133,134]. The short allele has been associated with reduced 5HTT binding in lymphoblasts [134], although one postmortem study found increased 5HTT binding in the frontal cortex among depressed suicide victims homozygous for that allele [135], and another larger postmortem study observed no association between 5HTTLPR genotype and 5HTT binding in the prefrontal cortex [136]. Genetic association analyses of this polymorphism have been inconsistent. An initial report did show a significant association between the short allele and MDD [131]; a subsequent analysis which combined results from three European centers was unable to identify a significant association between this allele and MDD, but did identify a significant association when bipolar and MDD patients were pooled. (OR: 1.23; 95% CI: 1.02–1.49).[137]. In the meta-analysis by Furlong and colleagues, described above, the association between the short allele and MDD did reach statistical significance (OR 1.23; 95% CI 1.01–1.42)[132]. Of note, two preliminary investigations in Parkinson's disease also suggest a relationship between the 5HTTLPR short allele and greater degree of depressive symptomatology [138,139]. However, a number of other studies have been unable to replicate the association between the short allele and MDD [136,140–144]. In some cases, negative findings may be attributable to limited statistical power, particularly if the relative risk conferred by the short allele is less than 1.5, as the meta-analysis suggests [132]. Interestingly, in one small study, the long allele was more common in depressed suicide victims than in controls [135].

In addition to the serotonin transporter, several of the genes encoding serotonin receptors have been examined. These include the 5HT2a receptor, another target of action for serotonergic antidepressants. A single base substitution (T102C) is relatively common, although it is believed to be a silent mutation—that is, one which does not change the structure of the protein which is expressed. Although one case-control study [145] reported a significant association between depression and the 102C allele, three more recent well-powered studies did not find that association [143,146,147]. Interestingly, one of these studies [143] did find that at least one copy of the 102C allele was associated with greater likelihood of antidepressant response at 4 weeks, and Arias and colleagues found a significant association between the 102C allele and a seasonal illness pattern [147]. These results await replication. An association between carrier status for a polymorphism in the 5HT2c receptor and MDD was reported recently in a large European sample [148] after a smaller study found no association [140]. Other serotonergic genes have been investigated in candidate gene studies, but thus far none has been associated with depression. These include the genes encoding the 5HT1b receptor [149], the 5HT5a receptor [150], the 5HT6 receptor [151,152], and tryptophan hydroxylase, the rate-limiting enzyme in serotonin synthesis [140,153,154].

Other Candidate Gene Studies

The efficacy of nonserotonergic interventions for MDD suggests that other neurobiological systems may be important in the pathophysiology or treatment response in MDD. In particular, the role of other monoamine neurotransmitter systems in depression is being investigated in many candidate gene studies. Two studies failed to detect an association between MDD and polymorphisms in the monoamine oxidase A gene, which is located on the X chromosome and encodes the enzyme inhibited by one of the earliest identified classes of antidepressants (MAOIs) [155,156]. One of these did report a significant association between homozygosity for an allele in the promoter region and recurrent MDD among female patients. A polymorphism in the norepinephrine transporter has also been investigated in a single negative association study [157]. Initial work on dopaminergic genes was driven by findings implicating dopamine receptors in antipsychotic effects (reviewed in Ref. 158); the early characterization of a number of dopaminergic genes probably accounts for the number of studies in MDD rather than the attractiveness of the dopamine system as a candidate per se. An early study of dopamine-related candidate genes failed to find an association with MDD among 49 patients and 100 controls for the D2 and D3 receptors and the dopamine transporter, but did identify an association with the D4 receptor [159]. However, a subsequent examination of both the D4 receptor and the tyrosine hydroxylase gene, the rate-limiting step in dopamine synthesis, found no association. [160]. Several other loci have been associated with MDD in preliminary studies; including a GABA-A receptor subunit (GABRA5) [161], the G-protein beta-3 subunit, which is important in intracellular second-messenger systems [162], and the nicotinic receptor alpha-7 gene [163]. Many other candidate genes have been examined with negative results to date, including the *clock* gene, believed to be important in regulation of circadian rhythms [164], and the cytotoxic T-lymphocyte antigen-4 gene [165]. Other negative studies are probably underreported.

In summary, a variety of candidate genes have been investigated in MDD but with mixed and often inconsistent results. Replication of results is essential to rule out chance findings or false positives (e.g., due to population stratification). And, just as individual studies reporting positive results can rarely establish an association, those with negative results may not rule out an association. Because the effect of individual susceptibility genes involved in MDD may be modest, many studies may lack sufficient power to detect association or linkage; in addition, many of the polymorphisms studied are not known to be functional, and the possibility remains that positive results might be found with other polymorphisms in the same genes. In any event, none of the genes examined thus far can be considered to have an established role in the etiology of MDD.

Pharmacogenomics

In addition to the search for genes involved in the pathogenesis of unipolar depression, the tools of genetics are also being applied to examine the molecular basis of treatment response. In current clinical practice, selection of an appropriate antidepressant is largely empirical. The ability to predict whether an individual will respond to and tolerate a particular antidepressant would be an extremely valuable tool for providing more rapid and safe treatment of MDD. Because the molecular targets of many antidepressant drugs are known (e.g., neurotransmitter receptors and transporters), genes encoding these targets are obvious candidates for pharmacogenomic studies. Despite the limited number of such studies to date, initial findings have been intriguing (for a review, see Ref. 166). A particularly appealing candidate has been the gene encoding the serotonin transporter (5HTT), the site of action for SSRI antidepressants. The hypothesis that genetic differences in 5HTT expression or functionality could account for differential responsiveness to SSRIs is intuitively reasonable. Two investigations of the 5HTTLPR promoter polymorphism found an association between the short allele and poorer response to fluvoxamine [167,168] or paroxetine [169]. Similarly, in a study of patients with late-life depression, homozygosity for the long allele was associated with more rapid response to paroxetine [170]. Conversely, another report found a *better* response to fluoxetine or paroxetine in depressed subjects homozygous for the short allele [171]. The latter study comprised an Asian sample in contrast to the European-Caucasian samples examined in studies reporting poorer response among patients with the short allele, raising the possibility that there may be ethnic differences in the effect of 5HTTLPR genotype. Interestingly, a preliminary study [172] recently suggested an association between homozygosity for the short allele and anti-depressant-induced mania among bipolar patients. Pharmacogenomic studies have not been limited to the 5HT transporter; for example, one recent report suggests an association between homozygosity for a tryptophan hydroxylase polymorphism and slower response to fluvoxamine (without pindolol augmentation) among MDD or bipolar patients [173]; in another study, 5HT2a genotype influenced degree of change in HAM-D-17 over 4 weeks of antidepressant treatment [143].

Pharmacogenomic studies to date have suffered from some of the same limitations that apply to candidate gene studies of susceptibility to MDD (discussed below). The definition of the phenotype (treatment response) often varies across studies. Genetic and allelic heterogeneity can reduce the power to detect genetic associations. An additional problem particular to treatment studies is that of placebo response: controlled trials in MDD may yield placebo response rates up 30–40% [174]. The inclusion of placebo responders, who could be considered "phenocopies," decreases the statistical power of these studies to detect an association between genetic polymorphisms and response to treatment. The placebo response may itself be a reasonable target for future association studies.

THE CHALLENGE OF COMPLEXITY

As reviewed in the preceding sections and summarized in Figure 1, there is substantial evidence that genes contribute to the etiology of MDD, but the specific genes involved remain unknown. In the search for susceptibility genes for MDD and other psychiatric disorders, there is perhaps no greater challenge than addressing the issue of "complexity." This complexity can be found at two levels. First, there is the problem of *genetic* complexity. Although segregation analyses have not excluded the possibility that there are genes of major effect involved, most cases of MDD are not transmitted in a simple mendelian fashion. The likelihood is that there are many genes involved in the susceptibility to MDD, that some of them will have relatively modest effects, and that interactions among these genes (epistasis) may be necessary for their expression as a clinical phenotype. In addition, several studies have supported the widely held assumption that gene-environment interactions are involved in the pathogenesis of MDD [51,52]. (Further complicating the picture is evidence that genes influencing MDD act in part by increasing an individuals' likelihood of selecting themselves into stressful environments [49].) Moreover, if the susceptibility

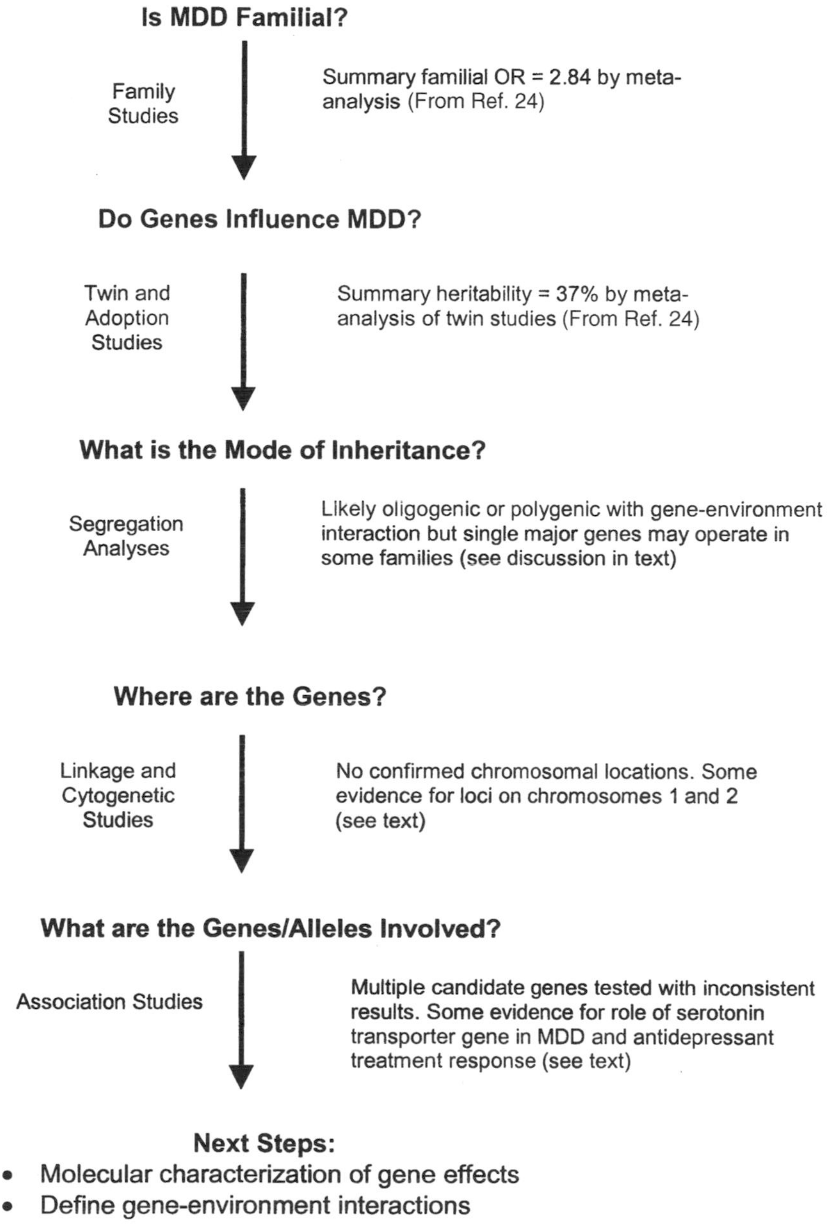

Is MDD Familial?

Family
Studies

Summary familial OR = 2.84 by meta-analysis (From Ref. 24)

Do Genes Influence MDD?

Twin and
Adoption
Studies

Summary heritability = 37% by meta-analysis of twin studies (From Ref. 24)

What is the Mode of Inheritance?

Segregation
Analyses

Likely oligogenic or polygenic with gene-environment interaction but single major genes may operate in some families (see discussion in text)

Where are the Genes?

Linkage and
Cytogenetic
Studies

No confirmed chromosomal locations. Some evidence for loci on chromosomes 1 and 2 (see text)

What are the Genes/Alleles Involved?

Association Studies

Multiple candidate genes tested with inconsistent results. Some evidence for role of serotonin transporter gene in MDD and antidepressant treatment response (see text)

Next Steps:
- Molecular characterization of gene effects
- Define gene-environment interactions

FIGURE 1   Chain of psychiatric genetic research. (After Ref. 3.) Questions and selected findings about the genetic basis of MDD.

alleles are incompletely penetrant, individuals with the "affected genotype" may not appear to have the affected phenotype. There is also the possibility that different alleles of a particular gene can influence the phenotype (allelic heterogeneity) or that different sets of susceptibility genes can produce the phenotype (locus heterogeneity). Each of these issues complicates linkage and association studies.

Second, and perhaps even more challenging, is the problem of *phenotypic* complexity. The DSM-IV diagnosis of MDD may not be the most fruitful phenotypic definition for genetic studies. In fact, in an analysis of their female twin sample, Kendler and Gardner [59] found little evidence that the DSM-IV criteria for defining MDD capture a discrete syndrome. Subsyndromal depressive symptoms appeared to be on a continuum with the major depression in terms of predicting recurrent episodes of depression in an index twin or familial risk of depression in a cotwin, leading the authors to suggest that, "our current DSM-IV diagnostic conventions for major depression ... may be arbitrary and not reflective of a natural discontinuity in depressive symptoms as experienced in the general population" (p. 177). We have also seen that family and twin studies have sometimes challenged the view that there are sharp boundaries between MDD and other disorders (e.g., bipolar disorder, alcoholism, anxiety disorders). If the liability to MDD can be variably expressed, individuals who are not affected with the clinical phenotype may nevertheless be expressing the genetic diathesis and might be misclassified as unaffected in genetic studies. Conversely, individuals may have the MDD phenotype for reasons unrelated to the genes under study (phenocopies) and may be misclassified as affected in a genetic study. In general, within a given sample of depressed individuals, there is likely to be etiologic heterogeneity—that is to say, the genetic and environmental factors causing depression are likely to vary among the sample.

How can we hope to find genes in the face of this kind of complexity? Success may require moving beyond the clinical diagnosis of depression to define more genetically homogeneous or less genetically complex phenotypes. This may include focusing on those phenotypic features or subtypes of depression that appear to be most familial. As we discussed above, family and twin studies have suggested that recurrent, early-onset, severe forms of depression may be under strongest genetic influence. Large-scale linkage studies of early-onset recurrent depression are currently underway, so we can expect to see soon whether this ascertainment strategy will yield susceptibility genes for depression. The depression phenotype may also be dissected into components or subtypes that have distinct genetic determinants. For example, suicidal ideation appears to be associated with familial depression [62], and suicidality itself may be under genetic influence [175]. Several recent studies suggest an association between suicide attempts and polymorphisms of the gene for tryptophan hydroxylase, the rate-limiting enzyme in serotonin synthesis [154,176,177].

Progress may also come from the study of "intermediate" traits—that is, personality traits and temperaments that may reflect "depression proneness." Analyses of quantitative traits may incorporate more information than those that rely on categorical diagnoses and minimize the problem of diagnostic misclassification. "Neuroticism," which refers to the predisposition to experience psychological distress and negative affects [178], appears to be associated with the risk of both anxiety disorders and depression (i.e., "neurotic disorders") [108,178–180] Numerous large twin studies have demonstrated that genes influence neuroticism, with heritability estimates consistently in the range of 30–60% [181–183]. Furthermore, twin studies of depression indicate that the genetic basis of neuroticism overlaps substantially with that of major depression [109,184]. A number of linkage and association studies have attempted to identify genes influencing this trait, beginning with a report by Lesch and colleagues [134], which documented an association between neuroticism and the functional promoter polymorphism in the serotonin transporter gene (5HTTLPR). Since then a series of studies have attempted to replicate this finding with mixed results. Although some studies have found evidence of an association between the 5HTTLPR and neuroticism [185,186], a larger number have not [187–192]. Differences in populations, assessment methods, and statistical power may account for some of these discrepancies. "Behavioral inhibition," a temperamental profile involving shyness and withdrawal in unfamiliar or novel situations [193], appears to be associated with parental MDD (particularly when comorbid panic disorder is present) [110]. Like neuroticism, behavioral inhibition is a heritable trait [194], and studies are underway to identify susceptibility loci [195].

Another approach to reducing the genetic complexity has been to search for biological or neuropsychological traits, or "endophenotypes," that may more closely reflect the expression of genes related to MDD. Endophenotypes may have a simpler genetic architecture than the disorder itself, facilitating molecular genetic searches for genes related to the disorder. To be useful for genetic studies, such endophenotypes should (1) co-occur with the disorder of interest among affected individuals; (2) be relatively stable traits rather than state-dependent concomitants of illness or treatment; (3) cosegregate with the disorder in affected family members; (4) be heritable; and (5) be more prevalent in unaffected relatives of affected probands than in the general population [196]. Although several biological traits have been associated with MDD, few studies of the familiality or heritability of such traits have been reported. Notably, in several studies, polysomnographic abnormalities characteristic of depressed individuals have been found at elevated rates in their nondepressed ("high-risk") relatives [11,197–199]. The search for and validation of biological endophenotypes for depression is in its early stages, but may be an important mechanism for overcoming some of the complexities that have slowed gene identification.

CLINICAL IMPLICATIONS AND FUTURE DIRECTIONS

Our burgeoning understanding of the genetics of MDD may have important implications for the future of both clinical care and research. For example, as genetic knowledge advances, mental health clinicians may be increasingly called upon to provide a kind of genetic counseling to psychiatric patients and their families [200]. As we have seen, family studies indicate that first-degree relatives of depressed individuals have a nearly threefold excess risk of the disorder. At this point, however, providing precise risk estimates in the clinical setting is problematic, because the recurrence risk estimates derived from epidemiological studies may not apply to the constellation of affected members in a particular family. Nevertheless, informing patients about the state of knowledge of the familial and genetic basis of depression can provide a useful psychoeducational function. Some patients and their families may overestimate the familial risk of illness and may find such information reassuring. Understanding the multifactorial etiology of MDD (i.e., that both genetic and environmental factors contribute) may also relieve unwarranted guilt or blame within an affected family. In addition, studies implicating features of depressive disorders or childhood temperament that increase the familial and developmental risk of depression (discussed above) may provide a means of identifying and targeting interventions to individuals at greater risk.

The insights gained from genetic research on MDD may also inform the nosology of mood disorders. As we have emphasized, family and genetic studies have highlighted the heterogeneity and complexity of the phenotype of depression. The boundaries among mood, anxiety, alcohol-related, and even psychotic disorders have not been fully delineated and may not be isomorphic with the diagnostic categories found in DSM-IV. Even within the domain of unipolar depression, the distinction between MDD, subsyndromal depressive symptoms, and temperamental/dimensional traits has been debated. By clarifying which phenotypes "breed true" in families and which are variable expressions of a shared genetic diathesis, genetic studies may allow us to refine our definitions of depressive illness.

Perhaps the most important dividend of molecular genetic research on MDD will be to enhance our understanding of the biological substrate of the disorder. Although psychiatric research has already made substantial advances in elucidating the neurobiology of mood disorders, we still have a limited understanding of the pathogenesis of MDD. The identification of even a single gene that contributes to MDD might provide a window onto unexpected pathways involved in the disorder. The examples of obesity and Alzheimer's disease, where molecular genetics has opened new avenues in biological research and treatment, provide a proof of this principle (200a,b). Identifying susceptibility genes and their protein products, in turn, can provide novel pharmacological treatment targets. At the same time, pharmacogenomic research may identify genetic variants which predict treatment response [158].

Actual identification of susceptibility genes for MDD will require advances in statistical and molecular genetics. Powerful analytic methods will be needed to identify susceptibility loci whose effects are likely to be modest and are probably mediated through gene-gene and gene-environment interactions. The construction of a genomewide map of single nucleotide polymorphisms (SNPs) and haplotypes, currently underway, may allow association studies in which allelic variants in any and all genes could be tested. DNA microarray ("chip") technology is making the requirements of high-throughput genotyping tractable [201]. However, even with these tools, there are statistical problems of multiple testing that remain to be solved before genomewide association analysis would be readily interpretable. And, as we have emphasized throughout this chapter, the successful application of these technologies will also require careful attention to phenotypic definition.

REFERENCES

1. Blazer DG, Kessler RC, McGonagle KA, Swartz MS. The prevalence and distribution of major depression in a national community sample: the National Comorbidity Survey. Am J Psychiatry 1994; 151(7):979–986.
2. Michaud CM, Murray CJ, Bloom BR. Burden of disease—implications for future research. JAMA 2001; 285(5):535–539.
3. Faraone S, Tsuang M. Methods in psychiatric genetics. In: Tsuang M, Tohen M, Zahner G, eds. Textbook in Psychiatric Epidemiology. New York: Wiley-Liss, 1995, pp 81–134.
4. Risch N, Merikangas K. The future of genetic studies of complex human diseases. Science 1996; 273:1516–1517.
5. Gershon E, Hamovit J, Guroff J, Dibble E, Leckman J, Sceery W, Targum S, Nurnberger J, Goldin L, Bunney W. A family study of schizoaffective, bipolar I, bipolar II, unipolar, and normal control probands. Arch Gen Psychiatry 1982; 39:1157–1167.
6. Winokur G, Tsuang M, Crowe R. The Iowa 500: affective disorder in relatives of manic and depressive patients. Am J Psychiatry 1982; 139:209–212.

7. Weissman MM, Gershon ES, Kidd KK, Prusoff BA, Leckman JF, Dibble E, Hamovit J, Thompson D, Pauls DL, Guroff JJ. Psychiatric disorders in the relatives of probands with affective disorders: the Yale University–National Institute of Mental Health Collaborative Study. Arch Gen Psychiatry 1984; 41(1):13–21.

8. Bland RC, Newman SC, Orn H. Recurrent and nonrecurrent depression: a family study. Arch Gen Psychiatry 1986; 43(11):1085–1089.

9. McGuffin P, Katz R, Bebbington P. Hazard, heredity and depression: a family study. J Psychiat Res 1987; 21(4):365–375.

10. Merikangas KR, Prusoff BA, Weissman MM. Parental concordance for affective disorders: psychopathology in offspring. J Affect Disord 1988; 15: 279–290.

11. Giles DE, Biggs MM, Rush AJ, Roffwarg HP. Risk factors in families of unipolar depression I. Psychiatric illness and reduced REM latency. J Affect Disord 1988; 14:51–59.

12. Kupfer DJ, Frank E, Carpenter LL, Neiswanger K. Family history in recurrent depression. J Affect Disord 1989; 17:113–119.

13. Andreasen NC, Rice J, Endicott J, Coryell W, Grove WM, Reich T. Familial rates of affective disorder: a report from the National Institute of Mental Health Collaborative Study. Arch Gen Psychiatry 1987; 44(5):461–469.

14. Puig-Antich J, Goetz D, Davies M, Kaplan T, Davies S, Ostrow L, Asnis L, Twomey J, Iyengar S, Ryan ND. A controlled family history study of prepubertal major depressive disorder. Arch Gen Psychiatry 1989; 46(5):406–418.

15. Mitchell J, McCauley E, Burke P, Calderon R, Schloredt K. Psychopathology in parents of depressed children and adolescents. J Am Acad Child Adolesc Psychiatry 1989; 28(3):352–357.

16. Kutcher S, Marton P. Affective disorders in first-degree relatives of adolescent onset bipolars, unipolars, and normal controls. J Am Acad Child Adolesc Psychiatry 1991; 30(1):75–78.

17. Weissman MM, Wickramaratne P, Adams PB, Lish JD, Horwath E, Charney D, Woods SW, Leeman E, Frosch E. The relationship between panic disorder and major depression: a new family study. Arch Gen Psychiatry 1993; 50(10):767–780.

18. Sadovnick AD, Remick RA, Lam R, Zis AP, Yee IML, Huggins MJ, Baird PA. Mood Disorder Service Genetic Database: morbidity risks for mood disorders in 3,942 first- degree relatives of 671 index cases with single depression, recurrent depression, bipolar I, or bipolar II. Am J Med Genet 1994; 54:132–140.

19. Williamson DE, Ryan ND, Birmaher B, Dahl RE, Kaufman J, Rao U, Puig-Antich J. A case-control family history study of depression in adolescents. J Am Acad Child Adolesc Psychiatry 1995; 34(12):1596–1607.

20. Harrington R, Rutter M, Weissman M, Fudge H, Groothues C, Bredenkamp D, Pickles A, Rende R, Wickramaratne P. Psychiatric disorders in the

relatives of depressed probands I. Comparison of prepubertal, adolescent and early adult onset cases. J Affect Disord 1997; 42:9–22.

21. Farmer A, Harris T, Redman K, Sadler S, Mahmood A, McGuffin P. Cardiff depression study. A sib-pair study of life events and familiality in major depression. Br J Psychiatry 2000; 176:150–155.

22. Warner V, Mufson L, Weissman MM. Offspring at high and low risk for depression and anxiety: mechanisms of psychiatric disorder. J Am Acad Child Adolesc Psychiatry 1995; 34(6):786–797.

23. Andreasen NC, Rice J, Endicott J, Reich T, Coryell W. The family history approach to diagnosis. How useful is it? Arch Gen Psychiatry 1986; 43(5): 421–429.

24. Sullivan PF, Neale MC, Kendler KS. Genetic epidemiology of major depression: review and meta-analysis. Am J Psychiatry 2000; 157(10): 1552–1562.

25. Tsuang MT, Winokur G, Crowe RR. Morbidity risks of schizophrenia and affective disorders among first degree relatives of patients with schizophrenia, mania, depression and surgical conditions. Br J Psychiatry 1980; 137:497–504.

26. Maier W, Lichtermann D, Minges J, Hallmayer J, Heun R, Benkert O, Levinson DF. Continuity and discontinuity of affective disorders and schizophrenia. Results of a controlled family study. Arch Gen Psychiatry 1993; 50(11):871–883.

27. Kendler K. Twin studies of psychiatric illness. Arch Gen Psychiatry 1993; 50:905–915.

28. Von Knorring A, Cloninger R, Bohman M, Sigvardsson S. An adoption study of depressive disorders and substance abuse. Arch Gen Psychiatry 1983; 40(9):943–950.

29. Cardoret RJ, O'Gorman TW, Heywood E, Troughton E. Genetic and environmental factors in major depression. J Affect Disord 1985; 9(2):155–164.

30. Wender PH, Kety SS, Rosenthal D, Schulsinger F, Ortmann J, Lunde I. Psychiatric disorders in the biological and adoptive families of adopted individuals with affective disorders. Arch Gen Psychiatry 1986; 43(10):923–929.

31. Tsuang M, Faraone S. The Genetics of Mood Disorders. Baltimore, MD: Johns Hopkins University Press, 1990.

32. Bierut LJ, Heath AC, Bucholz KK, Dinwiddie SH, Madden PA, Statham DJ, Dunne MP, Martin NG. Major depressive disorder in a community-based twin sample: are there different genetic and environmental contributions for men and women? Arch Gen Psychiatry 1999; 56(6):557–563.

33. Lyons M, Eisen S, Goldberg J, True W, Lin N, Meyer J, Toomey R, Faraone S, Merla-Ramos M, Tsuang M. A registry-based twin study of depression in men. Arch Gen Psychiatry 1998; 55:468–472.

34. Kendler K, Prescott C. A population-based twin study of lifetime major depression in men and women. Am J Psychiatry 1999; 56:39–44.

35. Kendler KS, Gardner CO, Prescott CA. Corrections to 2 prior published articles. Arch Gen Psychiatry 2000; 57(1):94–95.
36. McGuffin P, Katz R, Watkins S, RUtherford J. A hospital-based twin register of the heritability of DSM-IV unipolar depression. Arch Gen Psychiatry 1996; 53:129–136.
37. Kendler KS, Pedersen NL, Neale MC, Mathe AA. A pilot Swedish twin study of affective illness including hospital- and population-ascertained subsamples: results of model fitting. Behav Genet 1995; 25(3):217–232.
38. Crowe RR, Namboodiri KK, Ashby HB, Elston RC. Segregation and linkage analysis of a large kindred of unipolar depression. Neuropsychobiology 1981; 7(1):20–25.
39. Goldin LR, Gershon ES, Targum SD, Sparkes RS, McGinniss M. Segregation and linkage analyses in families of patients with bipolar, unipolar, and schizoaffective mood disorders. Am J Hum Genet 1983; 35(2): 274–287.
40. Tsuang MT, Bucher KD, Fleming JA, Faraone SV. Transmission of affective disorders: an application of segregation analysis to blind family study data. J Psychiatr Res 1985; 19(1):23–29.
41. Price RA, Kidd KK, Weissman MM. Early onset (under age 30 years) and panic disorder as markers for etiologic homogeneity in major depression. Arch Gen Psychiatry 1987; 44:434–440.
42. Cox N, Reich T, Rice J, Elston R, Schober J, Keats B. Segregation and linkage analysis of bipolar and major depressive illness in multigenerational pedigrees. J Psychiat Res 1989; 23:109–123.
43. Marazita ML, Neiswanger K, Cooper M, Zubenko GS, Giles DE, Frank E, Kupfer DJ, Kaplan BB. Genetic segregation analysis of early-onset recurrent unipolar depression. Am J Hum Genet 1997; 61:1370–1378.
43a. Maher BS, Marazita ML, Zubenko WN, Spiker DG, Giles DE, Kaplan BB, Zubenko GS. Genetic segregation analysis of recurrent, early-onset major depression: evidence for single major locus transmission. Am J Med Genet 2002; 114(2):214–221.
44. Paykel ES. Stress and affective disorders in humans. Semin Clin Neuropsychiatry 2001; 6(1):4–11.
45. Kendler KS, Karkowski LM, Prescott CA. Causal relationship between stressful life events and the onset of major depression. Am J Psychiatry 1999; 156(6):837–841.
46. McGuffin P, Katz R, Bebbington P. The Camberwell Collaborative Depression Study. III. Depression and adversity in the relatives of depressed probands. Br J Psychiatry 1988; 152:775–782.
47. Thapar A, McGuffin P. Genetic influences on life events in childhood. Psychol Med 1996; 26(4):813–820.
48. Rijsdijk FV, Sham PC, Sterne A, Purcell S, McGuffin P, Farmer A, Goldberg D, Mann A, Cherny SS, Webster M, Ball D, Eley TC, Plomin R. Life events and depression in a community sample of siblings. Psychol Med 2001; 31(3):401–410.

49. Kendler KS, Karkowski-Shuman L. Stressful life events and genetic liability to major depression: genetic control of exposure to the environment? Psychol Med 1997; 27(3):539–547.
50. Thapar A, Harold G, McGuffin P. Life events and depressive symptoms in childhood-shared genes or shared adversity? A research note. J Child Psychol Psychiat 1998; 39:1153–1158.
51. Kendler KS, Kessler RC, Walters EE, MacLean C, Neale MC, Heath AC, Eaves LJ. Stressful life events, genetic liability, and onset of an episode of major depression in women. Am J Psychiatry 1995; 152(6):833–842.
52. Silberg J, Rutter M, Neale M, Eaves L. Genetic moderation of environmental risk for depression and anxiety in adolescent girls. Br J Psychiatry 2001; 179:116–121.
53. Kendler KS, Thornton LM, Gardner CO. Genetic risk, number of previous depressive episodes, and stressful life events in predicting onset of major depression. Am J Psychiatry 2001; 158(4):582–586.
54. Weissman MM, Bland R, Joyce PR, Newman S, Wells JE, Wittchen HU. Sex differences in rates of depression: cross-national perspectives. J Affect Disord 1993; 29(2–3):77–84.
55. Weissman MM, Merikangas KR, Wickramaratne P, Kidd KK, Prusoff BA, Leckman JF, Pauls DL. Understanding the clinical heterogeneity of major depression using family data. Arch Gen Psychiatry 1986; 43(5):430–434.
56. Kendler KS, Neale MC, Kessler RC, Heath AC, Eaves LJ. A population-based twin study of major depression in women. Arch Gen Psychiatry 1992; 49(4):257–266.
57. Kendler KS, Gardner CO, Neale MC, Prescott CA. Genetic risk factors for major depression in men and women: similar or different heritabilities and same or partly distinct genes? Psychol Med 2001; 31(4):605–616.
57a. Zubenko GS, Hughes HB, 3rd, Maher BS, Stiffler JS, Zubenko WN, Marazita ML. Genetic linkage of region containing the CREB1 gene to depressive disorders in women from families with recurrent, early-onset, major depression. Am J Med Genet 2002; 114(8):980–987.
57b. Zubenko GS, Hughes HB, Stiffler JS, Zubenko WN, Kaplan BB. Genome survey for susceptability loci for recurrent, early-onset major depression: results at 10cM resolution. Am J Med Genet 2002; 114(4):413–422.
58. Kendler KS, Neale MC, Kessler RC, Heath AC, Eaves LJ. A population-based twin study of major depression in women: the impact of varying definitions of illness. Arch Gen Psychiatry 1992; 49:257–266.
59. Kendler K, Gardner C. Boundaries of major depression: an evaluation of DSM-IV criteria. Am J Psychiatry 1998; 155:172–177.
60. Kendler K, Eaves L, Walters E, Neale M, Heath A, Kessler R. The identification and validation of distinct depressive syndromes in a population-based sample of female twins. Arch Gen Psychiatry 1996; 53: 391–399.
61. Gershon ES, Weissman MM, Guroff JJ, Prusoff BA, Leckman JF. Validation of criteria for major depression through controlled family study. J Affect Disord 1986; 11:125–131.

62. Kendler K, Gardner C, Prescott C. Clinical characteristics of major depression that predict risk of depression in relatives. Arch Gen Psychiatry 1999; 56:322–327.
63. Weissman MM, Wickramaratne P, Merikangas KR, Leckman JF, Prusoff BA, Caruso KA, Kidd KK, Gammon D. Onset of major depression in early adulthood: increased familial loading and specificity. Arch Gen Psychiatry 1984; 41(12):1136–1143.
64. Weissman MM, Warner V, Wickramratne P, Prusoff BA. Early-onset major depression in parents and their children. J Affect Disord 1988; 15: 269–277.
65. Kovacs M, Devlin B, Pollock M, Richards C, Mukerji P. A controlled family history study of childhood-onset depressive disorder. Arch Gen Psychiatry 1997; 54(7):613–623.
65a. Zubenko GS, Zubenko WN, Spiker DG, Giles DE, Kaplan BB. Malignancy of recurrent, early-onset major depression: a family study. Am J Med Genet 2001; 105(8):690–699.
66. Blacker D, Tsuang M. Contested boundaries of bipolar disorder and the limits of categorical diagnosis in psychiatry. Am J Psychiatry 1992; 149:1473–1483.
67. Blacker D, Lavori P, Faraone S, Tsuang M. Unipolar relatives in bipolar pedigrees: a search for indicators of underlying bipolarity. Am J Med Genet 1993; 48:192–199.
68. Blacker D, Faraone SV, Rosen AE, Guroff JJ, Adams P, Weissman MM, Gershon ES. Unipolar relatives in bipolar pedigrees: a search for elusive indicators of underlying bipolarity. Am J Med Genet 1996; 67(5):445–454.
69. Adams LJ, Mitchell PB, Fielder SL, Rosso A, Donald JA, Schofield PR. A susceptibility locus for bipolar affective disorder on chromosome 4q35. Am J Hum Genet 1998; 62(5):1084–1091.
70. Detera-Wadleigh SD, Badner JA, Berrettini WH, Yoshikawa T, Goldin LR, Turner G, Rollins DY, Moses T, Sanders AR, Karkera JD, Esterling LE, Zeng J, Ferraro TN, Guroff JJ, Kazuba D, Maxwell ME, Nurnberger JI, Jr., Gershon ES. A high-density genome scan detects evidence for a bipolar-disorder susceptibility locus on 13q32 and other potential loci on 1q32 and 18p11.2. Proc Natl Acad Sci U S A 1999; 96(10):5604–5609.
71. Winokur G, Coryell W. Familial subtypes of unipolar depression: a prospective study of familial pure depressive disease compared to depression spectrum disease. Biol Psychiatry 1992; 32(11):1012–1018.
72. Winokur G. All roads lead to depression: clinically homogeneous, etiologically heterogeneous. J Affect Disord 1997; 45(1–2):97–108.
73. Merikangas KR, Leckman JF, Prusoff BA, Pauls DL, Weissman MM. Familial transmission of depression and alcoholism. Arch Gen Psychiatry 1985; 42(4):367–372.
74. Merikangas KR, Risch NJ, Weissman MM. Comorbidity and co-transmission of alcoholism, anxiety and depression. Psychol Med 1994; 24:69–80.
75. Rende R, Weissman M, Rutter M, Wickramaratnc P, Harrington R, Pickles A. Psychiatric disorders in the relatives of depressed probands II. Familial

loading for comorbid non-depressive disorders based upon age of onset. J Affect Disord 1997; 42:23–28.

76. Grant BF, Hasin DS, Dawson DA. The relationship between DSM-IV alcohol use disorders and DSM-IV major depression: examination of the primary-secondary distinction in a general population sample. J Affect Disord 1996; 38(2–3):113–28.

77. Kendler KS, Davis CG, Kessler RC. The familial aggregation of common psychiatric and substance use disorders in the National Comorbidity Survey: a family history study. Br J Psychiatry 1997; 170:541–548.

78. Kendler KS, Heath AC, Neale MC, Kessler RC, Eaves LJ. Alcoholism and major depression in women. A twin study of the causes of comorbidity. Arch Gen Psychiatry 1993; 50(9):690–698.

79. Prescott CA, Aggen SH, Kendler KS. Sex-specific genetic influences on the comorbidity of alcoholism and major depression in a population-based sample of US twins. Arch Gen Psychiatry 2000; 57(8):803–811.

80. Cadoret RJ, Winokur G, Langbehn D, Troughton E, Yates WR, Stewart MA. Depression spectrum disease, I: The role of gene-environment interaction. Am J Psychiatry 1996; 153(7):892–899.

81. Nurnberger JI, Jr., Foroud T, Flury L, Su J, Meyer ET, Hu K, Crowe R, Edenberg H, Goate A, Bierut L, Reich T, Schuckit M, Reich W. Evidence for a locus on chromosome 1 that influences vulnerability to alcoholism and affective disorder. Am J Psychiatry 2001; 158(5):718–724.

82. Brier A, Charney D, Heninger G. The diagnostic validity of anxiety disorders and their relationship to depressive illness. Am J Psychiatry 1985; 142: 787–797.

83. Maier W, Minges J, Lichtermann D. The familial relationship between panic disorder and unipolar depression. J Psychiatr Res 1995; 29(5):375–388.

84. Munjack D, Moss H. Affective disorder and alcoholism in families of agoraphobics. Arch Gen Psychiatry 1981; 38:869–871.

85. Noyes R, Jr., Clancy J, Crowe R, Hoenk PR, Slymen DJ. The familial prevalence of anxiety neurosis. Arch Gen Psychiatry 1978; 35:1057–1059.

86. Cloninger C, Martin R, Clayton P, Guze S. A blind follow-up and family study of anxiety neurosis: preliminary analysis of the St. Louis 500. In: Klein D, Rabkin J, eds. Anxiety: New Research and Changing Concepts. New York: Raven Press, 1981; 137–150.

87. Crowe RR, Noyes R, Pauls DL, Slymen D. A family study of panic disorder. Arch Gen Psychiatry 1983; 40:1065–1069.

88. Harris EL, Noyes R, Jr., Crowe RR, Chaudry DR. Family study of agoraphobia: report of a pilot study. Arch Gen Psychiatry 1983; 40:1061–1064.

89. Noyes R, Jr., Crowe RR, Harris EL, Hampa BJ, McChesney CM, Chaudry DR. Relationship between panic disorder and agoraphobia: a family study. Arch Gen Psychiatry 1986; 43:227–232.

90. Mendlewicz J, Papdimitriou G, Wilmotte J. Family study of panic disorder: comparison with generalized anxiety disorder, major depression and normal subjects. Psychiatric Genet 1993; 3:73–78.

91. Goldstein RB, Weissman MM, Adams PB, Horwath E, Lish JD, Charney D, Woods SW, Sobin C, Wickramaratne PJ. Psychiatric disorders in relatives of probands with panic disorder and/or major depression. Arch Gen Psychiatry 1994; 51:383–394.

92. Mannuzza S, Chapman TF, Klein DF, Fyer AJ. Familial transmission of panic disorder: effect of major depression comorbidity. Anxiety 1994/1995; 1:180–185.

93. Leckman J, Weissman M, Merikangas K, Pauls D, Prusoff B. Panic disorder and major depression: increased risk of depression, alcoholism, panic, and phobic disorders in families of depressed probands with panic disorder. Arch Gen Psychiatry 1983; 40:1055–1060.

94. Weissman M, Leckman J, Merikangas K, Gammon G, Prusoff B. Depression and anxiety disorders in parents and children: results from the Yale Family Study. Arch Gen Psychiatry 1984; 41:845–852.

95. Coryell W, Endicott J, Andreasen N, Keller M, Clayton P, Hirschfeld R, Scheftner W, Winokur G. Depression and panic attacks: the significance of overlap as reflected in follow-up and family study data. Am J Psychiatry 1988; 145:293–300.

96. Coryell W, Endicott J, Winokur G. Anxiety syndromes as epiphenomena of primary major depression: outcome and familial psychopathology. Am J Psychiatry 1992; 149:100–107.

97. Breslau N, Davis GC, Prabucki K. Searching for evidence on the validity of generalized anxiety disorder: psychopathology in children of anxious mothers. Psychiatry Res 1987; 20(4):285–297.

98. Biederman J, Rosenbaum J, Bolduc E, Faraone S, Hirshfeld D. A high risk study of young children of parents with panic disorder and agoraphobia with and without comorbid major depression. Psychiatry Res 1991; 37:333–348.

99. Biederman J, Faraone SV, Hirshfeld-Becker DR, Friedman D, Robin JA, Rosenbaum JF. Patterns of psychopathology and dysfunction in high-risk children of parents with panic disorder and major depression. Am J Psychiatry 2001; 158(1):49–57.

100. Fyer A, Mannuzza S, Chapman T, Liebowitz M, Klein D. A direct interview family study of social phobia. Arch Gen Psychiatry 1993; 50:286–293.

101. Noyes RJ, Clarkson C, Crowe R, Yates W, McChesney C. A family study of generalized anxiety disorder. Am J Psychiatry 1987; 144:1019–1024.

102. Horwath E, Wolk SI, Goldstein RB, Wickramaratne P, Sobin C, Adams P, Lish JD, Weissman MM. Is the comorbidity between social phobia and panic disorder due to familial cotransmission or other factors? Arch Gen Psychiatry 1995; 52:574–582.

103. Stein MB, Chartier MJ, Hazen AL, Kozak MV, Tancer ME, Lander S, Furer P, Chubaty D, Walker JR. A direct-interview family study of generalized social phobia. Am J Psychiatry 1998; 155(1):90–97.

104. Kendler KS, Neale MC, Kessler RC, Heath AC, Eaves LJ. Major depression and generalized anxiety disorder: same genes, (partly) different environments? Archives of General Psychiatry 1992; 49:716–722.

105. Kendler K, Neale M, Kessler R, Heath A, Eaves L. Major depression and phobias: the genetic and environmental sources of comorbidity. Psychol Med 1993; 23:361–371.

106. Kendler KS, Walter EE, Neale MC, Kessler RC, Heath AC, Eaves LJ. The structure of the genetic and environmental risk factors for six major psychiatric disorders in women. Arch Gen Psychiatry 1995; 52:374–383.

107. Roy MA, Neale MC, Pedersen NL, Mathe AA, Kendler KS. A twin study of generalized anxiety disorder and major depression. Psychol Med 1995; 25(5):1037–1049.

108. Andrews G, Stewart G, Allen R, Henderson A. The genetics of six neurotic disorders: a twin study. J Affect Disord 1990; 19:23–29.

109. Kendler KS, Neale MC, Kessler RC, Heath AC, Eaves LJ. A longitudinal twin study of personality and major depression in women. Arch Gen Psychiatry 1993; 50(11):853–862.

110. Rosenbaum JF, Biederman J, Hirshfeld-Becker DR, Kagan J, Snidman N, Friedman D, Nineberg A, Gallery DJ, Faraone SV. A controlled study of behavioral inhibition in children of parents with panic disorder and depression. Am J Psychiatry 2000; 157(12):2002–2010.

111. Maier W, Minges J, Lichtermann D, Franke P, Gansicke M. Personality patterns in subjects at risk for affective disorders. Psychopathology 1995; 28(Suppl 1):59–72.

112. Venter JC, Adams MD, Myers EW, et al. The sequence of the human genome. Science 2001; 291(5507):1304–1351.

113. Lander ES, Linton LM, Birren B, et al. Initial sequencing and analysis of the human genome. Nature 2001; 409(6822):860–921.

114. Klein DN, Riso LP, Donaldson SK, Scwartz JE, Anderson RL, Ouimette PC, Lizardi H, Aronson TA. Family study of early-onset dysthymia: mood and personality disorders in relatives of outpatients with dysthymia and episode major depression and normal controls. Arch Gen Psychiatry 1995; 52(6):487–496.

115. Klein DN. Depressive personality in the relatives of outpatients with dysthymic disorder and episodic major depressive disorder and normal controls. J Affect Disord 1999; 55(1):19–27.

116. Lander E, Kruglyak L. Genetic dissection of complex traits: guidelines for interpreting and reporting linkage results. Nat Genet 1995; 11:241–247.

117. Spielman. The TDT and other family-based tests for linkage disequilibrium and association. Am J Hum Genet 1996; 59:983–989.

118. Winokur G. The division of depressive illness into depression spectrum disease and pure depressive disease. Int Pharmacopsychiatry 1974; 9(1):5–13.

119. Tanna VL, Wilson AF, Winokur G, Elston RC. Linkage analysis of pure depressive disease. J Psychiatr Res 1989; 23:99–107.

120. Balciuniene J, Yuan QP, Engstrom C, Lindblad K, Nylander PO, Sundvall M, Schalling M, Pettersson U, Adolfsson R, Jazin EE. Linkage analysis of candidate loci in families with recurrent major depression. Mol Psychiatry 1998; 3:162–168.

121. Neiswanger K, Zubenko G, Giles D, Frank E, Kupfer D, Kaplan B. Linkage and association analysis of chromosomal regions containing genes related to neuroendocrine or serotonin function in families with early-onset, recurrent major depression. Am J Med Genet (Neuropsychiatr Genet) 1998; 81:443–449.

122. Blackwood DH, Fordyce A, Walker MT, St Clair DM, Porteous DJ, Muir WJ. Schizophrenia and affective disorders—cosegregation with a translocation at chromosome 1q42 that directly disrupts brain-expressed genes: clinical and P300 findings in a family. Am J Hum Genet 2001; 69(2):428–433.

123. Millar JK, Wilson-Annan JC, Anderson S, Christie S, Taylor MS, Semple CA, Devon RS, Clair DM, Muir WJ, Blackwood DH, Porteous DJ. Disruption of two novel genes by a translocation co-segregating with schizophrenia. Hum Mol Genet 2000; 9(9):1415–1423.

124. Devon RS, Anderson S, Teague PW, Burgess P, Kipari TM, Semple CA, Millar JK, Muir WJ, Murray V, Pelosi AJ, Blackwood DH, Porteous DJ. Identification of polymorphisms within Disrupted in Schizophrenia 1 and Disrupted in Schizophrenia 2, and an investigation of their association with schizophrenia and bipolar affective disorder. Psychiatr Genet 2001; 11(2):71–78.

124a. Zubenko GS, Hughes IH, Stiffler JS, Zubenko WN, Kaplan BB. D2S2944 identifies a likely susceptibility locus for recurrent, early-onset, major depression in women. Mol Psychiatry 2002; 7(5):460–467.

125. Ioannidis JP, Ntzani EE, Trikalinos TA, Contopoulos-Ioannidis DG. Replication validity of genetic association studies. Nat Genet 2001; 29(3):306–9.

126. Lesch KP, Balling U, Gross J, Strauss K, Wolozin BL, Murphy DL, Riederer P. Organization of the human serotonin transporter gene. J Neural Transm Gen Sect 1994; 95(2):157–162.

127. Battersby S, Ogilvie AD, Smith CA, Blackwood DH, Muir WJ, Quinn JP, Fink G, Goodwin GM, Harmar AJ. Structure of a variable number tandem repeat of the serotonin transporter gene and association with affective disorder. Psychiatr Genet 1996; 6(4):177–181.

128. MacKenzie A, Quinn J. A serotonin transporter gene intron 2 polymorphic region, correlated with affective disorders, has allele-dependent differential enhancer-like properties in the mouse embryo. Proc Natl Acad Sci USA 1999; 96(26):15251–15255.

129. Mellerup E, Bennike B, Bolwig T, Dam H, Hasholt L, Jorgensen MB, Plenge P, Sorensen SA. Platelet serotonin transporters and the transporter gene in control subjects, unipolar patients and bipolar patients. Acta Psychiatr Scand 2001; 103(3):229–233.

130. Ogilvie AD, Battersby S, Bubb VJ, Fink G, Harmar AJ, Goodwim GM, Smith CA. Polymorphism in serotonin transporter gene associated with susceptibility to major depression. Lancet 1996; 347(9003):731–733.

131. Gutierrez B, Pintor L, Gasto C, Rosa A, Bertranpetit J, Vieta E, Fananas L.

Variability in the serotonin transporter gene and increased risk for major depression with melancholia. Hum Genet 1998; 103(3):319–322.

132. Furlong RA, Ho L, Walsh C, Rubinsztein JS, Jain S, Paykel ES, Easton DF, Rubinsztein DC. Analysis and meta-analysis of two serotonin transporter gene polymorphisms in bipolar and unipolar affective disorders. Am J Med Genet 1998; 81(1):58–63.

133. Heils A, Teufel A, Petri S, Stober G, Riederer P, Bengel D, Lesch KP. Allelic variation of human serotonin transporter gene expression. J Neurochem 1996; 66(6):2621–2624.

134. Lesch K-P, Bengel D, Heils A, Sabol S, Greenberg B, Petri S, Benjamin J, Muller C, Hamer D, Murphy D. Association of anxiety-related traits with a polymorphism in the serotonin transporter gene regulatory region. Science 1996; 274:1527–1531.

135. Du L, Faludi G, Palkovits M, Demeter E, Bakish D, Lapierre YD, Sotonyi P, Hrdina PD. Frequency of long allele in serotonin transporter gene is increased in depressed suicide victims. Biol Psychiatry 1999; 46(2):196–201.

136. Mann JJ, Huang YY, Underwood MD, Kassir SA, Oppenheim S, Kelly TM, Dwork AJ, Arango V. A serotonin transporter gene promoter polymorphism (5-HTTLPR) and prefrontal cortical binding in major depression and suicide. Arch Gen Psychiatry 2000; 57(8):729–738.

137. Collier DA, Stober G, Li T, Heils A, Catalano M, Di Bella D, Arranz MJ, Murray RM, Vallada HP, Bengel D, Muller CR, Roberts GW, Smeraldi E, Kirov G, Sham P, Lesch KP. A novel functional polymorphism within the promoter of the serotonin transporter gene: possible role in susceptibility to affective disorders. Mol Psychiatry 1996; 1(6):453–460.

138. Menza MA, Palermo B, DiPaola R, Sage JI, Ricketts MH. Depression and anxiety in Parkinson's disease: possible effect of genetic variation in the serotonin transporter. J Geriatr Psychiatry Neurol 1999; 12(2):49–52.

139. Mossner R, Henneberg A, Schmitt A, Syagailo YV, Grassle M, Hennig T, Simantov R, Gerlach M, Riederer P, Lesch KP. Allelic variation of serotonin transporter expression is associated with depression in Parkinson's disease. Mol Psychiatry 2001; 6(3):350–352.

140. Frisch A, Postilnick D, Rockah R, Michaelovsky E, Postilnick S, Birman E, Laor N, Rauchverger B, Kreinin A, Poyurovsky M, Schneidman M, Modai I, Weizman R. Association of unipolar major depressive disorder with genes of the serotonergic and dopaminergic pathways. Mol Psychiatry 1999; 4(4):389–392.

141. Bellivier F, Henry C, Szoke A, Schurhoff F, Nosten-Bertrand M, Feingold J, Launay JM, Leboyer M, Laplanche JL. Serotonin transporter gene polymorphisms in patients with unipolar or bipolar depression. Neurosci Lett 1998; 255(3):143–146.

142. Ohara K, Nagai M, Tsukamoto T, Tani K, Suzuki Y. Functional polymorphism in the serotonin transporter promoter at the SLC6A4 locus and mood disorders. Biol Psychiatry 1998; 44(7):550–554.

143. Minov C, Baghai TC, Schule C, Zwanzger P, Schwarz MJ, Zill P, Rupprecht

R, Bondy B. Serotonin-2A-receptor and -transporter polymorphisms: lack of association in patients with major depression. Neurosci Lett 2001; 303(2): 119–122.

144. Hoehe MR, Wendel B, Grunewald I, Chiaroni P, Levy N, Morris-Rosendahl D, Macher JP, Sander T, Crocq MA. Serotonin transporter (5-HTT) gene polymorphisms are not associated with susceptibility to mood disorders. Am J Med Genet 1998; 81(1):1–3.

145. Du L, Bakish D, Lapierre YD, Ravindran AV, Hrdina PD. Association of polymorphism of serotonin 2A receptor gene with suicidal ideation in major depressive disorder. Am J Med Genet 2000; 96(1):56–60.

146. Bondy B, Kuznik J, Baghai T, Schule C, Zwanzger P, Minov C, de Jonge S, Rupprecht R, Meyer H, Engel RR, Eisenmenger W, Ackenheil M. Lack of association of serotonin-2A receptor gene polymorphism (T102C) with suicidal ideation and suicide. Am J Med Genet 2000; 96(6):831–835.

147. Arias B, Gutierrez B, Pintor L, Gasto C, Fananas L. Variability in the 5-HT(2A) receptor gene is associated with seasonal pattern in major depression. Mol Psychiatry 2001; 6(2):239–242.

148. Lerer B, Macciardi F, Segman RH, Adolfsson R, Blackwood D, Blairy S, Del Favero J, Dikeos DG, Kaneva R, Lilli R, Massat I, Milanova V, Muir W, Noethen M, Oruc L, Petrova T, Papadimitriou GN, Rietschel M, Serretti A, Souery D, Van Gestel S, Van Broeckhoven C, Mendlewicz J. Variability of 5-HT2C receptor cys23ser polymorphism among European populations and vulnerability to affective disorder. Mol Psychiatry 2001; 6(5):579–585.

149. Fehr C, Grintschuk N, Szegedi A, Anghelescu I, Klawe C, Singer P, Hiemke C, Dahmen N. The HTR1B 861G > C receptor polymorphism among patients suffering from alcoholism, major depression, anxiety disorders and narcolepsy. Psychiatry Res 2000; 97(1):1–10.

150. Arias B, Collier DA, Gasto C, Pintor L, Gutierrez B, Valles V, Fananas L. Genetic variation in the 5-HT5A receptor gene in patients with bipolar disorder and major depression. Neurosci Lett 2001; 303(2):111–114.

151. Hong CJ, Tsai SJ, Cheng CY, Liao WY, Song HL, Lai HC. Association analysis of the 5-HT(6) receptor polymorphism (C267T) in mood disorders. Am J Med Genet 1999; 88(6):601–602.

152. Liu HC, Hong CJ, Liu CY, Lin KN, Tsai SJ, Liu TY, Chi CW, Wang PN. Association analysis of the 5-HT6 receptor polymorphism C267T with depression in patients with Alzheimer's disease. Psychiatry Clin Neurosci 2001; 55(4):427–429.

153. Du L, Bakish D, Hrdina PD. Tryptophan hydroxylase gene 218A/C polymorphism is associated with somatic anxiety in major depressive disorder. J Affect Disord 2001; 65(1):37–44.

154. Souery D, Van Gestel S, Massat I, Blairy S, Adolfsson R, Blackwood D, Del-Favero J, Dikeos D, Jakovljevic M, Kaneva R, Lattuada E, Lerer B, Lilli R, Milanova V, Muir W, Nothen M, Oruc L, Papadimitriou G, Propping P, Schulze T, Serretti A, Shapira B, Smeraldi E, Stefanis C, Thomson M, Van Broeckhoven C, Mendlewicz J. Tryptophan hydroxylase polymorphism and

suicidality in unipolar and bipolar affective disorders: a multicenter association study. Biol Psychiatry 2001; 49(5):405–409.

155. Syagailo YV, Stober G, Grassle M, Reimer E, Knapp M, Jungkunz G, Okladnova O, Meyer J, Lesch KP. Association analysis of the functional monoamine oxidase A gene promoter polymorphism in psychiatric disorders. Am J Med Genet 2001; 105(2):168–171.

156. Schulze TG, Muller DJ, Krauss H, Scherk H, Ohlraun S, Syagailo YV, Windemuth C, Neidt H, Grassle M, Papassotiropoulos A, Heun R, Nothen MM, Maier W, Lesch KP, Rietschel M. Association between a functional polymorphism in the monoamine oxidase A gene promoter and major depressive disorder. Am J Med Genet 2000; 96(6):801–803.

157. Owen D, Du L, Bakish D, Lapierre YD, Hrdina PD. Norepinephrine transporter gene polymorphism is not associated with susceptibility to major depression. Psychiatry Res 1999; 87(1):1–5.

158. Pickar D, Rubinow K. Pharmacogenomics of psychiatric disorders. Trends Pharmacol Sci 2001; 22(2):75–83.

159. Manki H, Kanba S, Muramatsu T, Higuchi S, Suzuki E, Matsushita S, Ono Y, Chiba H, Shintani F, Nakamura M, Yagi G, Asai M. Dopamine D2, D3 and D4 receptor and transporter gene polymorphisms and mood disorders. J Affect Disord 1996; 40(1–2):7–13.

160. Oruc L, Verheyen GR, Furac I, Jakovljevic M, Ivezic S, Raeymaekers P, Van Broeckhoven C. Analysis of the tyrosine hydroxylase and dopamine D4 receptor genes in a Croatian sample of bipolar I and unipolar patients. Am J Med Genet 1997; 74(2):176–178.

161. Oruc L, Verheyen GR, Furac I, Ivezic S, Jakovljevic M, Raeymaekers P, Van Broeckhoven C. Positive association between the GABRA5 gene and unipolar recurrent major depression. Neuropsychobiology 1997; 36(2):62–64.

162. Zill P, Baghai TC, Zwanzger P, Schule C, Minov C, Riedel M, Neumeier K, Rupprecht R, Bondy B. Evidence for an association between a G-protein beta3-gene variant with depression and response to antidepressant treatment. Neuroreport 2000; 11(9):1893–1897.

163. Lai I, Hong C, Tsai S. Association study of nicotinic-receptor variants and major depressive disorder. J Affect Disord 2001; 66(1):79–82.

164. Desan PH, Oren DA, Malison R, Price LH, Rosenbaum J, Smoller J, Charney DS, Gelernter J. Genetic polymorphism at the CLOCK gene locus and major depression. Am J Med Genet 2000; 96(3):418–421.

165. Jun TY, Pae CU, Chae JH, Bahk WM, Kim KS. Polymorphism of CTLA-4 gene for major depression in the Korean population. Psychiatry Clin Neurosci 2001; 55(5):533–537.

166. Weizman A, Weizman R. Serotonin transporter polymorphism and response to SSRIs in major depression and relevance to anxiety disorders and substance abuse. Pharmacogenomics 2000; 1(3):335–341.

167. Smeraldi E, Zanardi R, Benedetti F, Di Bella D, Perez J, Catalano M. Polymorphism within the promoter of the serotonin transporter gene

and antidepressant efficacy of fluvoxamine. Mol Psychiatry 1998; 3(6): 508–511.

168. Zanardi R, Serretti A, Rossini D, Franchini L, Cusin C, Lattuada E, Dotoli D, Smeraldi E. Factors affecting fluvoxamine antidepressant activity: influence of pindolol and 5-HTTLPR in delusional and nondelusional depression. Biol Psychiatry 2001; 50(5):323–330.

169. Zanardi R, Benedetti F, Di Bella D, Catalano M, Smeraldi E. Efficacy of paroxetine in depression is influenced by a functional polymorphism within the promoter of the serotonin transporter gene. J Clin Psychopharmacol 2000; 20(1);105–107.

170. Pollock BG, Ferrell RE, Mulsant BH, Mazumdar S, Miller M, Sweet RA, Davis S, Kirshner MA, Houck PR, Stack JA, Reynolds CF, Kupfer DJ. Allelic variation in the serotonin transporter promoter affects onset of paroxetine treatment response in late-life depression. Neuropsychopharmacology 2000; 23(5):587–590.

171. Kim DK, Lim SW, Lee S, Sohn SE, Kim S, Hahn CG, Carroll BJ. Serotonin transporter gene polymorphism and antidepressant response. Neuroreport 2000; 11(1):215–219.

172. Mundo E, Walker M, Cate T, Macciardi F, Kennedy JL. The role of serotonin transporter protein gene in antidepressant-induced mania in bipolar disorder: preliminary findings. Arch Gen Psychiatry 2001; 58(6):539–544.

173. Serretti A, Zanardi R, Cusin C, Rossini D, Lorenzi C, Smeraldi E. Tryptophan hydroxylase gene associated with paroxetine antidepressant activity. Eur Neuropsychopharmacol 2001; 11(5):375–380.

174. Trivedi MH, Rush H. Does a placebo run-in or a placebo treatment cell affect the efficacy of antidepressant medications? Neuropsychopharmacology 1994; 11(1):33–43.

175. Oquendo MA, Mann JJ. The biology of impulsivity and suicidality. Psychiatr Clin North Am 2000; 23(1):11–25.

176. Mann JJ, Malone KM, Nielsen DA, Goldman D, Erdos J, Gelernter J. Possible association of a polymorphism of the tryptophan hydroxylase gene with suicidal behavior in depressed patients. Am J Psychiatry 1997; 154(10):1451–1453.

177. Abbar M, Courtet P, Bellivier F, Leboyer M, Boulenger JP, Castelhau D, Ferreira M, Lambercy C, Mouthon D, Paoloni-Giacobino A, Vessaz M, Malafosse A, Buresi C. Suicide attempts and the tryptophan hydroxylase gene. Mol Psychiatry 2001; 6(3):268–273.

178. Clark L, Watson D, Mineka S. Temperament, personality and the mood and anxiety disorders. J Abnorm Psychol 1994; 103:103–116.

179. Andrews G, Stewart G, Morris-Yates A, Holt P, Henderson S. Evidence for a general neurotic syndrome. Br J Psychiatry 1990; 157:6–12.

180. Bienvenu OJ, Nestadt G, Samuels JF, Costa PT, Howard WT, Eaton WW. Phobic, panic, and major depressive disorders and the five-factor model of personality. J Nerv Ment Dis 2001; 189(3):154–161.

181. Floderus-Myrhed B, Pedersen N, Rasmuson I. Assessment of heritability for personality, based on a short-form of the Eysenck Personality Inventory: a study of 12,898 twin pairs. Behav Genet 1980; 10:153–162.

182. Mackinnon A, Henderson A, Andrews G. Genetic and environmental determinants of the liability of trait neuroticism and the symptoms of anxiety and depression. Psychol Med 1990; 20:581–590.

183. Rose R, Koskenvuo M, Kaprio J, Sarna S, Langinvainio H. Shared genes, shared experiences, and similarity of personality: data from 14,288 adult Finnish co-twins. J Pers Soc Psychol 1988; 54:161–171.

184. Roberts SB, Kendler KS. Neuroticism and self-esteem as indices of the vulnerability to major depression in women. Psychol Med 1999; 29(5): 1101–1109.

185. Du L, Bakish D, Hrdina PD. Gender differences in association between serotonin transporter gene polymorphism and personality traits. Psychiatr Genet 2000; 10(4):159–164.

186. Jang KL, Hu S, Livesley WJ, Angleitner A, Riemann R, Ando J, Ono Y, Vernon PA, Hamer DH. Covariance structure of neuroticism and agreeableness: a twin and molecular genetic analysis of the role of the serotonin transporter gene. J Pers Soc Psychol 2001; 81(2):295–304.

187. Flory JD, Manuck SB, Ferrell RE, Dent KM, Peters DG, Muldoon MF. Neuroticism is not associated with the serotonin transporter (5-HTTLPR) polymorphism. Mol Psychiatry 1999; 4(1):93–96.

188. Gelernter J, Kranzler H, Coccaro EF, Siever LJ, New AS. Serotonin transporter protein gene polymorphism and personality measures in African American and European American subjects. Am J Psychiatry 1998; 155(10):1332–1338.

189. Gustavsson JP, Nothen MM, Jonsson EG, Neidt H, Forslund K, Rylander G, Mattila-Evenden M, Sedvall GC, Propping P, Asberg M. No association between serotonin transporter gene polymorphisms and personality traits. Am J Med Genet 1999; 88(4):430–436.

190. Ball D, Hill L, Freeman B, Eley T, Strelau J, Riemann R, Spinath F, Angleitner A, Plomin R. The serotonin transporter gene and peer-rated neuroticism. Neuroreport 1997; 8:1301–1304.

191. Jorm AF, Henderson AS, Jacomb PA, Christensen H, Korten AE, Rodgers B, Tan X, Easteal S. An association study of a functional polymorphism of the serotonin transporter gene with personality and psychiatric symptoms. Mol Psychiatry 1998; 3(5):449–451.

192. Deary IJ, Battersby S, Whiteman MC, Connor JM, Fowkes FG, Harmar A. Neuroticism and polymorphisms in the serotonin transporter gene. Psychol Med 1999; 29(3):735–739.

193. Kagan J. Galen's Prophecy. New York: Basic Books, 1994.

194. Robinson J, Kagan J, Reznick J, Corley R. The heritability of inhibited and uninhibited behavior: a twin study. Dev Psychol 1992; 28:1030–1037.

195. Smoller JW, Rosenbaum JF, Biederman J, Susswein LS, Kennedy J, Kagan J, Snidman N, Laird N, Tsuang MT, Faraone SV, Schwarz A, Slaugenhaupt

SA. Genetic association analysis of behavioral inhibition using candidate loci from mouse models. Am J Med Genet 2001; 105(3):226–235.

196. Tsuang M, Faraone S, Lyons M. Identification of the phenotype in psychiatric genetics. Eur Arch Psychiatry Clin Neurosci 1993; 243:131–142.

197. Giles DE, Kupfer DJ, Roffwarg HP, Rush AJ, Biggs MM, Etzel BA. Polysomnographic parameters in first-degree relatives of unipolar probands. Psychiatry Res 1989; 27:127–136.

198. Fulton MK, Armitage R, Rush AJ. Sleep electroencephalographic coherence abnormalities in individuals at high risk for depression: a pilot study. Biol Psychiatry 2000; 47(7):618–625.

199. Krieg JC, Lauer CJ, Schreiber W, Modell S, Holsboer F. Neuroendocrine, polysomnographic and psychometric observations in healthy subjects at high familial risk for affective disorders: the current state of the 'Munich vulnerability study'. J Affect Disord 2001; 62(1–2):33–37.

200. Faraone S, Tsuang M, Tsuang D. Genetics of Mental Disorders: A Guide for Students, Clinicians, and Researchers. New York: Guilford Press, 1999.

200a. Ravussin E, Bouchard C. Human genomics and obesity: finding appropriate drug targets. Eur J Pharmacol 2000; 410(2–3):131–145.

200b. Selkoe DJ, Podlisny MB. Deciphering the genetic basis of Alzheimer's disease. Annu Rev Genomics Hum Genet 2002; 3:67–99.

201. Sklar P. The genomic approach to candidate genes. Harv Rev Psychiatry 2001; 9(4):197–207.

6

Psychopharmacology of Dysthymia

Robert H. Howland
Western Psychiatric Institute and Clinic
University of Pittsburgh School of Medicine
Pittsburgh, Pennsylvania, U.S.A.

INTRODUCTION

By contrast with major depression, dysthymic disorder (dysthymia) is characterized by the combination of chronicity and milder depressive symptoms. Because of its typically early age of onset, chronic course, mild symptoms, and association with longstanding psychosocial and personality problems, psychotherapy historically was viewed as the most appropriate treatment approach [1,2]. This common perception contributed to a paucity of empirical data on the utility of antidepressant drugs in the treatment of dysthymia until the 1980s when the concept of dysthymia as a mood disorder began to evolve and pharmacotherapy studies began to appear in the literature [3,4]. This chapter reviews the psychopharmacology of dysthymia, emphasizing the results of randomized controlled clinical trials of heterocyclic antidepressants, monoamine oxidase inhibitors (MAOIs), serotonin reuptake inhibitors (SRIs), atypical antidepressant drugs, and atypical antipsychotic drugs. Because of their similarities to dysthymia, recent treatment studies of chronic major depression and double depression (i.e., major depression superimposed on dysthymia) will

139

also be reviewed. In addition, long-term treatment studies of dysthymia and other chronic depressions will be reviewed. Finally, some important methodological issues, areas for further study, and general clinical principles for treating dysthymia will be discussed.

SHORT-TERM PHARMACOTHERPY FOR DYSTHYMIA

Heterocyclic Antidepressants

Various tricyclic antidepressants (TCAs), such as imipramine, desipramine, amitriptyline, doxepin, and dothiepin, have been well studied in the treatment of dysthymia. Open-label studies [1,5] and placebo-controlled studies [1,6–10] have clearly demonstrated the efficacy of these drugs. In addition, controlled comparisons between TCAs and other psychotropic antidepressant drugs, such as tianeptine [11,12], phenelzine [7], moclobemide [10,13], sertraline [8], ritanserin [6], reboxetine [14], minaprine [15], and amisulpride [9,16], have also shown them to be effective in the treatment of dysthymia. Some of these studies are discussed in more detail in later sections.

Tianeptine is an unusual TCA drug whose mechanism of action is uncertain. Unlike the pharmacological effects of most other standard antidepressant drugs, it increases serotonin reuptake and may also affect dopamine metabolism. An open-label study of 20 patients with dysthymia suggested that tianeptine was effective and well tolerated [17]. Several other open-label studies, which included patients with dysthymia or major depression, supported its efficacy [18–20]. One randomized controlled 6-week study of 265 dysthymic patients found that tianeptine was as effective as amitriptyline [12]. Several other randomized controlled studies that included patients with dysthymia or major depression found comparable efficacy between tianeptine and other antidepressants [11,21].

Amineptine is another unusual TCA drug that appears to act primarily on dopamine systems. A large randomized double-blind placebo-controlled 12-week study of 323 patients with dysthymia found that amineptine and the atypical antipsychotic amisulpride were equally effective and superior to placebo [22].

A randomized double-blind study of maprotiline, a tetracyclic antidepressant, and fluvoxamine, an SRI, in 48 patients with dysthymia or major depression found comparable and significant improvements with both drugs after 6 weeks of treatment, although the clinical effects were modest [23]. Another randomized double-blind 4-week study found that the tetracyclic antidepressant mianserin was slightly more effective than maprotiline in 35 patients with dysthymia or major depression, but the difference was not significant [24].

Monoamine Oxidase Inhibitors

The MAOIs have not been as well studied in the treatment of dysthymia compared to the TCAs. Several earlier controlled studies suggested that the older irreversible nonspecific MAOIs are effective in the treatment of dysthymia [1]. In a reanalysis of data from a 6-week randomized double-blind study, focusing on 153 patients with chronic depressive symptoms, Stewart and colleagues [7] found that phenelzine was significantly more effective than imipramine, and that both drugs were significantly more effective than placebo. Of particular interest, patients with early-onset mild chronic depression (akin to dysthymia) showed the same differential treatment response as patients with more severe chronic depression. A caveat of this study, however, is that these patients had predominantly atypical symptoms of depression, which have been shown to be relatively more responsive to treatment with MAOIs than to TCAs [25].

The MAOI moclobemide is a reversible inhibitor of MAO type A, and it does not require the dietary restrictions necessary for use with the older MAOIs. An open-label randomized 4-week study comparing moclobemide and imipramine in 40 patients with dysthymia or major depression found these drugs to be equally effective [13]. A randomized double-blind 6-week study of 42 patients with double depression found a relatively greater response rate to moclobemide (71%) compared to fluoxetine (38%), although the drugs were equally effective on other outcome measures of depression, and both were well tolerated [26]. A limitation of this study, however, was the use of a low fixed dose of fluoxetine (20 mg/day), which may not be an optimal dose for treating all patients with double depression. Versiani and colleagues [10] studied moclobemide and imipramine in an 8-week placebo-controlled trial of 315 patients with dysthymia. Both active compounds were significantly more effective than placebo and not significantly different from each other in terms of efficacy. Moclobemide (mean dose 675 mg/day) was generally better tolerated than imipramine (mean dose 225 mg/day), although insomnia was more common in the group receiving moclobemide. Finally, a randomized controlled trial comparing moclobemide and moclobemide plus interpersonal psychotherapy (IPT) in 35 dysthymic patients found that both groups showed significant improvement over time [27]. There was only a nonsignificant trend for additional improvement in the IPT group, but they were also less likely to drop out of treatment; suggesting that psychotherapy may enhance treatment adherence. Unfortunately, the sample size of this study may have been too small to demonstrate a clinically significant advantage for combination treatment.

Serotonin Reuptake Inhibitors

More recent studies of the psychopharmacology of dysthymia have focused on the use of SRI drugs, which are the most commonly used antidepressants for the treatment of all types of depression. Open-label studies of various SRIs, such as fluoxetine [28–31], sertraline [32], and citalopram [33,34], have suggested that they are effective in a majority of patients. In addition, open-label studies of adolescents with dysthymia have suggested that SRIs are effective and well tolerated [35–38].

Placebo-controlled studies have demonstrated the efficacy of fluoxetine [39,40], sertraline [8,41,42], and paroxetine [43,44], although a study by Burrows and colleagues [45] did not find a significant difference between paroxetine and placebo in 24 very elderly nursing home patients with dysthymia.

Hellerstein and colleagues [39] conducted one of the first prospective placebo-controlled studies of "pure" dysthymia (i.e., the patients did not have double depression). This small (n = 32) study found that fluoxetine (20–60 mg/day) was an effective and well-tolerated treatment. Approximately 60% of patients responded to treatment with fluoxetine compared to a placebo response rate of 19%.

The largest controlled clinical trial of pure dysthymia included 410 patients who were randomly assigned to 12 weeks of double-blind treatment with imipramine (mean dose 190 mg/day), sertraline (mean dose 154 mg/day), or placebo [8]. Both active drugs were significantly more effective than placebo, although side effects and attrition due to adverse events were significantly more common in imipramine-treated patients. Interestingly, women responded significantly better to sertraline than to imipramine, whereas men responded equally well to both drugs [46]. Successful drug treatment in these patients also resulted in improved psychosocial and personality functioning [47,48]. Similarly, a recent randomized double-blind study of 310 patients with pure dysthymia found that sertraline was more effective than placebo in improving depression symptoms, and it was also associated with greater improvement in psychosocial functioning and quality of life [42].

Vanelle and colleagues [40] conducted a three-part, 6-month placebo-controlled study of fluoxetine in 140 patients with pure dysthymia. During the first 3-month acute phase, 66% of 91 fluoxetine patients (20 mg/day) and only 31% of 49 placebo patients responded to double-blind treatment. In the second part of the study, those patients who had responded to acute phase treatment (which included 42 fluoxetine patients and 13 placebo patients) entered a 3-month continuation phase. The proportion of these patients achieving full remission by the end of the continuation phase was significantly greater in the fluoxetine group. In the third part of the study, those patients who had not responded during acute phase treatment (31 nonresponders) entered a new treatment phase in which patients who had received placebo initially were treated with fluoxetine (20 mg/day) and those who had received fluoxetine 20 mg/day initially had their dosage increased to 40 mg/day. Response rates of 53% (in the group whose dosage was increased) and 69% (in those switched from placebo to fluoxetine) further documented the efficacy of fluoxetine in the treatment of dysthymia.

More recently, Barrett and colleagues [49] conducted a large randomized controlled study comparing paroxetine, problem-solving therapy (PST), and placebo in primary care patients with minor depression or dysthymia. Among the subgroup of 211 elderly patients (60 years and older) with dysthymia, paroxetine was somewhat more effective than placebo or PST, although the differences were relatively modest [43]. Among the subgroup of 127 patients (ages 18–59 years) with dysthymia, paroxetine and PST were significantly more effective than placebo [44], with a nonsignificant trend favoring paroxetine over PST. Additional analyses of the results from this study found that the difference between active treatments (either paroxetine or PST) and placebo were significantly greater in younger patients than in older patients [50]. This finding is consistent with the results from the study by Burrows and colleagues [45], which did not find a significant difference between paroxetine and placebo in elderly patients (80 years and older) with dysthymia. There was also evidence from the primary care study that the difference between active treatments and placebo was significantly greater in men than in women [50].

Controlled comparisons between SRIs and other psychotropic antidepressant drugs, such as maprotiline [23], moclobemide [26], venlafaxine [51], and amisulpride [52–56], have also shown them to be effective in the treatment of dysthymia. Some of these studies were discussed previously and others are discussed in more detail below.

Dunner and colleagues [57] randomly assigned 31 dysthymic patients to 16 weeks of treatment with either fluoxetine (20–40 mg/day) or cognitive therapy. Attrition was greater in the fluoxetine group, and a consistent pattern of differences suggested that pharmacotherapy had somewhat better outcomes, but most of these differences were not statistically significant in this small study. Another randomized controlled trial comparing fluoxetine and fluoxetine plus group psychotherapy in 40 dysthymic patients found that both groups showed significant improvement over time [58]. There was only a nonsignificant trend for additional improvement in the psychotherapy group, but the sample size of this study may have been too small to demonstrate a clinically significant advantage for combination treatment.

Ravindran and colleagues [41] conducted a placebo-controlled study comparing sertraline and group cognitive therapy, singly and in combination, among 97 patients with dysthymia. Sertraline was significantly more effective than placebo, whereas group therapy was not. The combined treatment condition produced significantly greater improvements on several psychosocial outcome measures. The remission rate was also 18% higher in the combined group compared to sertraline alone, although this difference was not statistically significant.

Atypical Antidepressants

As a group, the most commonly used atypical antidepressants (i.e., venlafaxine, bupropion, mirtazapine, and nefazodone) have not been well studied in the treatment of dysthymia. Several open-label studies have suggested that venlafaxine [59–62], bupropion [63], and mirtazapine [64] are effective in a majority of patients. A randomized double-blind comparison of venlafaxine and paroxetine in patients with dysthymia or major depression found them to be effective, with nonsignificant trends for greater response rates with venlafaxine [51]. Viloxazine is an atypical bicyclic antidepressant that inhibits the reuptake of norepinephrine and may enhance the release of serotonin. Several studies have shown that it is effective in the treatment of dysthymia [65,66].

Ritanserin is a $5-HT_2$ receptor antagonist with antidepressant and anxiolytic effects. In a randomized double-blind study of 23 dysthymic patients, ritanserin was more effective than placebo [67]. Bakish and colleagues [6] compared ritanserin and imipramine in a placebo-controlled study of 50 patients with dysthymia. The active drugs had comparable efficacy, and both were significantly more effective than placebo. A randomized double-blind study of 70 dysthymic patients found that ritanserin and the atypical antipsychotic flupenthixol were equally effective [68].

Reboxetine is a selective norepinephrine reuptake inhibitor. Several open-label and placebo-controlled studies that included patients with dysthymia suggested that reboxetine is effective and relatively well tolerated [69,70]. A randomized double-blind study of 129 patients with dysthymia found that reboxetine and imipramine were both effective, although imipramine showed a modest but significant advantage [14].

Minaprine is an atypical antidepressant drug that enhances serotonin and dopamine function. One randomized double-blind study of 67 patients with dysthymia found it to be as effective as imipramine but somewhat better tolerated [15].

Atypical Antipsychotics

Amisulpride is an atypical antipsychotic drug that, at low doses, is a relatively selective D_2 and D_3 antagonist for presynaptic dopamine receptors, which leads to increased dopamine activity in the limbic system and clinical antidepressant effects [71,72]. In a randomized controlled 6-month study of 219 patients with dysthymia, double depression, or major depression in partial remission, amisulpride (50 mg/day) was as effective as imipramine (100 mg/day), and both active treatments were significantly more effective than placebo [9]. In addition, amisulpride was generally better tolerated than imipramine. In another placebo-controlled study of 323 dysthymic patients, amisulpride (50 mg/day) and amineptine (200 mg/day) were significantly more effective than placebo [22].

Randomized controlled comparison studies have also found amisulpride to be as effective as amitriptyline [16], fluoxetine [52,54,55], sertraline [53,56], and viloxazine [66]. Although generally well tolerated, these studies found that women treated with amisulpride more often experienced one or more endocrine or gynecological symptoms likely due to secondary hyperprolactinemia. Because amisulpride blocks postsynaptic D_2 receptors at higher doses, which increases prolactin release, the optimal dose might be lower than 50 mg/day for some women. Future studies with amisulpride should investigate the efficacy and tolerability of a lower dose range (i.e., 25 mg/day and higher) in the treatment of dysthymia.

Sulpiride and flupenthixol are other atypical antipsychotics that have been shown to be effective in the treatment of dysthymia in some [68,73,74] but not all studies [75]. Unfortunately, olanzapine and risperidone have not been well studied in dysthymia [76–78], although these drugs appear to have antidepressant effects [79]. Because of the pronounced interactions of serotonin and dopamine in the limbic system and prefrontal cortex, it would be interesting and important to study the use of various atypical antipsychotics, including amisulpride, olanzapine, and risperidone, alone and in combination, to treat patients with chronic depression who have failed to respond to SRI drugs [80].

CHRONIC MAJOR DEPRESSION AND DOUBLE DEPRESSION

Two large randomized multicenter research studies have been conducted in patients with chronic major depression and double depression. Although these studies excluded patients with pure dysthymia, the results are relevant to reviewing the psychopharmacology of dysthymia because of evidence suggesting that dysthymia, double depression, and chronic major depression have more similarities than differences [81–83].

The first randomized controlled study of 635 patients with chronic major depression or double depression found that sertraline and imipramine were equally effective (showing response rates of approximately

50%), but sertraline was better tolerated [84]. Successful antidepressant treatment was also associated with improved psychosocial functioning in these patients [85]. Interestingly, women responded relatively better to sertraline than to imipramine, whereas men responded relatively better to imipramine than to sertraline [86]. Moreover, premenopausal women responded relatively better to sertraline than to imipramine, whereas postmenopausal women responded equally well to sertraline and to imipramine [86].

In another phase of this study, patients who had failed to respond to 12 weeks of double-blind treatment with either imipramine (n = 51) or sertraline (n = 117) were crossed over to receive the alternative drug [87]. Patients crossed over from imipramine to sertraline were significantly more likely to respond than those switched from sertraline to imipramine (60 vs 44%, respectively). Sertraline was again better tolerated, and significantly fewer patients dropped out because of side effects. Although less than half of the imipramine-treated patients responded to crossover therapy, a 44% response rate is clinically significant among patients who had not benefited from 12 weeks of sertraline therapy. Thus, failure to respond to one class of antidepressant drug should not preclude trials of alternative classes of medication. Indeed, the overall cumulative treatment response rate for patients completing this study (i.e., the response during the initial phase together with the response during the crossover phase) was approximately 80% [84,87]; suggesting that rational sequential trials of rigorously applied alternative medications (having different pharmacological structures) may ultimately be effective in a large proportion of chronically depressed patients.

A second large randomized study comparing nefazodone alone, a modified form of cognitive therapy alone, and their combination in 681 patients with chronic major depression or double depression found that the treatment response rate to nefazodone or to psychotherapy alone was approximately 50% after 12 weeks [88]. This response rate was impressive for a very chronically depressed group of patients (the average duration of their current episode of dysthymia was approximately 23 years and for their current episode of major depression approximately 8 years), but was significantly less than the astounding 70% response rate seen in the combination group [88]. Those patients receiving nefazodone (either alone or in combination) responded to treatment significantly earlier than the psychotherapy alone group. The results from a crossover phase of this study (in which subjects who do not respond to drug or psychotherapy alone are switched to the alternative therapy) are not yet available, but should be of particular clinical interest in comparison to the sertraline-imipramine crossover study [87].

LONG-TERM PHARMACOTHERAPY FOR
CHRONIC DEPRESSION

A 4- to 6-month period of continuation pharmacotherapy is now recommended for virtually all antidepressant responders to help consolidate response and prevent relapse. Thereafter, an indefinite course of maintenance pharmacotherapy may be recommended to lower the risk of a future recurrence. An important clinical assumption has been that chronic depressive disorders, including dysthymia, warrant such maintenance pharmacotherapy, but long-term treatment has not been well studied compared to short-term therapies. Several open-label studies have suggested that long-term treatment of dysthymia is effective [18,19,30,89].

Kocsis and colleagues [90] found that 16–20 weeks of continuation therapy with desipramine was effective in maintaining remission and preventing relapse in a large majority of patients with dysthymia or double depression, which also contributed to improved psychosocial functioning [91,92]. Those patients remaining well after continuation therapy (n = 51) were enrolled in a randomized double-blind placebo-controlled 24-month maintenance therapy study with desipramine [5]. This study found that 52% of the patients in the placebo condition relapsed compared to only 15% of the patients taking desipramine. Among the 27 patients with pure dysthymia in this study, 46% of the placebo patients relapsed compared to none of the desipramine-treated patients [93].

Stewart and colleagues [94] conducted a randomized double-blind placebo-controlled maintenance phase study of 60 patients with chronic atypical depression [7] who had responded to acute and continuation phase therapy with either imipramine or phenelzine. Surprisingly, this study found that phenelzine had significant prophylactic efficacy but imipramine did not. As noted previously, however, these patients had predominantly atypical depressive symptoms, which are relatively more responsive to treatment with MAOIs than to TCAs [25].

In the sertraline-imipramine chronic depression study described above, 16 weeks of continuation therapy with these drugs was effective in maintaining remission and preventing relapse in a large majority of patients with chronic major depression or double depression [95]. The sertraline-treated patients who remained well after continuation therapy were enrolled in a randomized double-blind placebo-controlled 76-week maintenance therapy study [96]. Sertraline was significantly more effective than placebo in preventing a recurrence of depression. Moreover, successful prophylaxis was associated with the maintenance of improved psychosocial functioning in these patients [97]. Similarly, in the nefazodone-psychotherapy chronic depression study described above, preliminary findings from the 16-week continuation phase [98] and 52-week double-blind placebo-controlled maintenance phase [99] have shown that nefazodone is effective in maintaining a treatment response and preventing relapse and recurrence in a majority of patients with chronic major depression or double depression.

CONCLUSION

The results from open-label studies and controlled clinical trials clearly demonstrate that pharmacotherapy is effective in the acute treatment of dysthymia, and successful pharmacotherapy also is associated with improvements in psychosocial functioning and quality of life. In addition, long-term treatment appears to be effective, but has not been studied as extensively as short-term therapy. Although many treatment-resistant patients ultimately become chronically depressed, these findings prove that the majority of people with chronic depression are not treatment resistant. Unfortunately, these studies have primarily focused on the use of TCAs and, more recently, the SRIs. Given some evidence suggesting that there might be differences in efficacy between different classes of antidepressant drugs [100], there is a clear need for additional short-term and long-term efficacy and tolerability studies in dysthymia comparing the SRIs in particular to the atypical antidepressants venlafaxine, bupropion, mirtazapine, and nefazodone. Similar studies should also investigate their effectiveness in comparison to and in combination with such depression-focused psychotherapies as IPT and cognitive therapy. Moreover, there is an important need to identify and understand various clinical, demographic, and biological variables that might lead to more informed decisions about whether to use pharmacotherapy, psychotherapy, or their combination; how to select the most effective treatment from among different classes of antidepressants and different forms of psychotherapy; and determining the need for long-term treatment. For example, age and gender may be important variables that predict a differential response to antidepressant therapies [46,50,86,101].

One problem in reviewing the literature and interpreting the results of treatment studies on the pharmacotherapy of dysthymia is that research investigators often group together patients with pure dysthymia, double depression, chronic major depression, and partially remitted major depression. This ultimately may not prove to be much of a problem, however, because of the arbitrary nature of the distinctions among these diagnostic categories and because of developing evidence that they may have more similarities than differences [81–83]. Nonetheless, a sufficient number of studies focusing on pure dysthymia have been conducted to conclude that pharmacotherapy is indeed effective.

Another problem is the definition and appropriate measurement of an acceptable treatment response in patients with dysthymia. Rating scales that are commonly used in controlled trials of antidepressants, such as the Hamilton [102] and the Montgomery-Åsberg [103] Rating Scales, were developed for use in studies of more severely depressed patients. These scales also are weighted heavily by the presence of melancholic symptoms, and they do not adequately measure atypical depressive symptoms, which may characterize many patients with early-onset dysthymia. Thus, using threshold scores or change ratios that have been standardized in studies of more severely depressed patients might not be sensitive enough to detect a significant treatment response in dysthymia. The Comell Dysthymia Rating Scale [104] was developed to address these problems, but it has not been widely used or extensively evaluated in comparison to other rating scales.

A surprisingly large proportion of chronically depressed patients have never been treated with antidepressant medications [88,105]. The selection of an SRI as a first-line treatment is appropriate for most patients given that they have been well studied in chronic depression (especially fluoxetine, sertraline, and paroxetine), are safer and better tolerated than the TCAs, and are already widely used for virtually all depressive disorders. Compared to the more noradrenergically active TCAs, serotonergic SRIs may be more appropriate for early-onset dysthymic patients (who often present with hypersomnia, increased appetite, or weight gain), and especially among younger patients in whom SRIs are relatively more effective [50,101]. Because of their different pharmacological effects and side effect profiles, the atypical antidepressants venlafaxine, bupropion, mirtazapine, and nefazodone may also be considered for first-line treatment as an alternative to the SRIs depending on the patient's clinical symptoms and treatment history. For example, some of these drugs are less likely to cause sexual dysfunction (e.g., bupropion, nefazodone, and mirtazapine) or weight gain (e.g., bupropion, venlafaxine, and nefazodone), and some may be relatively more beneficial for insomnia (e.g., nefazodone and mirtazapine) or prominent anxiety (e.g., venlafaxine, nefazodone, and mirtazapine). Of these drugs, only nefazodone has been specifically and systematically studied in chronic depression. Clinical experience and extrapolation from their demonstrated efficacy in nonchronic depression would suggest, however, that the other atypical antidepressants might also prove to be effective in controlled studies of chronic depression.

In patients who do not have an adequate or acceptable response to treatment, several options should be considered. For those patients with a partial response, maximizing their antidepressant dosage and/or augmenting with a second drug may be the most effective approach [40,106]. For those patients with minimal or no response, switching to a different antidepressant therapy may be more appropriate [87,107]. Alternative antidepressant choices for SRI nonresponders include the atypical antidepressants, TCAs, and MAOIs. Among the group of atypical antidepressants, venlafaxine has the best evidence for efficacy in treatment-resistant depression [108]. In contemporary clinical practice, the TCAs and MAOIs are usually reserved for patients who have failed to respond to multiple trials of SRIs, atypical antidepressants, psychotropic drug combinations, and combined pharmacotherapy-psychotherapy.

Proper acute phase pharmacotherapy of dysthymia and other chronic depressive disorders is guided by several principles. Full doses of antidepressant drugs should be used as necessary, with the goal of achieving a complete remission of depressive symptoms. Chronic depressions may respond more slowly to treatment, and patients may therefore require longer courses of acute phase therapy (i.e., 8- to 12-week trials rather than 4- to 6-week trials). Comorbid disorders should be identified and appropriately treated [109]. The need for psychotherapy should be evaluated in all patients. The treatment plan should be periodically modified and revised to achieve complete remission, handle relapses and recurrences, and maintain treatment adherence. During long-term therapy, full doses of the antidepressant should be maintained.

Whether chronically depressed patients who have achieved a complete remission (and maintained it for longer than 6 months) require long-term therapy is not clearly known. A conservative strategy would be to recommend maintenance phase treatment routinely for patients with chronic major depression or double depression. Patients with persistent residual symptoms, especially those associated with significant psychosocial impairment or comorbidity [109], have the greatest need for long-term pharmacotherapy, and they may be appropriate candidates for using a combination of pharmacotherapy and psychotherapy [110,111].

REFERENCES

1. RH Howland. Pharmacothempy of dysthymia: a review. J Clin Psychopharmacol 11:83–92, 1991.
2. RH Howland. Psychosocial therapies for dysthymia. In: FF Flach, ed. The Hatherleigh Guide to Managing Depression. New York: Hatherleigh Press, 1996, pp 225–241.
3. RH Howland, ME Thase. Biological studies of dysthymia. Biol Psychiatry 30:283–304, 1991.
4. RH Howland. Chronic depression. Hosp Commun Psychiatry 44:633–639, 1993.
5. JH Kocsis, RA Friedman, JC Markowitz, AC Leon, NL Miller, L Gniwesch,

M Parides. Maintenance therapy for chronic depression: a controlled clinical trial. Arch Gen Psychiatry 53:769–774, 1996.

6. D Bakish, YD Lapierre, R Weinstein, J Klein, A Wiens, B Jones, E Horn, M Browne, D Bourget, A Blanchard, C Thibaudeau, C Waddell, D Raine. Ritanserin, imipramine and placebo in the treatment of dysthymic disorder. J Clin Psychopharmacol 13:409–414, 1993.

7. JW Stewart, PJ McGrath, FM Quitkin, W Harrison, S Wager, E Nunes, K Ocepek-Welikson, E Tricamo. Chronic depression: Response to placebo, imipramine, and phenelzine. J Clin Psychopharmacol 13:391–396, 1993.

8. ME Thase, M Fava, U Halbreich, JH Kocsis, L Koran, J Davidson, J Rosenbaum, W Harrison. A placebo-controlled, randomized clinical trial comparing sertraline and imipramine for the treatment of dysthymia. Arch Gen Psychiatry 53:777–784, 1996.

9. Y Lecrubier, P Boyer, S Turjanski, W Rein, Amisulpride Study Group. Amisulpride versus imipramine and placebo in dysthymia and major depression. J Affect Disord 43:95–103, 1997.

10. M Versiani, R Amrein, M Stabl. Moclobemide and imipramine in chronic depression (dysthymia): An international double-blind, placebo-controlled trial. Int Clin Psychopharmacol 12:183–193, 1997.

11. H Loo, R Malka, R Defrance, D Barrucand. Tianeptine and amitriptyline: Controlled double-blind trial in depressed alcoholic patients. Neuropsychobiology 19:79–85, 1988.

12. JD Guelfi, P Pichot, JF Dreyfus. Efficacy of tianeptine in anxious-depressed patients: Results of a controlled multicenter trial versus amitriptyline. Neuropsychobiology 22:41–48, 1989.

13. M Casacchia, A Rossi. A comparison of moclobemide and imipramine in treatment of depression. Pharmacopsychiatry 22:152–155, 1989.

14. C Katona, E Bercoff, E Chiu, P Tack, M Versiani, H Woelk. Reboxetine versus imipramine in the treatment of elderly patients with depressive disorders: A double-blind randomized trial. J Affect Disord 55:203–213, 1999.

15. E Salzmann, JL Robin. Multicentric double-blind study comparing efficacy and safety of minaprine and imipramine in dysthymic disorders. Neuropsychobiology 31:68–75, 1995.

16. L Ravizza, AMILONG investigators. Amisulpride in medium-term treatment of dysthymia: a six-month, double-blind safety study versus amitriptyline. J Psychopharmacol 13:248–254, 1999.

17. D de Maio, A Levi Minzi. Considerations on the efficacy of tianeptine, a new antidepressant drug. G Neuropsicofarmacol 12:83–87, 1990.

18. H Loo, H Ganry, C Marey, G Briole. Acceptability of tianeptine in 170 depressed patients treated during a one year period. Encephale 16:445–452, 1990.

19. A Souche, L Duclaud, JR Zekri, G Yzombard. Patients treated for a one-year period with tianeptine: presentation of results obtained at one of the Centers of South-East France. Encephale 16:181–187, 1990.

20. JS Ruiz, JM Montes, E Alvarez, S Cervera, J Giner, J Guerrero, F Dourdil, A Seva. Tianeptine treatment for depression in the elderly. Actas Luso Esp Neurol Psiquiatr Cienc Afines 25:79–83, 1997.
21. JD Guelfi. Efficacy of tianeptine in comparative trials versus reference antidepressants: An overview. Br J Psychiatry 160(Suppl 15):72–75, 1992.
22. P Boyer, Y Lecrubier, A Stalla-Bourdillon, O Fleurot. Amisulpride versus amineptine and placebo for the treatment of dysthymia. Pharmacopsychiatry 39:25–32, 1999.
23. F de Jonghe, J Swinkels, H Tuynman-Qua. Randomized double-blind study of fluvoxamine and maprotiline in treatment of depression. Pharmacopsychiatry 24:21–27, 1991.
24. F Schifano, A Garbin, V Renesto, MG de Dominicis. A double-blind comparison of mianserin and maprotiline in depressed medially ill elderly people. Acta Psychiatr Scand 81:289–294, 1990.
25. JW Stewart, PJ McGrath, FM Quitkin. Relevance of DSM-III depressive subtype and chronicity to antidepressant efficacy in atypical depression. Arch Gen Psychiatry 46:1080–1087, 1989.
26. A Duarte, H Mikkelsen, A Delini-Stula. Moclobemide versus fluoxetine for double depression: A randomized double-blind study. J Psychiatry Res 30:453–458, 1996.
27. MF de Mello, LM Myczcowisk, PR Menezes. A randomized controlled trial comparing moclobemide and moclobemide plus interpersonal psychotherapy in the treatment of dysthymic disorder. J Psychother Pract Res 10:117–123, 2001.
28. D Bakish, A Ravindran, C Hooper, Y Lapierre. Psychopharmacological treatment response of patients with a DSM-III diagnosis of dysthymic disorder. Psychopharmacol Bull 30:53–59, 1994.
29. AV Ravindran, RJ Bialik, YD Lapierre. Therapeutic efficacy of specific serotonin reuptake inhibitors (SSRIs) in dysthymia. Can J Psychiatry 39: 21–26, 1994.
30. DJ Hellerstein, L Wallner Samstag, M Cantillon, M Maurer, J Rosenthal, P Yanowitch, A Winston. Follow-up assessment of medication-treated dysthymia. Prog Neuropsychopharmacol Biol Psychiatry 20:427–442, 1996.
31. MS Nobler, DP Devanand, MK Kim, LM Fitzsimons, TM Singer, N Turret, HA Sackeim, SP Roose. Fluoxetine treatment of dysthymia in the elderly. J Clin Psychiatry 57:254–256, 1996.
32. A Chinchilla, A Cebollada, M Vega, M Diaz, G Guzman, JM Montes. Treatment of dysthymia with sertraline. Actas Luso Esp Neurol Psiquiatr Cien Afines 25:3–9, 1997.
33. E Zanalda, M Scotta, P Rocca, M Mazzucco, L Ravizza. The efficacy and tolerance of citalopram in dysthymia. G Neuropsicofarmacol 20:79–82, 1998.
34. DL Dunner, HE Hendrickson, C Bea, CB Budech, SD Friedman. Dysthymic disorder: Treatment with citalopram. Depression Anxiety 15:18–22, 2002.
35. BD Waslick, BT Walsh, LL Greenhill, M Eilenberg, L Capasso, D Lieber. Open trial of fluoxetine in children and adolescents with dysthymic disorder or double depression. J Affect Disord 56:227–236, 1999.

36. M Nobile, B Bellotti, C Marino, M Molteni, M Battaglia. An open trial of paroxetine in the treatment of children and adolescents diagnosed with dysthymia. J Child Adolesc Psychopharmacol 10:103–109, 2000.
37. J Rabe-Jablonska. Therapeutic effects and tolerability of fluvoxamine treatment in adolescents with dysthymia. J Child Adolesc Psychopharmacol 10:9–18, 2000.
38. MK Nixon, R Milin, JG Simeon, P Cloutier, W Spenst. Sertraline effects in adolescent major depression and dysthymia: a six-month open trial. J Child Adolesc Psychopharmacol 11:131–142, 2001.
39. DJ Hellerstein, P Yanowitch, J Rosenthal, L Wallner Samstag, M Maurer, K Kasch, L Burrows, M Poster, M Cantillon, A Winston. A randomized double-blind study of fluoxetine versus placebo in the treatment of dysthymia. Am J Psychiatry 150:1169–1175, 1993.
40. JM Vanelle, D Attar-Levy, MF Poirier, M Bouhassira, P Blin, JP Olié. Controlled efficacy study of fluoxetine in dysthymia. Br J Psychiatry 171:345–350, 1997.
41. AV Ravindran, H Anisman, Z Merali, Y Charbonneau, J Telner, RJ Bialik, A Wiens, J Ellis, J Griffiths. Treatment of primary dysthymia with group cognitive therapy and pharmacotherapy: clinical symptoms and functional impairments. Am J Psychiatry 156:1608–1617, 1999.
42. AV Ravindran, JD Guelfi, RM Lane, GB Cassano. Treatment of dysthymia with sertraline: a double-blind, placebo-controlled trial in dysthymic patients without major depression. J Clin Psychiatry 61:821–827, 2000.
43. JW Williams, J Barrett, T Oxman, E Frank, W Katon, M Sullivan, J Cornell, A Sengupta. Treatment of dysthymia and minor depression in primary care: a randomized controlled trial in older adults. JAMA 284:1519–1526, 2000.
44. JE Barrett, JW Williams, TE Oxman, E Frank, W Katon, M Sullivan, MT Hegel, JE Cornell, AS Sengupta. Treatment of dysthymia and minor depression in primary care: a randomized trial in patients aged 18 to 59 years. J Fam Pract 50:405–412, 2001.
45. AB Burrows, C Salzman, A Satlin, K Noble, BG Pollock, T Gersh. A randomized, placebo-controlled trial of paroxetine in nursing home residents with non-major depression. Depression Anxiety 15:102–110, 2002.
46. ME Thase, E Frank, S Kornstein, KA Yonkers. Gender differences in response to treatments of depression. In: E Frank, ed. Gender and Its Effects on Psychopathology. Washington, DC: American Psychiatric Press, 2000, pp 103–129.
47. JH Kocsis, S Zisook, J Davidson, R Shelton, K Yonkers, DJ Hellerstein, J Rosenbaum, U Halbreich. Double-blind comparison of sertraline, imipramine, and placebo in the treatment of dysthymia: psychosocial outcomes. Am J Psychiatry 154:390–395, 1997.
48. DJ Hellerstein, JH Kocsis, D Chapman, J Stewart, W Harrison. Double-blind comparison of sertraline, imipramine, and placebo in the treatment of dysthymia: effects on personality. Am J Psychiatry 157:1436–1444, 2000.

49. JE Barrett, JW Williams, TE Oxman, W Katon, E Frank, MT Hegel, M Sullivan, HC Schulberg. The treatment effectiveness project. A comparison of the effectiveness of paroxetine, problem-solving therapy, and placebo in the treatment of minor depression and dysthymia in primary care patients: background and research plan. Gen Hosp Psychiatry 21:260–273, 1999.

50. W Katon, J Russo, E Frank, J Barrett, JW Williams, T Oxman, M Sullivan, J Cornell. Predictors of nonresponse to treatment in primary care patients with dysthymia. Gen Hosp Psychiatry 24:20–27, 2002.

51. C Ballus, G Quiros, T de Flores, J de la Torre, D Palao, L Rojo, M Gutierrez, L Casais, Y Riesgo. The efficacy and tolerability of venlafaxine and paroxetine in outpatients with depressive disorder or dysthymia. Int Clin Psychopharmacol 15:43–48, 2000.

52. E Smeraldi, E Haefele, G Crespi, GL Casadei, F Biondi, E Vigorelli. Amisulpride versus fluoxetine in dysthymia: preliminary results of a double-blind comparative study. Eur Psychiatry 11(Suppl 3):141S–143S, 1996.

53. S Bellino, G Barzega, F Bogetto, G Maina, S Venturello, L Ravizza. An open-label, randomized, prospective comparison of sertraline and amisulpride in the treatment of dysthymia in the elderly. Curr Ther Res 58:798–808, 1997.

54. F Bogetto, G Barzega, S Bellino, G Maina, L Ravizza. Drug treatment of dysthymia: A clinical study. Riv Psichiatria 32:1–5, 1997.

55. E Smeraldi. Amisulpride versus fluoxetine in patients with dysthymia or major depression in partial remission: a double-blind, comparative study. J Affect Disord 48:47–56, 1998.

56. M Amore, MC Jori. Faster response on amisulpride 50 mg versus sertraline 50–100 mg in patients with dysthymia or double depression: a randomized, double-blind, parallel group study. Int Clin Psychopharmacol 16:317–324, 2001.

57. DL Dunner, KB Schmaling, H Hendrickson, J Becker, A Lehman, C Bea. Cognitive therapy versus fluoxetine in the treatment of dysthymic disorder. Depression 4:34–41, 1996.

58. DJ Hellerstein, SAS Little, L Wallner Samstag, S Batchelder, JC Muran, M Fedak, D Kreditor, RN Rosenthal, A Winston. Adding group psychotherapy to medication treatment in dysthymia: a randomized prospective pilot study. J Psychother Pract Res 10:93–103, 2001.

59. DL Dunner, HE Hendrickson, C Bea, CB Budech. Venlafaxine in dysthymic disorder. J Clin Psychiatry 58:528–531, 1997.

60. AV Ravindran, Y Charbonneau, MD Zaharia, K Al-Zaid, A Wiens, H Anisman. Efficacy and tolerability of venlafaxine in the treatment of primary dysthymia. J Psychiatry Neurosci 23:288–292, 1998.

61. DJ Hellerstein, ST Batchelder, SAS Little, MJ Fedak, D Kreditor, J Rosenthal. Venlafaxine in the treatment of dysthymia: an open-label study. J Clin Psychiatry 60:845–849, 1999.

62. G Perugi, G Ruffolo, C Torti, I Maremmani. Venlafaxine XR in the long-term treatment of comorbidity among generalized anxiety disorder and major depression or dysthymia: a naturalistic study. Riv Psichiatria 36:337–343, 2001.

63. DJ Hellerstein, ST Batchelder, D Kreditor, M Fedak. Bupropion sustained-release for the treatment of dysthymic disorder: an open-label study. J Clin Psychopharmacol 21:325–329, 2001.

64. DL Dunner, HE Hendrickson, C Bea, CB Budech, E O'Connor. Dysthymic disorder: treatment with mirtazapine. Depression Anxiety 10:68–72, 1999.

65. S Cairoli, P Tosca, G Somenzino, F Zeebi. Considerations on the utility of an atypical bicyclic antidepressive (viloxazine) administered intravenously in depressed patients: plasma levels, tolerance, and clinical response. Psichiatria Psicoter Analit 6:341–350, 1987.

66. CA Leon, J Vigoya, S Conde, G Campo. Efficacy of amisulpride and viloxazine in the treatment of dysthymia: a comparison. Acta Psiquiatrica Psicol America Latina 40:41–49, 1994.

67. G Bersani, F Pozzi, S Marini, A Grispini. 5-HT-sub-2 receptor antagonism in dysthymic disorder: a double-blind placebo-controlled study with ritanserin. Acta Psychiatr Scand 83:244–248, 1991.

68. A Geisler, S Mygind, OR Knudsen, M Sloth-Nielson. Ritanserin and flupenthixol in dysthymic disorder: a controlled double-blind study in general practice. Nordic J Psychiatry 46:237–243, 1992.

69. GD Burrows, KP Maguire, TR Norman. Antidepressant efficacy and tolerability of the selective norepinephrine reuptake inhibitor reboxetine: a review. J Clin Psychiatry 59(Suppl 14):4–7, 1998.

70. V Andreoli, G Carbognin, A Abati, G Vantini. Reboxetine in the treatment of depression in the elderly: pilot study. J Geriatr Psychiat Neurol 12:206–210, 1999.

71. GL Gessa. Dysthymia and depressive disorders: Dopamine hypothesis. Eur Psychiatry 11(Suppl 3):123S–127S, 1996.

72. L Pani, GL Gessa. The substituted benzamides and their clinical potential on dysthymia and on the negative symptoms of schizophrenia. Mol Psychiatry 7:247–253, 2002.

73. R Scarzella, L Scarzella, GG Rovera. Amisulpride versus sulpiride: double-blind clinical study in 68 patients with dysthymic disorder. G Neuropsicofarmacol 12:73–78, 1990.

74. W Maier, O Benkert. Treatment of chronic depression with sulpiride: Evidence of efficacy in placebo-controlled single case studies. Psychopharmacology 115:495–501, 1994.

75. SL Kivelae, E Lehtomaeki. Sulpiride and placebo in depressed elderly outpatients: a double-blind study. Int J Geriatr Psychiatry 2:255–260, 1987.

76. JA Bourgeois, M Klein. Risperidone and fluoxetine in the treatment of pedophilia with comorbid dysthymia. J Clin Psychopharmacol 16:257–258, 1996.

77. EM Szigethy, SC Schulz. Risperidone in comorbid borderline personality disorder and dysthymia. J Clin Psychopharmacol 17:326–327, 1997.

78. SC Schulz, KL Camlin, SA Berry, JA Jesberger. Olanzapine safety and efficacy in patients with borderline personality disorder and comorbid dysthymia. Biol Psychiatry 46:1429–1435, 1999.

79. ME Thase. What role do atypical antipsychotic drugs have in treatment-resistant depression? J Clin Psychiatry 63:95–103, 2002.

80. RC Shelton, GD Tollefson, M Tohen, S Stahl, KS Gannon, TC Jacobs, WR Buras, FP Bymaster, W Zhang, KA Spencer, PD Feldman, HY Meltzer. A novel augmentation strategy for treating resistant major depression. Am J Psychiatry 158:131–134, 2001.

81. RA Remick, AD Sadovnick, RW Lam, AP Zis, IML Yee. Major depression, minor depression, and double depression: are they distinct clinical entities? Am J Med Genet 67:347–353, 1996.

82. JP McCullough, DN Klein, MB Keller, CE Holzer, SM Davis, SG Kornstein, RH Howland, ME Thase, WM Harrison. Comparison of DSM-III chronic major depression and major depression superimposed on dysthymia (double depression): validity of the distinction. J Abnorm Psychol 109:419–427, 2000.

83. T Yang, DL Dunner. Differential subtyping of depression. Depression Anxiety 13:11–17, 2001.

84. MB Keller, AJ Gelenberg, RMA Hirschfeld, AJ Rush, ME Thase, JH Kocsis, JC Markowitz, JA Fawcett, LM Koran, DN Klein, JM Russell, SG Kornstein, JP McCullough, SM Davis, WM Harrison. The treatment of chronic depression. Part 2: A double-blind, randomized trial of sertraline and imipramine. J Clin Psychiatry 59:598–607, 1998.

85. IW Miller, AF Schatzberg, DN Klein, ME Thase, AJ Rush, JC Markowitz, DS Schlager, SG Kornstein, SM Davis, MB Keller. The treatment of chronic depression, Part 3: Psychosocial functioning before and after treatment with sertraline or imipramine. J Clin Psychiatry 59:608–619, 1998.

86. SG Kornstein, AF Schatzberg, ME Thase, KA Yonkers, JP McCullough, GI Keitner, AJ Gelenberg, SM Davis, WM Harrison, MB Keller. Gender differences in treatment response to sertraline versus imipramine in chronic depression. Am J Psychiatry 157:1445–1452, 1998.

87. ME Thase, AJ Rush, RH Howland, SG Kornstein, JH Kocsis, AJ Gelenberg, AF Schatzberg, LM Koran, MB Keller, JM Russell, RMA Hirschfeld, LM LaVange, DN Klein, J Fawcett, WM Harrison. Double-blind switch study of imipramine or sertraline treatment of antidepressant-resistant chronic depression. Arch Gen Psychiatry 59:233–239, 2002.

88. MB Keller, JP McCullough, DN Klein, B Arnow, DL Dunner, AJ Gelenberg, JC Markowitz, CB Nemeroff, JM Russell, ME Thase, MH Trivedi, J Zajecka. A comparison of nefazodone, the cognitive behavioral-analysis system of psychotherapy, and their combination for the treatment of chronic depression. N Engl J Med 342:1462–1470, 2000.

89. RF Haykal, HS Akiskal. The long-term outcome of dysthymia in private practice: clinical features, temperament, and the art of management. J Clin Psychiatry 60:508–518, 1999.

90. JH Kocsis, RA Friedman, JC Markowitz, N Miller. Stability of remission during tricyclic antidepressant continuation therapy for dysthymia. Psychopharmacol Bull 31:213–216, 1995.

91. RA Friedman, JC Markowitz, M Parides, JH Kocsis. Acute response of social functioning in dysthymic patients with desipramine. J Affect Disord 34:85–88, 1995.

92. RA Friedman, JC Markowitz, M Parides, L Gniwesch, JH Kocsis. Six months of desipramine for dysthymia: can dysthymic patients achieve normal social functioning? J Affect Disord 54:283–286, 1999.

93. NL Miller, JH Kocsis, AC Leon, L Portera, S Dauber, JC Markowitz. Maintenance desipramine for dysthymia: a placebo-controlled study. J Affect Disord 64:231–237, 2001.

94. JW Stewart, E Tricamo, PJ McGrath, FM Quitkin. Prophylactic efficacy of phenelzine and imipramine in chronic atypical depression: likelihood of recurrence on discontinuation after 6 months' remission. Am J Psychiatry 154:31–36, 1997.

95. LM Koran, AJ Gelenberg, SG Kornstein, RH Howland, RA Friedman, C DeBattista, D Klein, JH Kocsis, AF Schatzberg, ME Thase, AJ Rush, RMA Hirschfeld, LM LaVange, MB Keller. Sertraline versus imipramine to prevent relapse in chronic depression. J Affect Disord 65:27–36, 2001.

96. MB Keller, JH Kocsis, ME Thase, AJ Gelenberg, AJ Rush, L Koran, A Schatzberg, J Russell, R Hirschfeld, D Klein, JP McCullough, JA Fawcett, S Kornstein, L LaVange, W Harrison. Maintenance phase efficacy of sertraline for chronic depression: a randomized controlled trial. JAMA 280:1665–1672, 1998.

97. JH Kocsis, A Schatzberg, AJ Rush, DN Klein, R Howland, L Gniwesch, SM Davis, W Harrison. Psychosocial outcomes following long-term, double-blind treatment of chronic depression with sertraline versus placebo. Arch Gen Psychiatry 59:723–728, 2002.

98. JH Kocsis, B Arnow, FE Borian, DL Dunner, AJ Gelenberg, G Kenner, DN Klein, L Koran, SG Kornstein, R Manber, JC Markowitz, I Miller, C Nemeroff, B Rothbaum, AJ Rush, AF Schatzberg, RH Howland, MH Trivedi, D Vivian, MB Keller. Nefazodone, CBAS-psychotherapy and their combination for the continuation treatment of chronic major depression. American Psychiatric Association Annual Meeting, New Orleans, May, 2001.

99. AJ Gelenberg, MH Trivedi, AJ Rush, ME Thase, R Howland, DN Klein, SG Kornstein, DL Dunner, JC Markowitz, RMA Hirschfeld, GI Keitner, J Zajecka, JH Kocsis, JM Russell, I Miller, R Mamber, B Arnow, B Rothbaum, M Munsaka, P Banks, FE Borian, MB Keller. Randomized, placebo-controlled trial of nefazadone maintenance treatment in preventing recurrence in chronic depression. Biol Psychiatry. In press.

100. ME Thase, AR Entsuah, RL Rudolph. Remission rates during treatment with venlafaxine or selective serotonin reuptake inhibitors. Br J Psychiatry 178:234–241, 2001.

101. GJ Emslie, TL Mayes. Mood disorders in children and adolescents: psychopharmacological treatment. Biol Psychiatry 49:1082–1090, 2001.

102. M Hamilton. A rating scale for depression. J Neurol Neurosurg Psychiatry 23:56–62, 1960.

103. SA Montgomery, M Åsberg. A new depression scale designed to be sensitive to change. Br J Psychiatry 134:382–389, 1979.

104. BJ Mason, JH Kocsis, AC Leon, S Thompson, AJ Frances, RO Morgan, MK Parides. Measurement of severity and treatment response in dysthymia. Psychiatr Ann 23:625–631, 1993.

105. RC Shelton, J Davidson, KA Yonkers, L Koran, ME Thase, T Pearlstein, U Halbreich. The undertreatment of dysthymia. J Clin Psychiatry 58:59–65, 1997.

106. ME Thase, RH Howland, ES Friedman. Treating antidepressant non-responders with augmentation strategies: an overview. J Clin Psychiatry 59(Suppl 5):5–15, 1998.

107. RH Howland, ME Thase. Switching strategies for the treatment of unipolar major depression. Mod Probl Pharmacopsychiatry 25:56–65, 1997.

108. ME Thase, ES Friedman, RH Howland. Venlafaxine and treatment-resistant depression. Depression Anxiety 12(Suppl 1):55–62, 2000.

109. RH Howland. General health, health care utilization, and medical comorbidity in dysthymia. Int J Psychiatry Med 23:211–238, 1993.

110. GA Fava, S Grandi, M Zielezny, R Canestrari, MA Morphy. Cognitive behavioral treatment of residual symptoms in primary major depressive disorder. Am J Psychiatry 151:1295–1299, 1994.

111. GA Fava, S Grandi, M Zielezny, C Rafanelli, R Canestrari. Four-year otucome for cognitive behavioral treatment of residual symptoms in major depression. Am J Psychiatry 153:945–947, 1996.

7

Psychotherapy for Chronic Depressive Disorders

Gabor I. Keitner
Brown University and Rhode Island Hospital
Providence, Rhode Island, U.S.A.

Esteban V. Cardemil
Clark University
Worcester, Massachusetts, U.S.A.

INTRODUCTION

Considerable research has demonstrated the efficacy of a wide range of different psychotherapies for acute major depression, including individual psychotherapies [1,2], group psychotherapies [3,4] and marital/family treatments [5,6]. Knowledge regarding the efficacy of psychosocial treatments for chronic depressive disorders, however, is lacking, as few studies have explicitly examined the efficacy of psychotherapy for them [7]. Moreover, with a few notable exceptions (e.g., see Ref. 8), the small sample sizes and methodological limitations in these studies constrain our ability to draw firm conclusions regarding the efficacy of individual psychotherapy as the sole treatment for chronic depressive disorders.

This dearth in psychotherapy research for chronic depressive disorders is problematic, since by definition, chronic depressive disorders rarely remit spontaneously [9], and even with treatment, they demonstrate low recovery and high relapse rates [10,11]. There are several reasons why the development of an effective psychotherapy for chronic depressive disorders is an important undertaking [12]. First, approximately half of patients with dysthymic disorder, one form of chronic depression, do not respond to antidepressant medication. Second, many others choose not to take medication for a variety of reasons, including intolerable side effects, and so would benefit from psychotherapy. Third, many patients who respond to pharmacotherapy may benefit from additional psychotherapy. Finally, evidence is emerging suggesting that treatments that combine both pharmacotherapy and psychotherapy may provide the best treatment option for chronic depression (e.g., see Refs. 8,13,14, and 15). Developing and evaluating effective psychotherapies for chronic depressive disorders to be used either alone or in combination with pharmacotherapy are clinically important.

In this chapter, we review the literature on psychotherapy for chronic depressive disorders, which are broadly defined. Given the limited research on chronic depression per se, we have expanded the definition of chronic depression to include dysthymic disorder and double depression. In addition, we also review the psychotherapy literature on recurrent and severe depression. Including other forms of chronic depressive disorders in our review allows us to expand the pool of information from which to find commonalities in the psychotherapy research. Given that there is considerable overlap in diagnostic categories, symptom presentation, and functional impairment among these chronic depressive conditions [16], it is likely that the psychotherapeutic issues will also have considerable overlap. Following this review of psychotherapy for chronic depressive disorders, we draw on the commonalities present across these studies to make general recommendations for clinicians and researchers. We conclude with research directions that would help the field better understand the psychotherapeutic treatment of chronic depression.

PSYCHODYNAMIC PSYCHOTHERAPY

Historically, psychoanalytic thinking considered chronic depression to be an expression of character pathology, and thus amenable to treatment with psychodynamic therapies. Unfortunately, very little empirical data exist to support this contention, leading some to argue that psychoanalytic thinking may be incompatible with treatment for chronic depression [17]. It is unclear, for example, whether patients with chronic depression might respond as well to a more passive therapeutic approach rather than the more proactive stance endorsed by advocates of nonpsychoanalytic therapies.

A recent study conducted by Luborsky and colleagues [18] investigated the effectiveness of treating chronic depression with supportive expressive dynamic psychotherapy, a specific form of psychodynamic psychotherapy [19]. Supportive-expressive therapy is a modern form of psychodynamic therapy in that it uses traditional psychodynamic principles in a time-limited and more present-oriented fashion than other psychodynamic therapies [19]. Supportive-expressive therapy addresses depressive symptoms by providing support via the therapeutic alliance, and by focusing on interpersonal conflictual themes through the transference that emerges in the patient-therapist relationship [19,20]. In this study, 25 patients with chronic depression and 24 patients with acute major depression were treated for 16–20 sessions with supportive-expressive psychotherapy. Results indicated very little difference between the chronic depression and acute depression groups. Patients in the chronic depression group reported significant improvement from intake to termination on both the Beck Depression Inventory (BDI) [21] (mean scores dropped from 27.91 to 14.28), the Hamilton Rating Scale for Depression (HAM-D) [22] (14.24 to 6.28), and the Global Assessment Scale (GAS) [23] (53.56 to 66.12). No data on percentage improved or recovered were presented.

This study was the only one that we were able to find that addressed the efficacy of psychodynamic psychotherapy in treating any chronic depressive disorder. The positive results are encouraging, but given the inherent limitations of the design (e.g., small sample size, no control group, or random assignment), they must be taken as preliminary. Nevertheless, they suggest that psychodynamic psychotherapy, at least in a time-limited fashion, can play a useful role in the treatment of chronic depression.

COGNITIVE-BEHAVIORAL THERAPY

Cognitive-behavioral therapy (CBT) treats depression by addressing the maladaptive and pessimistic thinking in which depressed individuals engage. Working collaboratively, the individual and therapist identify and then change those elements of a patient's thinking and behavior that are believed to be contributing to the depressive symptoms. Considerable evidence exists to support the efficacy of CBT in the treatment of acute depression [2,24] and in the prevention of relapse [25–28]. This strong support for treating acute depression with CBT has led researchers to investigate its efficacy in treating chronic depressive disorders.

To date, nine studies have presented data on the efficacy of CBT with chronic depressive disorders. We have divided these studies into two broad categories. The first category focuses on studies that analyzed the efficacy of CBT for chronic depressive disorders within a larger study of CBT for major depression. These research studies represent the field's first attempts to investigate psychosocial treatments for chronic depressive disorders. A strength of these studies is their reliance on standard psychosocial interventions that have been well-established with acute major depression. A weakness, however, is the assumption that standard treatments for acute major depression will translate into effective treatments for chronic depressive disorders.

The second category is limited to those studies that investigated the efficacy of CBT specifically for chronic depressive disorders. By not including patients with acute major depression, these studies are able to modify standard treatments so as to address better the difficulties encountered by patients with chronic depression. A weakness, however, is that the novel interventions do not have the extensive history of empirical validation of the standard interventions. Together, however, these two categories of research studies provide some useful information regarding the efficacy of CBT with chronic depressive disorders.

Cognitive-Behavioral Therapy for Mixed Samples: Chronic Depression and Acute Depression

Four studies have reported outcome data for CBT in which patients with chronic depression comprised some portion of the overall sample. These studies provide some index of the relative efficacy of CBT for chronic depression when compared to patients with acute depression. Generally, these studies found that patients with chronic depression have a worse response to CBT than patients with acute depression.

Gonzales, et al. [29] followed patients from three prior treatment outcome studies of CBT for depression. Of the 113 outpatients who participated in their longitudinal follow-up, 59 met Research Diagnostic Criteria (RDC) [30] criteria for major depression, 28 met RDC criteria for intermittent depression (i.e., dysthymia), and 26 met RDC criteria for double depression (i.e., major depression superimposed on dysthymia). All participants received 12 2-hour sessions of either group or individual therapy over a period of 2 months, with 1- and 6-month booster sessions added. Treatment focused on social interactions, relaxation skills, increasing pleasant activities, and managing negative cognitions. At 1-year follow-up, 70% of the major depressives, 43% of the chronic depressives, and 27% of the double depressives were rated as recovered. At the 1-year follow-up, relapse rates were 31% for the major depressives, 33% for the chronic depressives, and 14% for the double depressives.

Two studies reanalyzed existing data to compare the efficacy of CBT for acute depression and chronic depression. Like the Gonzales et al. [29]

results, these two studies found that chronic depressives had a worse outcome than acute depressives. Thase et al. [31] used data from two different research protocols to compare the efficacy of CBT for men with chronic depression (n = 22) with that of CBT for men with acute depression (n = 40). Of the men diagnosed with chronic depression, 15 met criteria for double depression and 7 met criteria for chronic depression alone. Therapy followed the Beck manual [32] and consisted of 16 weeks of treatment with a maximum of 20 sessions. In general, the results indicated that at the end of treatment, the chronic depression group was more symptomatic than the acute depressive group on most of the outcome measures, including the HAM-D, the GAS, and the BDI. No information was presented comparing the chronic depressives with and without the additional diagnosis of double depression.

Agosti and Ocepek-Welikson [33] reanalyzed the National Institute of Mental Health (NIMH) Treatment of Depression Collaborative Research Program (TCRCP) [34] to investigate the efficacy of imipramine, traditional CBT therapy, and interpersonal psychotherapy (IPT) in treating patients who met criteria for early-onset chronic depression (n = 65). Results indicated that there were no differences among the three conditions; moreover, there were no differences between the active treatment conditions and the placebo condition, with an approximate 50% reduction in depression severity for all patients. The 16 patients in the CBT condition demonstrated almost a 10 point drop in HAM-D scores (19.4 at pretreatment to 9.5 at posttreatment), whereas the 15 patients in the placebo condition demonstrated a 9-point drop in HAM-D scores (18.5 at pretreatment to 9.5 at posttreatment). This change was slightly worse than the improvement in depressive symptoms reported by those patients in the overall sample randomized to the CBT condition (19.2 at pretreatment to 7.6 at posttreatment) (see Ref. 34).

In a study with a smaller sample, Mercier et al. [35] found similar results. They treated 25 patients with cognitive therapy: 10 who met criteria for major depressive disorder alone, 8 who met criteria for dysthymia alone, and 7 who met criteria for both dysthymia and major depression (i.e., double depression). Participants received 12–16 sessions of individual cognitive therapy over 12–16 weeks. Treatment focused primarily on managing depression. Using the Clinical Global Impressions (CGI) scale criteria for "much improved" and "very much improved," three (38%) of the eight dysthymic patients and three (43%) of the seven double depression patients were deemed to have responded to the cognitive therapy. In addition, all responders had significantly greater change in depressive symptoms as measured by the BDI [34] and the HAM-D [35]. Moreover, of all the responders to cognitive therapy, nine (69%) maintained their gains over 6 months. This 6-month follow-up period included four preplanned booster sessions. No information was presented describing the six month follow-up results for the dysthymic and double-depression patients.

In summary, the four studies that presented chronic depression outcome data along with other results were fairly consistent in their findings. Cognitive-behavioral therapy appeared to produce approximately a 45% response rate with significant improvement in symptoms; however, this outcome was consistently worse than the response rate for the acute depressives. Unfortunately, our ability to understand the differences in outcome between the chronic depressive and acute depressives is limited by lack of information regarding the treatment provided. For example, we do not know the extent to which the CBT was modified on a patient-by-patient basis, and so may have systematically differed between the chronic depressives and the acute depressives.

Cognitive-Behavioral Therapy for Sample of Chronic Depression Only

The weaknesses of mixed sample studies can be overcome by studies that include only patients with chronic depressive disorders. If patients with chronic depressive disorders present with different concerns than do patients with episodic major depressive disorder, as has been theorized (e.g., see Refs. 16 and 36), then studies that utilize pure samples of chronic depression would be able to investigate adaptations of more traditional psychotherapy. To date, five studies reported in the literature have specifically investigated the application of traditional CBT to chronic depression. The results from these five studies have been mixed. All five studies were small-scale pilot studies, limiting the generalizability of their conclusions.

Three studies that did not describe adaptations to traditional CBT when investigating its efficacy with chronic depression found varying results. Fennell and Teasdale [37], in a pilot study of five chronic depressives who were refractory to pharmacotherapy, found that traditional CBT (e.g., see Ref. 32) produced a low response rate: Only one patient met the criteria for "marked improvement," two reported some improvement, and two remained unchanged. In contrast, Stravynski, et al. [38] presented more positive data from a small open trial of CBT for 6 patients diagnosed with dysthymia. All patients received 15 one-hour sessions of CBT, in which traditional CBT techniques were used to help manage negative thoughts. Results at six-month follow-up indicated that 83% (5/6) of the patients showed clinically meaningful improvement in their depressive symptoms and negative thinking. 66% (4/6) of the patients no longer met criteria for dysthymia. Given the limited description of the CBT that was used in both these studies, speculation regarding their differential success is difficult. Dunner et al. [39] randomized

31 dysthymic patients to treatment with either traditional CBT or fluoxetine (20 mg/day). Generally, there were no statistically significant group differences in response to treatment, although more patients assigned to fluoxetine dropped out (33%) than those assigned to CBT (9%). Of the 10 patients who completed the 16-week treatment of CBT, mean HAM-D scores improved from 15.4 to 10.8., and 2 patients met criteria for "asymptomatic" response (defined as HAM-D-17 $<= 7$ and BDI $<= 8$). Overall, the results from these three studies suggest that traditional CBT may be a useful starting point in treating chronic depression, but that specific therapeutic adaptations might yield stronger results.

Two other studies of CBT for chronic depression explicitly adapted the therapy in order to better address issues specific to chronic depression. Harpin et al. [40], in a wait-list control experiment with 12 chronically depressed patients, included four major components in their cognitive-behavioral therapy: (1) social skills training for patients and their significant others, (2) specific behavioral and cognitive skills, (3) modification of the social contingencies that reinforced the depressive behavior, and (4) anxiety management training. In addition, significant attention was devoted to psychoeducation and alliance-building prior to engaging in the more traditional cognitive-behavioral skills. While there were no significant differences between the experimental group and the wait-list control (most likely due to low statistical power), the experimental group demonstrated significant pre-post differences on both measures of depression and anxiety, while the control group did not. Moreover, the experimental group continued to demonstrate significant improvement on anxiety measures (but not measures of depression) at 6-month follow-up, while the control group did not. No categorical remission data was presented, but the authors noted that 33% (2/6) of the treated patients showed "major pre-post improvement" in depressive symptoms, and 17% (1/6) of the patients maintained these gains at the 6-month follow-up.

Similarly, de Jong, et al. [41] found positive results with another modification of traditional CBT. They treated 30 patients who met the criteria for major depressive disorder and had dysthymic disorder prior to the current episode of major depression. Patients who were assigned to CBT condition that combined individual therapy (activity scheduling and cognitive restructuring) and group therapy (social competence training) did significantly better (60% responders) than patients who were assigned to a CBT that focused exclusively on cognitive restructuring (30% responders) or a wait-list control condition (10% responders). A 6-month follow-up of 14 patients indicated that the gains were maintained.

Given the limitation of these five studies, including small sample size, lack of appropriate control conditions, and absence of blind raters, it is unclear what caused the different results. For example, it is possible that the emphasis on alliance-building and modification of social contingencies in the Harpin et al. [40] study played a significant role in the positive results they found. Perhaps the inclusion of the group therapy in the de Jong et al. [41] treatment contributed to their positive results. Unfortunately, we are unable yet to identify the ingredients that contributed to the discrepancy between these findings and the negative findings of Fennell and Teasdale [37]. To further complicate the picture, Stravynski et al. [38] found positive results without reporting modifications to traditional CBT in a manner that contrasted with Fennell and Teasdale's [37] findings.

INTERPERSONAL PSYCHOTHERAPY

Some researchers have investigated the efficacy of IPT in treating chronic depression. This is a time-limited, focused psychotherapeutic approach that helps patients change problematic feelings, thoughts, and behaviors in difficult interpersonal relationships [12,42]. After gathering information on the patient's interpersonal history, the therapist helps the patient link the depressive symptoms to one of four interpersonal problem areas that will be the focus of therapy: grief, interpersonal role disputes, role transitions, or interpersonal deficits. As with cognitive-behavioral therapy, considerable evidence exists highlighting the efficacy of IPT in treating episodic depression [43] and preventing relapse [44–46]. Efforts have been made to apply standard IPT to chronic depression [12,17,36].

Weissman, et al. [12] identified six adaptations of IPT for a dysthymic population that highlight the importance of (1) searching for past periods of euthymia, (2) the time-limited nature of treatment, (3) emphasizing the medical model of depression, (4) normalizing patient self-expression, including feelings of anger, (5) continuation therapy to maintain gains, and (6) therapist skill and confidence in working with these patients. In three separate pilot studies, IPT has been used to treat a total of 17 dysthymic patients [12,47–49]. Significant improvement in mean HAM-D scores from baseline to acute termination were found in all three studies. Moreover, 65% of the patients met criteria for remission (HAM-D < 8).

As already noted, Agosti and Ocepek-Welikson [34] reanalyzed the NIMH TCRCP to investigate the efficacy of imipramine, traditional CBT therapy, and IPT in treating patients who met the criteria for early-onset chronic depression (n = 65). The 14 patients with chronic depression who were treated with IPT demonstrated an 8-point drop in HAM-D scores (18.6 at pretreatment to 10.3 at posttreatment). As with those chronically depressed patients treated with CBT, this improvement was slightly worse than that reported for patients with episodic major depression (18.9 at pretreatment to 6.9 at posttreatment; see Ref. 34).

The preliminary success of these pilot studies has led to the implementation of three large independent trials that are currently examining the efficacy of IPT in treating chronic depression [12]. Although the results of two of these studies are still pending, Browne et al. [50] reported results from a study in which 707 patients with dysthymia were randomized to treatment for 6 months with either sertraline alone, IPT alone, or the combination of sertraline and IPT. Response rates for IPT alone were comparable to that of other outcome studies for chronic depression: Approximately 47% of patients reported a 40% improvement in depressive symptoms, as rated by the Montgomery-Asberg Depression Rating Scale. The response rate for sertraline alone was 60.2% and the response rate for the combination treatment was 57.5%. At 2-yr follow-up, no differences were found between the sertraline and the combination treatment in reducing depressive symptoms, although both were more effective than IPT alone. Interestingly, patients in the combination treatment had fewer health and social service costs over the 2-year period than patients in the sertraline alone condition.

COGNITIVE-BEHAVIORAL ANALYSIS SYSTEM OF PSYCHOTHERAPY

The research presented thus far has focused primarily on the application of existing psychotherapeutic modalities (e.g., CBT and IPT) to chronic depression. Two studies in the literature report on the efficacy of a psychotherapeutic orientation that was developed specifically to address the difficulties faced by chronically depressed patients: cognitive-behavioral analysis system of psychotherapy (CBASP) [51]. The fundamental premise upon which CBASP is based is the belief that chronic depression results from maladaptive social problem solving and the inability to recognize and understand the interpersonal effects of one's behavior [51].

CBASP integrates elements from cognitive, behavioral, and interpersonal therapies for depression and applies them in a time-limited, interactional fashion. Through a stages-of-change approach in which goals for therapy vary depending on the stage in which a patient is functioning, CBASP teaches patients to change refractory and problematic cognitive and behavioral patterns of functioning. Patients first learn to appreciate the role that they play in generating negative events in their life. Once they become aware of the situational consequences they produce, they can increase their sense of efficacy and mastery over their life. This increased sense of efficacy results in modification of problematic cognitions and behaviors that prevent effective situation management, which eventually leads to generalization to more effective management of real-world stressors [9,51].

A preliminary trial of CBSAP with 10 dysthymic patients conducted by McCullough [9] produced encouraging results: 90% (n = 9) were remitted at the 2-year follow-up, and significant change in depressive symptoms and sense of control were also reported. These preliminary results led to the inclusion of CBASP in a large-scale randomized-controlled treatment trial of chronic depression [8]. In this study, the efficacy of pharmacotherapy, CBASP, and their combination was compared in the treatment of chronic depression. Although the results of the study clearly demonstrated the advantages of combined treatment over single-modality treatment for chronic depression, the CBASP condition performed well and equaled the pharmacotherapy condition. Among the 519 subjects who completed the acute phase of the study, the rates of response after 12 weeks (as defined by either a complete remission or a significant reduction in depressive symptoms) were 55% in the nefazodone group, 52% in the CBASP group, and 85% in the combined treatment group. Moreover, patients in all three conditions reported significant improvement in depressive symptoms, as measured by the HAM-D [35].

GROUP TREATMENT

The majority of the psychotherapy outcome studies for dysthymia have focused on individual psychotherapy. This fact is puzzling, as several researchers have emphasized the role of dysfunctional interpersonal relationships in the maintenance of the disorder (e.g., see Refs. 36 and 51). It is plausible that psychotherapeutic approaches that target interpersonal processes in a more focused manner (e.g., group- or family-based treatments) might add significant benefit to the treatment of chronic depression.

We found one study that examined the efficacy of group therapy for dysthymia. Ravindran et al. [52] randomized 97 dysthymic patients to either sertraline or placebo treatment. In addition, they were also randomized to receive either group cognitive therapy (n = 49) or not. The group cognitive therapy was a mix of traditional group cognitive therapy [53] and CBASP [51]. This therapy consisted of 12 weekly 90-minute sessions that included cognitive skills (e.g., learning the relationship between thoughts and mood, identification of dysfunctional thinking), behavioral skills (e.g., behavioral activation via pleasure and mastery ratings), and interpersonal skills (e.g., assertiveness, situational analyses). Results indicated that the group cognitive therapy condition reduced depressive symptoms, but not significantly more than the placebo condition. When combined with the sertraline, the group cognitive treatment appeared to enhance patients' functional improvement.

Clearly, more research is needed before any adequate recommendations can be made with regard to the efficacy of group treatment for chronic depressive disorders. However, these results suggest that it might be more efficacious in combined treatment with pharmacotherapy than as a stand-alone treatment.

FAMILY-BASED TREATMENT

Family-based interventions for chronic depressive disorders have also not been tested systematically, but have the potential to play a significant role. Family-based interventions focus on psychosocial functioning, which is particularly relevant for individuals with chronic depressive disorders (Chap. 1). One of the more important aspects of psychosocial functioning is family relationships and interactions. Not surprisingly, a patient's illness exerts a major influence on significant others in the patient's social field. Moreover, the ways in which these significant others respond to the patient's illness has a measurable and clinically significant impact on the symptomatology and course of that illness.

Although few studies have assessed the functioning of families in patients with chronic depressive disorders and even fewer have examined change in family functioning in chronically depressed patients over the course of acute treatment, much research has demonstrated the importance of family functioning in major depression. For example, problematic family functioning has been associated with a worse course of the depressive illness and poorer response to treatment [54–58]. Given the strong evidence for the role of family functioning in acute major depression, and the evidence for the presence of significant psychosocial impairment in chronic depression (Chap. 1), it is reasonable to expect that chronicity and severity of depression may be associated with family burden and dysfunction, which in turn may influence the course of the illness and its response to treatment. Miller et al. [59] found that patients with chronic depression reported impaired family functioning prior to treatment but significant improvement following 12 weeks of pharmacological treatment. Interestingly, patients with better baseline psychosocial functioning had a better response to pharmacotherapy.

This study also showed that patients with chronic forms of major depression reported similar patterns of family dysfunction to patients with acute major depression. This finding suggests that adding a family intervention to standard treatment for chronic depression may increase the likelihood of a favorable treatment outcome. One study specifically investigated the efficacy of a family-based treatment for dysthymia. Waring et al. [60] randomized 17 dysthymic women and their nonsymptomatic husbands to either 10 sessions of cognitive marital therapy (CMT) or a clinical management condition. In addition, these same couples were randomized to either doxepin (up to 150 mg/day) or a pill placebo condition. The CMT focused on the role of intimacy between the partners, and included open discussions of topics such as motivation for marrying and their experiences of their parents' marriages. Of the 12 couples who completed the 10 weeks of treatment, all of the dysthymic women across all conditions reported significant improvement on depression measures. There was no reported difference between the CMT condition and the clinical management condition, although a nonsignificant trend favoring the CMT condition began to emerge on the depressive symptoms as measured by the BDI. Moreover, there were no differences between the doxepin and placebo conditions. However, the low number of patients in this pilot study prevented more detailed analyses from being conducted.

Apart from the Waring et al. [60] study, no other studies have examined the efficacy of family-based treatment in addressing chronic depression. A previous report from our research group demonstrated that adding family therapy and cognitive therapy to standard pharmacotherapy for the treatment of patients with the most severe forms of depression leads to significantly greater rates of remission than pharmacotherapy alone at 6 months of follow-up [61]. Another recent study compared the relative efficacy of couples therapy and antidepressant medication for the acute maintenance and treatment of depressed patients living with a critical partner [6]. Results from this study showed that couples therapy was more acceptable than the antidepressant medication, and was at least as efficacious, if not more so, both in the treatment and maintenance phase of episodic major depression. These findings suggest that it is reasonable to consider the inclusion of family treatment in the psychotherapeutic management of patients with chronic depressive disorders, particularly if they are not responding optimally to pharmacotherapy, psychotherapy, or the combination of the two.

REVIEW OF OTHER RELEVANT LITERATURE

Given the relatively few studies investigating psychotherapy for chronic depressive disorders, we expanded our review of the literature to include psychotherapy research on patients with severe and/or recurrent depression. As stated earlier, our rationale for expanding the review of chronic depression to include these other forms of depression was to expand the pool of information from which to find commonalities in the psychotherapy research. Since there is considerable overlap among these depressive conditions [62], it is likely that many of the psychotherapeutic issues will also be similar.

Severe Depression

The psychotherapeutic treatment of severe depression without pharmacotherapy is controversial, and there exist few studies that have specifically
examined this proposition [63]. However, there have been various studies
examining the added benefit of psychotherapy to pharmacotherapy, especially with depressed inpatients. The research on depressed inpatients represents a potentially useful area of information from which to draw when
reviewing the literature on chronic depression, since many depressed inpatients have experienced chronic, recurrent, and severe forms of depression.
The emerging body of research has found results similar to the chronic
depression literature: Psychosocial treatments for depressed inpatients can
be effective, often in conjunction with pharmacotherapy, albeit at lower rates
than for depressed outpatients (e.g., see Refs. 64 and 65). Specifically,
researchers have found that adding cognitive-behavioral outpatient treatment to standard pharmacological treatment significantly improves treatment response and long-term follow-up in depressed inpatients [64,65],
particularly in those depressed inpatients who demonstrate initial cognitive
dysfunction [66]. In another study of treatment following inpatient hospitalization, Miller et al. [61] reported improved outcome for depressed inpatients
when both cognitive therapy and family therapy were added to standard
pharmacotherapy; significantly so for those patients whose initial depressive
symptoms were the most severe.

Recurrent Depression

Research on psychotherapeutic treatment of recurrent depression can also
offer useful insights into the treatment of chronic depressive disorders.
Recurrent depression, although episodic in nature, nevertheless can be
considered a chronic condition that requires continuous treatment. Moreover, there exists support for the efficacy of both CBT and IPT in sustaining
recovery and/or remission in high-risk patients with recurrent depressions.
Some investigators have examined the efficacy of adding a relatively brief dose
of psychotherapy following successful pharmacotherapy for patients who
may be at risk for recurrence. For example, Fava and colleagues [25,26]
reported the successful use of CBT to treat residual symptoms in patients who
had been previously treated with antidepressant medication, with improved
prevention of relapse for up to 4 years following treatment. They recently
extended this success to patients with recurrent depression [27]. Paykel et al.
[28] provided 16 weeks of CBT plus two follow-up booster sessions, in
addition to maintenance pharmacotherapy, for 158 partially remitted
patients. Results demonstrated that cognitive therapy reduced relapse rates
and residual symptoms over 68 weeks of follow-up. Jarrett et al. [67] found

that 8 months of continuation cognitive therapy significantly reduced relapse and recurrence, particularly in patients with early-onset major depression (16 vs. 67%). Teasdale et al. [68] found that a variant of CBT that included mindfulness-based skills was also successful in reducing risk of relapse, but only in those patients with three or more previous episodes of depression.

Other researchers have investigated the efficacy of ongoing maintenance psychotherapy in preventing recurrence. Blackburn and Moore [69] reported that patients who received maintenance cognitive therapy (tapered toward monthly sessions) had consistently lower BDI and HAM-D scores than patients who received maintenance pharmacotherapy, although these differences were not significant. Similar success has been reported in preventing relapse/recurrence with maintenance interpersonal therapy [44–46]. Frank et al. [44], for instance, found that monthly IPT lengthened the time between episodes for patients not on prophylactic antidepressants. However, patients on antidepressants (irrespective of whether they were receiving psychotherapy or not) did better than those without. This research group also reported that patients who received high-quality IPT showed a longer period before having a recurrence: 2 years versus 5 months [45]. Reynolds et al. [46] found similar results with elderly patients with recurrent major depression: Patients receiving monthly maintenance IPT had rates of recurrence of 64%; patients receiving maintenance nortriptyline therapy had recurrence rates of 43%; and patients receiving combined maintenance therapy had recurrence rates of 20%.

CLINICAL RECOMMENDATIONS

Overall, the literature we reviewed suggests that between 30 and 50% of patients with chronic forms of depression will respond to various types of psychotherapies. Given that these response rates are quite similar to those reported in pharmacotherapy treatment studies, patients have a real choice in the kind of treatment that they would prefer. The first choice of treatment should be decided collaboratively by patient and therapist, taking into consideration patient preference and motivation for working in therapy, therapist skill level and availability, and financial restrictions. For psychologically minded patients who are interested in developing skills to help them exert some control over their depressive illness, who are able and willing to put in the required commitment of time and effort, and whose depression is not overly severe and incapacitating, psychotherapy is a reasonable first-choice treatment.

The current state of the evidence precludes us from differentiating among cognitive-behavioral, interpersonal, and cognitive-behavioral analysis system of psychotherapy. Moreover, given the similar outcomes reported by these psychotherapies, it may be that common, nonspecific characteristics are as important in their effectiveness as are therapy-specific content and techniques. Some of the common elements of these psychotherapies follow:

Time-Limited Psychotherapy

The psychotherapies reviewed have tended to be relatively short term. Typically, these therapies consist of weekly sessions for 12–24 weeks. The explicit time-limited nature of treatment is hypothesized to focus both the patients' and therapists' energies and provide greater motivation for behavior change. Time-limited psychotherapy may also send an implicit message that the psychotherapist believes that improvement can be achieved in a relatively short period of time in contrast to the chronically depressed patient's hopeless assumption that nothing will change [12].

Explicit Rationale for Treatment

All of the psychotherapies offer their patients an explicit rationale for the treatment approach. Although these rationales differ in their content (e.g., cognitive to interpersonal to behavioral), all of these psychotherapies present the patient with a well-formulated and coherent rationale for how treatment will help patients control their depressive symptoms.

Therapist Is Active and Directive

Therapists in all effective psychosocial treatments take an active stance during treatment. It is the therapist's responsibility to lead and direct the therapy session. This behavior is generally thought to overcome the lack of energy, passivity, and helplessness that characterizes depressed patients in general and chronically depressed patients in particular.

Focus on Current Problems

As opposed to traditional psychodynamic and psychoanalytic psychotherapies, current psychosocial treatments focus specifically on problems that the patient is experiencing. Childhood or other past experiences may be explored, but only when they directly affect the patient's current issues. Weissman et al. [12] do make the point that it is important to search for past periods of euthymia, but as a means of helping the patient in the present.

Emphasis on Changing Current Behavior and Interpersonal Interactions

This emphasis serves at least two purposes. First, changing patient's current behavior produces objective improvements in their situations, particularly their social support networks. This improvement in turn positively affects the depression. Second, these changes reinforce a sense of personal control and efficacy consistent with the rationale for treatment.

Self-Monitoring of Change and Progress

Since a common symptom of depression is the tendency to perceive events in an overly negative light, most depressed patients tend to minimize treatment gains. Psychotherapy can guard against this tendency by teaching patients to monitor their own behavior and mood. This monitoring counters the tendency to minimize treatment gains, and also reinforces the relationship between behavior change and mood.

Regular Homework Assignments

Most effective psychosocial treatments for depression do not solely rely on activity in the therapy session to provide symptomatic and behavior change. Instead, the therapist and patient typically agree upon between-session assignments that will be completed by the patient. This homework extends the treatment lessons and provides patients with a clearer sense of how to apply their treatment to real-world problems. Moreover, homework assignments further reinforce patients' sense of personal control and efficacy.

Continuation/Maintenance Therapy to Extend Gains

Given the increasing evidence pointing to the importance of dealing with residual symptoms (e.g., see Refs. 26 and 45), continuation or maintenance therapy will likely play an important role in preventing relapse and recurrence. This maintenance therapy will likely be less frequent and intense than the therapy provided during the acute episode, but should be ready to increase in frequency and intensity should the patient's symptoms deteriorate.

Combined Pharmacological and Psychotherapeutic Treatment

For those patients who do not respond to psychotherapy or who are responding too slowly, there is now evidence to suggest that combining psychotherapy with pharmacotherapy may be an appropriate course of treatment. A recent study [8] showed that not only does the combination of CBASP and pharmacotherapy produce a greater degree of improvement over 12 weeks of treatment than either treatment alone, but that the improvement occurs more rapidly. Symptoms such as insomnia and anxiety are particularly amenable to a more rapid reduction with pharmacotherapy, which is likely to make the patient more accessible to psycho-therapeutic interventions.

Family-Based Interventions

As noted above, the inclusion of the family, broadly defined as significant others interacting within the patient's social field, may be an additional important consideration for those patients who have significant interperso-nal and social difficulties and those who have not responded adequately to either psychotherapy or the combination of psychotherapy and pharmaco-therapy. One potentially useful model of family treatment that our research group has developed and tested is the Problem Centered Systems Therapy of the Family (PCSFT) [70]. The PCSFT is a highly structured, multidimen-sional and systems-oriented treatment that allows the integration and coordination of a number of different treatment approaches depending on the specific clinical presentation.

CONCLUSION

Historically, chronic depressive disorders were considered to be a reflection of personality dysfunction, and therefore much less amenable to treatment. More recently, however, the field has begun to appreciate that both pharmacological and psychosocial treatments can be effective in treating both the symptoms and the psychosocial sequelae of chronic depression, albeit with lower response rates than acute depression. We agree with this shift in thinking following our review of the literature, especially given the positive results obtained by some of the more recent studies. And yet, despite the considerable progress in our understanding of psychotherapies for chronic depression, there remain significant gaps in our knowledge. Part of the reason for this knowledge deficit lies in the limitations. The majority of the research designs have been pilot studies that included small num-bers of patients, nonrandom assignment to condition, and nonblind raters of treatment response.

Future studies should implement randomized controlled designs, larger sample sizes, and more careful regulation of both the treatment (e.g., consistent length of delivery) and the patients included in the study (e.g., more homogeneous in terms of length and severity of depressive illness). In addition, we know very little about the long-term efficacy of these psycho-therapies. Evaluating the efficacy of any treatment for chronic disorders necessarily requires follow-up evaluation beyond 2 years. Most of the stu-dies presented follow-up assessments of under 1 year. Treatments that produce a short-term alleviation of symptoms are important; however, more information regarding the staying power of treatment effects is needed, particularly for a condition that by definition has to last at least 2 years. Additional areas needing investigations include such issues as patient predictors of treatment response, active ingredients of psychosocial treatments, and the role of psychiatric and medical comorbidity.

We think that what will emerge from more stringently designed research studies will be confirmation of the preliminary results we present here. Psychosocial treatments will likely be moderately effective in treating chronic depressive disorders, especially when they are adapted to address the specific issues faced by individuals who have experienced a chronic condition for many years. We also think that future success will be found in combined treatment research for chronic depression. This combined treatment could follow the traditional pattern of pharmacotherapy and individual psychotherapy, but it can also integrate different modalities of psychosocial treatment simultaneously (e.g., individual, group, and family-based treatments).

In comparison with the research on psychotherapy for acute depressive disorders, the research base on psychotherapy for chronic depression is relatively young. Given the societal consequences of chronic depression (e.g., see Refs. 71–73), this is a gap in the literature that is well worth closing.

ACKNOWLEDGMENT

Preparation of this chapter was supported by National Institute of Mental Health Grant (NIMH) postdoctoral grant F32 MH12855 to Esteban V. Cardemil.

REFERENCES

1. R Brown, P Lewinsohn. A psychoeducational approach to the treatment of depression: Comparison of group, individual, and minimal contact procedures. J Consult Clin Psychol 52:774–783, 1984.
2. K Dobson. A meta-analysis of the efficacy of cognitive therapy for depression. J Consult Clin Psychol 57:414–419, 1989.
3. W McDermut, IW Miller, RA Brown. The efficacy of group psychotherapy for depression: A meta-analysis and review of the empirical research. Clin Psychol Sci Pract 8:98–116, 2001.
4. LA Robinson, JS Berman, RA Neimeyer. Psychotherapy for the treatment of depression: A comprehensive review of controlled outcome research. Psychol Bull 108:30–49, 1990.
5. N Jacobson, K Dobson, A Fruzzetti, K Schmaling, S Salusky. Marital therapy as a treatment for depression. J Consult Clin Psychol 59:547–557, 1991.

6. J Leff, S Vearnals, CR Brewin, G Wolff, B Alexander, E Asen, D Dayson, E Jones, D Chisholm, B Everitt. The London Depression Intervention Trial: randomised controlled trial of antidepressants v. couple therapy in the treatment and maintenance of people with depression living with a partner: clinical outcome and costs. Br J Psychiatry 17:95–100, 2000.

7. JC Markowitz. Psychotherapy of dysthymia. Am J Psychiatry 151:1114–121, 1994.

8. MB Keller, JP McCullough, DN Klein, B Arnow, DL Dunner, AF Gelenberg, JC Markowitz, CB Nemeroff, JM Russell, ME Thase, MH Trivedi, J Zajecka. A comparison of nefazodone, the cognitive-behavioral-analysis system of psychotherapy, and their combination for the treatment of chronic depression. New Engl J Med 342:1462–1470, 2000.

9. JP McCullough. Psychotherapy for dysthymia: A naturalistic study of ten patients. J Nerv Ment Dis 179:734–740, 1991.

10. DN Klein, KA Norden, T Ferro, JB Leader, KL Kasch, LM Klein, JE Schwartz, TA Aronson. Thirty-month naturalistic follow-up study of early-onset dysthymic disorder: Course, diagnostic stability, and prediction of outcome. J Abnorm Psychol 107:338–348, 1998.

11. DN Klein, JE Schwartz, S Rose, JB Leader. Five-year course and outcome of dysthymic disorder: a prospective, naturalistic follow-up study. Am J Psychiatry 157:931–939, 2000.

12. MM Weissman, JC Markowitz, GL Klerman. Comprehensive Guide to Interpersonal Psychotherapy. New York: Basic Books, 2000.

13. IW Miller, WH Norman, GI Keitner. Combined treatment for patients with double depression. Psychother Psychosom 68:180–185, 1999.

14. ME Thase. When are psychotherapy and pharmacotherapy combinations the treatment of choice for major depressive disorder? Psychiatr Qu 70:333–346, 1999.

15. ME Thase, JB Greenhouse, E Frank, CF Reynolds, PA Pilkonis, K Hurley, V Grochocinski, DJ Kupfer. Treatment of major depression with psychotherapy or psychotherapy-pharmacothempy combinations. Arch Gen Psychiatry 54:1009–1015, 1997.

16. JP McCullough, DN Klein, MB Keller, CE Holzer, SM Davis, SG Kornstein, RH Howland, ME Thase, WM Harrison. Comparison of DSM-III-R chronic major depression and major depression superimposed on dysthymia (double depression): validity of the distinction. J Abnorm Psychol 109:419–27, 2000.

17. JC Markowitz. Psychotherapy of dysthymic disorder. In: JH Kocsis & DN Klein, eds. Diagnosis and Treatment of Chronic Depression. New York: Guilford Press, 1995, pp 146–168.

18. L Luborsky, L Diguer, J Cacciola, J Barber, K Moras, K Schmidt, R DeRubeis. Factors in outcomes of short-term psychotherapy for chronic vs. nonchronic major depression. J Psychother Pract Res 5:152–159, 1996.

19. L Luborsky. Principles of Psychoanalytic Psychotherapy: A Manual for Supportive-Expressive Treatment. New York: Basic Books, 1984.

20. L Luborsky, D Mark, AV Hole, C Popp, B Goldsmith, J Cacciola. Supportive-

expressive dynamic psychotherapy of depression: a time-limited version. In: JP
Barber and P Crits-Cristoph, eds. Dynamic Therapies for Psychiatric Disorders
(Axis I). New York: Basic Books, 1995, pp 13–42.

21. AT Beck, CH Ward, M Mendelson, JE Mock, JK Erbaugh. An inventory for
measuring depression. Arch Gen Psychiatry 4:561–571, 1961.

22. MA Hamilton. A rating scale for depression. J of Neurol, Neurosurg,
Psychiatry 23:56–62, 1960.

23. J Endicott, RL Spitzer, JL Fliess, J Cohen. The Global Assessment Scale: A
procedure for measuring overall severity of psychiatric disturbance. Arch Gen
Psychiatry 33:766–771, 1976.

24. RJ DeRubeis, P Crits-Cristoph. Empirically supported individual and group
psychological treatments for adult mental disorders. J of Consult Clin Psychol
66:37–52, 1998.

25. GA Fava, S Grandi, M Zielezny, C Rafanelli, R Canestrari. Four-year
outcome for cognitive-behavioral treatment of residual symptoms in major
depression. Am J Psychiatry 153:945–947, 1996.

26. GA Fava, C Rafanelli, S Grandi, R Canestrari, MA Morphy. Six-year outcome
for cognitive behavioral treatment of residual symptoms in major depression.
Am J Psychiatry 155:1443–1445, 1998.

27. GA Fava, C Rafanelli, S Grandi, S Conti, P Belluardo. Prevention of recurrent
depression with cognitive behavioral therapy. Arch Gen Psychiatry 55:816–820,
1998.

28. ES Paykel, J Scott, JD Teasdale, AL Johnson, A Garland, R Moore, A
Jenaway, PL Cornwall, H Hayhurst, R Abbott, M Pope. Prevention of relapse
in residual depression by cognitive therapy. Arch Gen Psychiatry 56:829–835:
1999.

29. L Gonzales, P Lewinsohn, G Clarke. Longitudinal follow-up of unipolar
depressives: An investigation of predictors of relapse. J Consult Clin Psychol
53:461–469, 1985.

30. RL Spitzer, J Endicott, E Robins. Research Diagnostic Criteria: rationale and
reliability. Arch Gen Psychiatry 35:773–782, 1978.

31. ME Thase, CF Reynolds, E Frank, AD Simons, GD Garamoni, J McGeary, T
Harden, AL Fasiczka, JF Cahalane. Response to cognitive-behavioral therapy
in chronic depression. J Psychother Pract Res 3:204–214, 1994.

32. A Beck, A Rush, B Shaw, G Emery. Cognitive Therapy for Depression. New
York: Guilford Press, 1979.

33. V Agosti, K Ocepek-Welikson. The efficacy of imipramine and psychotherapy
in early-onset chronic depression: a reanalysis of the National Institute of
Mental Health Treatment of Depression Collaborative Research Program. J of
Affect Disord 43:181–186, 1997.

34. I Elkin, MT Shea, JT Watkins, SD Imber, SM Sotsky, JF Collins, DR Glass,
PA Pilkonis, WR Leber, JP Docherty, SJ Fiester, MB Parloff. National
Institute of Mental Health Treatment of Depression Collaborative Research
Program: General effectiveness of treatments. Arch Gen Psychiatry 46:971–982,
1989.

35. M Mercier, J Stewart, J Quitkin. A pilot sequential study of cognitive therapy and pharmacotherapy of atypical depression. J Clin Psychiatry 53:166–170, 1992.

36. JC Markowitz. Interpersonal Psychotherapy for Dysthymic Disorder. Washington, DC: American Psychiatric Press, 1998.

37. MJV Fennell, JD Teasdale. Cognitive therapy with chronic, drug-refractory depressed outpatients: a note of caution. Cog Ther Res 6:455–460, 1986.

38. A Stravynski, A Shahar, R Verreault. A pilot study of the cognitive treatment of dysthymic disorder. Behav Psychother 19:369–372, 1991.

39. DL Dunner, KB Schmaling, H Hendrickson, J Becker, A Lehman, C Bea. Cognitive therapy versus fluoxetine in the treatment of dysthymic disorder. Depression 4:34–41, 1996.

40. RE Harpin, RP Liberman, I Marks, R Stern, WE Bohannon. Cognitive-behavior therapy for chronically depressed patients: a controlled pilot study. J Nerv Men Dis 170:295–301, 1982.

41. R de Jong, R Treiber, G Henrich. Effectiveness of two psychological treatments for inpatients with severe and chronic depressions. Cog Ther Res 10:645–663, 1986.

42. G Klerman, M Weissman, B Rounsaville, E Chevron. Interpersonal Psychotherapy of Depression. New York: Basic Books, 1984.

43. MM Weissman, JC Markowitz. Interpersonal psychotherapy: current status. Arch Gen Psychiatry 51:599–606, 1994.

44. E Frank, DJ Kupfer, JM Perel, C Cornes, DB Jarrett, AG Mallinger, ME Thase, AB McEachran, VJ Grochocinski. Three-year outcomes for maintenance therapies in recurrent depression. Arch Gen Psychiatry 47:1093–1099, 1990.

45. E Frank, DJ Kupfer, EF Wagner, AB McEachran, C Cornes. Efficacy of interpersonal psychotherapy as a maintenance treatment of recurrent depression: contributing factors. Arch Gen Psychiatry 48:1053–1059, 1991.

46. CF Reynolds, E Frank, JM Perel, SD Imber, C Cornes, MD Miller, S Mazumdar, PR Houck, MA Dew, JA Stack, BG Pollock, DJ Kupfer. Nortriptyline and interpersonal psychotherapy as maintenance therapies for recurrent major depression: a randomized controlled trial in patients older than 59 years. JAMA 281:39–45, 1999.

47. B Mason, J Markowitz, G Klerman. Interpersonal psychotherapy for dysthymic disorders. In: G Klerman, M Weissman, eds. New Applications of Interpersonal Therapy. Washington, DC: American Psychiatric Association, 1993, pp 225–264.

48. JC Markowitz, GL Klerman, S Perry. Interpersonal therapy of depressed HIV-seropositive outpatients. Am J Psychiatry 152:1504–1509, 1992.

49. JC Markowitz, GL Klerman, SW Perry, KF Clougherty, LS Josephs. Interpersonal psychotherapy for depressed HIV-Seropositive patients. In: GL Klerman, MM Weissman, eds. New Applications of Interpersonal Psychotherapy. Washington, DC: American Psychiatric Press, 1993, pp 199–224.

50. G Browne, M Steiner, J Roberts, A Gafni, C Byrne, E Dunn, B Bell, M Mills, L

Chalkin, D Wallik, J Kraemer. Sertraline and/or interpersonal psychotherapy for patients with dysthymic disorder in primary care: 6-month comparison with longitudinal 2-yr follow-up of effectiveness and cost. J Affect Disord 68;317–330, 2002.

51. JP McCullough. Treatment for Chronic Depression: Cognitive Behavioral Analysis System of Psychotherapy. New York: Guilford Press, 2000.

52. AV Ravindran, H Anisman, Z Merali, Y Charbonneau, J Teiner, RJ Bialik, A Wiens, J Ellis, J Griffiths. Treatment of primary dysthymia with group cognitive therapy and pharmacotherapy: clinical symptoms and functional impairments. Am J Psychiatry 156:1608–1617, 1999.

53. SD Hollon, BF Shaw. Group cognitive therapy for depressed patients. In: AT Beck, AJ Rush, BF Shaw, G Emery, eds. Cognitive Therapy of Depression. New York: Guilford Press, 1979, pp 328–353.

54. JM Hooley, JD Teasdale. Predictors of relapse in unipolar depressives: expressed emotion, marital distress, and perceived criticism. J of Abnorm Psychol 98:229–235, 1989.

55. GI Keitner, CE Ryan, IW Miller, R Kohn, DS Bishop, NB Epstein. Role of the family in recovery and major depression. Am J Psychiatry 152:1002–1008, 1995.

56. GI Keitner, JW Miller, NB Epstein, DS Bishop, AE Fruzzetti. Family functioning and the course of major depression. Compre Psychiatry 28:54–64, 1987.

57. RW Swindle, RC Cronkite, RH Moos. Life stressors, social resources, coping, and the 4-year course of unipolar depression. J Abnorm Psycholo 98:468–477, 1989.

58. RH Moos. Depressed outpatients' life contexts, amount of treatment, and treatment outcome. J Nerv Ment Dis 178:105–12, 1990.

59. IW Miller, GI Keitner, AF Schatzberg, DN Klein, ME Thase, AJ Rush, JC Markowitz, DS Schlager, SG Kornstein, SM Davis, WM Harrison, MB Keller. The treatment of chronic depression, part 3: psychosocial functioning before and after treatment with sertraline or imipramine. J Clin Psychiatry 59:608–19, 1998.

60. EM Waring, CH Chamberlaine, EW McCrank, CA Stalker, C Carver, R Fry, S Barnes. Dysthymia: a randomized study of cognitive marital therapy and antidepressants. Can J Psychiatry 33:96–99, 1988.

61. IW Miller, GI Keitner, CE Ryan, DA Solomon. Matched vs Mismatched Treatment for Depressed Inpatients. Poster session presented at the annual meeting of the American Psychiatric Association, Toronto, May, 1998.

62. ME Thase, RH Howland. Refractory depression: relevance of psychosocial factors and therapies. Psychiatr Ann 24:232–240, 1994.

63. ME Thase, ES Friedman. Is psychotherapy an effective treatment for melancholia and other severe depressive states? J Affect Dis 54:1–19, 1999.

64. IW Miller, WH Norman, GI Keitner, SB Bishop, MG Dow. Cognitive-behavioral treatment of depressed inpatients. Behav Ther 20:25–47, 1989.

65. IW Miller, WH Norman, GI Keitner. Cognitive-behavioral treatment of depressed inpatients: Six- and twelve-month follow-up. Am J Psychiatry 146:1274–1279, 1989.

66. IW Miller, WH Norman, GI Keitner. Treatment response of high cognitive dysfunction depressed inpatients. Compre Psychiatry 31:62–71, 1990.

67. RB Jarrett, D Kraft, J Doyle, BM Foster, GG Eaves, PC Silver. Preventing recurrent depression using cognitive therapy with and without a continuation phase. Arch Gen Psychiatry 58:381–388, 2001.

68. JD Teasdale, ZV Segal, JMG Williams, VA Ridgeway, JM Soulsby, MA Lau, M.A. Prevention of relapse/recurrence in major depression by mindfulness-based cognitive therapy. J of Consult Clin Psychol 68:615–623, 2000.

69. IM Blackburn, RG Moore. Controlled acute and follow-up trial of cognitive therapy and pharmacotherapy in out-patients with recurrent depression. Br J Psychiatry 171:328–334, 1997.

70. NB Epstein, DS Bishop, GI Keitner, IW Miller. A systems therapy: problem-centered systems therapy of the family. In: RA Wells, VJ Giannetti, eds. Handbook of Brief Psychotherapies. New York: Plenum Press, 1988, pp 405–436.

71. ER Berndt, LM Koran, SN Finkelstein, AJ Gelenberg, SG Kornstein, IW Miller, GA Trapp, MB Keller. Lost human capital from early-onset chronic depression. Am J Psychiatry 157:940–947, 2000.

72. WE Broadhead, DG Blazer, LK George, CK Tse. Depression, disability and days lost from work in a prospective epidemiologic survey. JAMA 264:2524–2528, 1990.

73. G Klerman, M Weissman. The course, morbidity and costs of depression. Arch Gener Psychiatry 49:831–834, 1992.

8

Psychopharmacology and Psychotherapy of Subsyndromal Depressions

Rachel E. Maddux and Mark H. Rapaport
Cedars-Sinai Medical Center
Los Angeles, California, U.S.A.

INTRODUCTION

Our conceptualization and empirical understanding of the spectrum of depression has changed radically in recent years. This transition has been facilitated by refinements in our diagnostic nosology, data acquired from large-scale epidemiological surveys, longitudinal studies of the natural course of major depression, and the development of effective yet less "toxic" treatments for mood disorders. There is general consensus that people do present with and actually suffer from debilitating, persistent symptoms that fall short of our current clinical definitions of major depression and dysthymia. One of the major conceptual challenges we face is determining the relationship between these "less than major" forms of depression and our currently accepted construct of major depression. We will summarize existing evidence investigating this relationship in this chapter.

A second focus of this chapter is a critical review of the existing psychopharmacology and psychotherapy literature available for the treatment of depressive spectrum disorders. This section highlights some of the challenges faced by the field in developing treatment paradigms for these conditions. In this relatively new area of investigation there lacks consensus about how the diagnosis should be garnered, what types of existing measures are appropriate and sensitive enough to change to measure treatment effects in depressive spectrum disorders, and how to disentangle adverse treatment effects from lack of response in such studies.

This chapter begins with a historical overview and then contains sections summarizing data about the sociodemographics of depressive spectrum disorders, their prevalence, course, relationship to major depressive disorder, treatment, and longer term prognosis.

An ancillary yet important issue that presents when carefully reviewing the literature in this field is the relationship between mood disorders and aging. Epidemiological and clinical data suggest that subsyndromal mood disorders are of greater prevalence in older individuals than in the general adult population. We will specifically review the data investigating this relationship.

HISTORICAL OVERVIEW

The first edition of the American Psychiatric Association's (APA) *Diagnostic and Statistical Manual of Mental Disorders* (DSM) appeared in 1952. It subscribed to Adolf Meyer's psychobiological theory that mental illness was a reaction of the personality to social, psychological, and biological influences. The second edition of the DSM was published in 1968 and represented a shift in the classification system to one based on the International Classification of Diseases (ICD-8). The DSM-II discarded Meyer's psychobiological view and replaced it with a diagnostic system that failed to provide a theoretical framework for understanding mental disorders. Concern that the ninth revision of the ICD classification system might not incorporate new methodological developments nor serve the research and clinical needs of psychiatry in the United States stimulated the APA to appoint a Task Force on Nomenclature and Statistics whose job was to develop a classification system reflecting the most current research-based evidence while maintaining compatibility with the ICD-9.

The third edition of the *Diagnostic and Statistical Manual of Mental Disorders* (DSM-III) was published in 1980 and represented a major paradigm shift for psychiatry. It provided explicit criteria for the diagnosis of mental disorders. Until this point, the clinician defined the boundaries of the diagnostic categories. Operationalized diagnostic criteria introduced a new model for standardizing the recognition and classification of mental disorders. The DSM-III was a transition from a psychological approach to diagnosis toward a descriptive medical model using objective criteria with specific thresholds designed to increase reliability, sensitivity, and specificity. Such a standardized system facilitated communication for both clinicians and researchers. The DSM-III stipulated that diagnosis is contingent upon three factors: the quality of symptoms present, the duration of time symptoms have been present, and the number of symptoms [1]. Failure to meet any one of these criteria resulted in a failure to qualify for a diagnosis of a mental disorder. Until recently, the presence of symptoms failing to meet full syndromal criteria have been regarded as clinically benign.

Over the years, clinicians and researchers have encountered many patients with depressive symptoms that were insufficient in number or duration to satisfy diagnostic criteria but resulted in significant social dysfunction and impairment [2–4]. These "subthreshold" symptoms are typified by depressive symptoms where the quality, duration, or number of symptoms are insufficient to qualify for the DSM-III, DSM-III revised (DSM-III-R), or DSM-IV criteria for major depressive disorder. The recognition of dysthymia in DSM-III-R represented the first extension of the conceptualization of depressive disorders by the APA beyond the nosology for major depressive disorder. Although minor depression (MinD) lasting less than 2 years was found listed under Atypical Depression in DSM-III-R, the increasing importance of depressive spectrum disorders was acknowledged in DSM-IV. Although MinD and recurrent brief depression (RBD) were not included in the body of the DSM-IV, they were included in Appendix B. This suggests that both concepts were recognized as entities that merited more extensive investigation. The working DSM-IV definition of minor depressive disorder is the presence of at least two, but fewer than five, depressive symptoms, including depressed mood or anhedonia, during the same 2-week period. Patients may not have a history of a major depressive episode or dysthymic disorder. Recurrent brief depression is defined as the presence of depressed mood or anhedonia with at least four of the eight depressive symptoms, and distress or impairment in occupational or social activities lasting *less than* two weeks in duration, recurring at least once a month over the course of 1 year [5].

The newest revision of the International Classification of Diseases, ICD-10, has also begun to expand its conceptualization of depressive disorders. In particular, the ICD-10 includes the category of mild depressive disorder. This is defined as the presence of two or three symptoms of depression for at least 2 weeks [6].

Judd and colleagues have suggested there might be credence to investigating even milder forms of depression. They found that two-thirds to three-fourths of respondents with subthreshold depressive symptoms ascertained in epidemiological studies do not satisfy any of the proposed diagnostic categories [7]. These individuals have depressive symptoms but do not report having depressed mood and anhedonia; DSM-IV Criterion A for depressive disorders. These subjects have been identified as having "subsyndromal symptomatic depression" (SSD). The working definition of SSD is the presence of two or more symptoms of depression of the same quality as major depression disorder (MDD), excluding symptoms of depressed mood and anhedonia, present for at least 2 weeks and associated with social dysfunction (Table 1).

This brief historical overview demonstrates the influence that transitions in our diagnostic nosology has had on the development and acceptance of depressive spectrum disorders. As commonly accepted diagnostic schema has progressed from a Meyerian psychobiological conceptualization to our current more "evidence-based" nosology, there has been a reemergence of interest in the concept of depression as part of a continuum extending from a few but disabling depressive symptoms to double depression. This more expanded view of depressive disorders suggests that we need to evaluate critically the validity of currently accepted rules about the number of symptoms required to meet criteria for a depressive syndrome as well as the length of time that such symptoms need to be present.

PREVALENCE

SSD

A secondary analysis of community respondents from the National Institute of Mental Health (NIMH) Epidemiological Catchment Area (ECA) study revealed the 1-month prevalence of SSD in the general population to be 3.9%. This is remarkably greater than the 1-month prevalence of MDD (2.3%), and MinD (1.5%) [7]. The 1-year point prevalence in the general population for SSD was 8.4%, and 3.5% for minor depression [8]. The combined prevalence for MinD and SSD is 11.9%, which is greater than the 1-year prevalence of all other mood disorders combined (9.5%).

MinD

As previously discussed, the 1-month prevalence for MinD reported for the ECA study population is 1.5%, and the 1-year prevalence is 3.5%. More recent epidemiological data from the National Comorbidity Study reported by Kessler and colleagues found that the lifetime prevalence of MinD was 10.0% [9]. The prevalence of MinD in populations of patients seeking care in primary care settings may be as high as 15.6%.

TABLE 1 Diagnostic Classification of Depression and Depressive Subtypes

Depressive disorder	DSM-IV location	Symptoms required	Depression or anhedonia?	Functional impairment?	Duration
Subsyndromal symptomatic depression (SSD)[8]	Not recognized	2 or >	No	Yes	At least 2 weeks
Minor depression (MinD)	Folded into Depression NOS Also Appendix B	2 but < 5	Yes	Yes	At least 2 weeks
Recurrent brief depression (RBD)	Folded into Depression NOS Also Appendix B	4	Yes	Yes	At least 2 days but < 2 weeks, recurring once a month for 12 consecutive months
Dysthymic disorder	Mood disorders	2	Depressed mood	Yes	At least 2 years, never having been without symptoms longer than 2 months
Major depressive episode (MDE)	Mood disorders	5	Yes	Yes	At least 2 weeks
Double depression (DD)	Not recognized	2, Dysthymia + 5, MDE	Yes	Yes	At least 2 years dysthymic + at least 2 weeks MDE

Source: Refs. 5 and 8.

RBD

The majority of the work characterizing RBD has been performed in Europe. This is not surprising since this conceptualization was developed from Jules Angst's analysis of a longitudinal community epidemiological study of the citizens of Zurich, Switzerland. Angst and Hochstrasser reported the 1-year prevalence of recurrent brief depression between 5 and 9% among probands 20–30 years old [10]. This replicated a previous study of a selected sample of 28-year-olds from the Zurich cohort that found the 1-year prevalence of RBD to be 7.2% [11]. Maier examined a cohort of subjects 18–65 years old in Germany, and reported a prevalence to be 5.8% for RBD [10]. However, he found that 16% of the general population indicated that they had suffered from RBD for at least one period of time during their lives. Weiller interviewed 405 subjects in Paris and reported a current prevalence rate for RBD of 9.9% [12].

CHALLENGES POSED BY OUR CURRENT NOSOLOGY

The taxonomy of subthreshold depressions that has emerged since the introduction of the DSM-III rather' arbitrarily defined different categories of depressive spectrum disorders. For research purposes these categories have, at times, been conceptualized as representing distinct and discrete clinical entities. However, at this time, we do no know what the most accurate conceptualization of depressive disorders is. Some proponents have argued that depressive spectrum disorders merely represent transitional stages that people with unipolar disorder pass through as they go between MDD and euthymia and then back again to major depression. Others contend that depressive spectrum disorders are discrete, discontinuous states (Figure 1). It is possible that the depressive spectrum actually encompasses both of these propositions. For some people, at a certain point in time of their illness, a spectrum condition may be a transitional state, whereas other individuals may only suffer from a discrete depressive spectrum state like MinD. In the following section, we will review data describing the relationships between the spectrum disorders as well as the relationship between the spectrum disorders and MDD.

COMMON CHARACTERISTICS

This section summarizes findings investigating the phenomenology of depressive spectrum disorders, its course and relationship to major depression, and biological similarities between depressive spectrum disorders and major depression (MD).

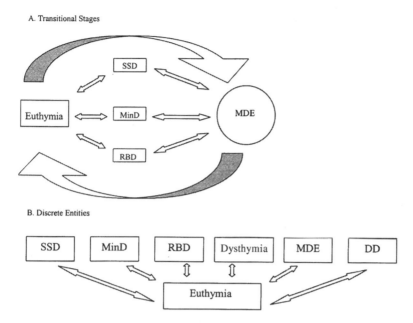

FIGURE 1 Conceptualization of depressive disorders. SSDA, subsyndromal symptomatic depression; MinD, minor depression; RBD, recurrent brief depression; MDE, major depressive episode; DD, double depression.

Sherbourne compared the demographic and clinical characteristics of 1420 subsyndromal depressive patients to 775 depressive disorder patients from the Medical Outcomes Study [3]. Fifty-two percent of subsyndromal patients and 55% of depressive disorder patients had a family history of depression. Both groups also had similar levels of medical and psychiatric comorbidity. They found that patients with subsyndromal depression more closely resembled depressive disorder patients than the non-depressed cohort.

Research examining the relationship of clinical characteristics among subthreshold depressive disorders has demonstrated a variety of common characteristics. Kessler used data from the National Comorbidity Survey to study lifetime prevalence, correlates, course, and impairment associated with MinD, major depression (MD) five to six symptoms, and MD seven or greater symptoms [9]. (In this analysis, a prior history of MDD was an exclusion criteria for MinD.) The estimated lifetime prevalences of MinD, MD 5–6, and MD 7–9 were 10.0, 8.3, and 7.5%, respectively. Sociodemographic correlates show that lifetime prevalences among all three categories are elevated among women, nonhispanic whites, and those defined as "other" with regard to employment status; namely, the disabled and unemployed. Nearly three-fourths of those with lifetime MinD and lifetime MD (72.1 and 72.3%) reported having more than one episode of the respective disorder. Only 0.5% of those with MinD and 0.2% of those with MDD reported that their depression persisted without any periods of remission. Social and economic impairment was found to be on a gradient with severity of illness. Forty-two percent of those with MinD, 49.7% with MD 5–6, and 68.2% with MD 7–9 reported either interference with life activities, sought help from a medical professional, or received and took medication for their depression. Data examining days lost from work in the past 30 days were similar in pattern: Lost work days per month were 0.17 for MinD, 0.17 for MD 5–6, and 0.48 for those with MD 7–9. Thus epidemiological data suggest (1) the sociodemographic characteristics of patients with MinD and MDD are similar, (2) the disorders have similar patterns for their course of illness, and (3) that there seems to be a continuous gradient of disability extending from MinD through severe MDD. It is particularly striking that MinD and MDD 5–6 symptoms have overlapping ranges of disability. These data suggest that the current threshold criteria for MDD may be arbitrary and may not hold up to empirical scrutiny. Such findings are in agreement with work by Kendler and Gardner [13].

There are less data investigating the relationship between RBD and other depressive and psychiatric conditions. Pretorius and colleagues investigated the relationship between personality traits, attempted suicide, and RBD in a study of 307 patients hospitalized for suicide attempts [14]. Patients meeting DSM-III-R criteria for RBD were investigated initially and in a 1-year follow-up assessment. RBD was found to be more common in women (32.1%) than in men (14.8%). Antisocial personality traits were found to occur most often among men in both assessments: 17.9% at initial assessment and 26.4% at follow-up assessment compared to women (5.1 and 8.3%). Women most commonly demonstrated histrionic personality traits at both initial assessment (24.4%) and follow-up assessment (21.5%) versus men (14.3 and 9.4%). These finding indicate a relationship between suicidal behavioral and recurrent brief depression, which was found to be related to the presence of antisocial personality traits in men and histrionic personality traits in women.

Angst and Merikangas performed one of the first longitudinal analyses of the course of subthreshold categories of depression with the Zurich Cohort Study of Young Adults [15]. They found that individuals frequently met multiple depressive subtypes over time. There was little stability within the diagnostic categories. Approximately half of those subjects suffering from MD continued to meet criteria for MD at follow-up, whereas the majority of the rest met criteria for subthreshold forms of depression. They found that one-third of subjects initially diagnosed with subthreshold depression developed MDD at follow-up. Again, the findings suggest that depression is fluid and encompasses a variety of phases.

This review of epidemiological data suggests that depressive spectrum disorders have a complex longitudinal course. Some individuals clearly worsen, others seem to recover, whereas a third group remains unchanged. Although these data cannot unequivocally clarify the relationship between these spectrum disorders and MD, they do support two related propositions. For some people a spectrum diagnosis represents a transitional state on the larger continuum of depression. Yet for others, the spectrum diagnosis may represent the stable, most severe form of a mood disorder that the individual may have.

LONGITUDINAL COURSE OF DEPRESSIVE SPECTRUM DISORDERS

There have been at least six large longitudinal epidemiological analyses demonstrating that the presence of depressive symptoms at the initial interview increases the likelihood that an individual will develop MDD. In 1990, Broadhead and colleagues reported that 10% of interviewees with MinD at Wave 1 of the ECA study had developed a fullblown MDD at Wave 2 [16]. Horwath was one of the first investigators to apply the concepts of relative risk and attributable risk to a psychiatric epidemiological study [17]. The relative risk of developing MD during the subsequent year was increased both for those with a history of depressive symptoms (odds ratio 4.4) and those subjects with a history of dysthymic disorder (odds ratio 5.5). The attributable risk of developing a first-onset major depression in the group with prior depressive symptoms is 55.3%. In contrast, since dysthymic disorder has a low prevalence rate, its attributable risk is only 7.8%. These findings suggest that depressive symptoms are predictive of a substantial proportion of first-onset cases of MD.

Judd performed a secondary analysis of 10,526 community respondents from the ECA study who participated in Wave 1 (the initial interview) and a follow-up interview, Wave 2, 1 year later [7]. Of 201 respondents diagnosed with MDD at Wave 1, 28% continued to meet criteria at Wave 2, whereas 23% met criteria for dysthymic disorder, 15% met criteria for MinD, 20% met criteria for SSD, and 14% resolved to asymptomatic status. Of those who at Wave 1 received a diagnosis of minor depression, 17% continued to meet criteria for MinD, 22% reported that their symptoms decreased to SSD, 5% had an increase in symptomology to either MD or dysthymia, whereas 28% resolved to asymptomatic status. Three hundred and fifty respondents met criteria for SSD at Wave 1 and at Wave 2, 17% continued to meet criteria for SSD, 10% met criteria for MinD, 2% for dysthymia, 4% for MD, whereas

48% of these respondents became asymptomic. This remarkable amount of fluidity over the course of 1 year suggests that the clinical picture of depression is dynamic. Symptoms wax and wane in severity over time and individuals traversed across the spectrum of depressive subtypes during 1-year follow-up.

Angst used data from two periods of time to study the longitudinal course of depressive spectrum disorders. The first was a 2-year span during which subjects were interviewed twice [15]. The second was a 7-year follow-up period where subjects were interviewed at three time points. Twenty-nine percent of those with a subthreshold depression diagnosis at initial interview had developed MDD at follow-up. Interestingly, 17% of those with any symptoms of depression at initial interview developed MDD. This, again, suggests that subthreshold depression is a positive predictor of subsequent major depression.

Wells reported that one-quarter of the individuals with depressive symptoms at baseline developed MDD by the time of the 2-year follow-up interview [18]. Similar findings have been reported by Maier, who performed initial evaluations and subsequent 1-year follow-up evaluations in a general medical practice cohort [19]. The risk for MDD during the follow-up period was 15.8% for patients who initially were diagnosed with minor or subsyndromal depression, 11.7% for subjects who had had RBD versus 3.8% for those with no affective symptoms at time 1. Finally, some of the most powerful data demonstrating that the presence of at least five symptoms of depression for 2 weeks might not be a valid construct was Kendler and Gardner's analysis of the Virginia twin registry [13]. Their data demonstrated that depressive symptoms at the initial interview were as strong a predictor of subsequent MDD as the presence of mild (five to six symptoms) MD. They also demonstrated that the positive predictive value of having symptoms for greater than 2 weeks was not statistically different than the positive predictive power of the presence of symptoms for 5–13 days.

In summary, the data suggest that depressive spectrum disorders may be a harbinger of future MDD for at least some patients. These data argue that at least some patients with subthreshold mood disorders are at risk of developing MDD.

RELATIONSHIP BETWEEN RESIDUAL SYMPTOMS, DEPRESSIVE SPECTRUM DISORDER, AND MD

Researchers and clinicians have found that residual depressive symptoms following recovery from a MD episode are an important clinical marker associated with an increase risk of relapse into MD. Patients with residual symptoms of MD relapsed to MD more than three times faster than patients who achieved a complete recovery to asymptomatic status (68 vs 231 weeks) [20]. They were five and a half times more likely to develop a depressive spectrum syndrome. These results agree with work by Thase, who found that patients who remitted during a short course of cognitive-behavioral therapy (CBT) but had residual symptoms were four times more likely to relapse than patients who had achieved an asymptomatic status [21].

Paykel has also focused on the detrimental effects of residual symptoms after remission from an episode of MD [22]. Subjects meeting Research Diagnostic Criteria (RDC) for primary unipolar MD were followed every 3 months to remission, which was defined as 2 consecutive months, retrospectively rated, below the inclusion criterion of MD. Patients who remitted were followed up at similar 3-month interviews and Beck Depression Inventory (BDI) assessments for 12–15 months. Relapse to major depressive episode (MDE) was defined as a return to RDC criteria for MD for at least 1 month. Sixty-four subjects participated in this study and 60 met criteria for remission at some point during this study. Seventy-five percent of patients with residual symptoms relapsed during the 12–15 month follow-up period compared to 25% of patients who did not have residual symptoms at recovery. There was a correlation between the severity of the index episode of depression and the presence of residual symptoms, and it is possible that patients who have just recovered from a more severe depression may be the ones at greatest risk of relapse. Family history, length of the current episode, and personality did not increase the risk of relapse or account for the presence of correlate with residual symptoms.

Faravelli and colleagues investigated predictors of relapse into MDE. One hundred and one patients suffering from primary unipolar depression were followed for 1 year after episode recovery [23]. Recovery was defined as the presence of no more than one RDC symptom of major depressive disorder, and the symptom-free status was defined as 2 months or more without any symptoms. At the 12-month point, 51 patients had relapsed into a new depressive episode. An analysis of relapsers versus nonrelapsers found that better psychosocial functioning and a greater degree of "social wellness" at the time of remission seemed to protect against relapse. Sociodemographic variables, severity of illness, and type of treatment did not correlate with relapse.

Data suggest that many patients do not fully recover from an episode of major depression but rather they traverse along the continuum of spectrum mood states. These patients with residual symptoms of their episode might meet operational criteria for MinD, SSD, or even RBD. One of the major challenges facing the field is what to do with these patients. Fava performed a prospective study investigating the efficacy of pharmacotherapy augmentation of antidepressant treatment [24]. Forty-nine outpatients meeting RDC criteria for MDD were treated with aggressive pharmacotherapy and were assessed as being "better" or "much better" on the CGI improvement scale. Six patients reported no residual symptoms of depression and were excluded from further participation in the study. The 43 remaining patients were randomly assigned to pharmacotherapy and CBT, or pharmacotherapy and clinical management. Both treatment groups received 10 40-min sessions every 2 weeks. Antidepressant medication was tapered by 25 mg every 2 weeks until it was withdrawn. Forty patients remained in the study until the end. Patients who received the CBT intervention had continued improvement on objective measures at the end of the 10 sessions. However, the most important finding was that at 2-year follow-up, 35% of patients in the clinical management group had relapsed compared to 15% of patients who received the behavioral intervention. Although this study requires replication, it suggests that a short-term cognitive-behavioral intervention after successful pharmacotherapy may decrease residual symptoms and protect against relapse.

In summary, data from both epidemiological and clinical studies demonstrate that many patients may traverse across a continuum of the symptoms spectrum from asymptomatic to MD. Patients who are identified and treated for MD will have a better long-term prognosis if the treatment intervention can help those patients reach full asymptomatic status. Patients who are unable to reach complete remission status and are arrested in some subsyndromal mood state are at much greater risk of relapse. Whether the presence of these residual symptoms reflects a more treatment-resistant form of depression in these individuals or merely the inadequacy of their current treatment is yet to be determined.

BIOLOGICAL STUDIES

There are very few biological investigations of depressive spectrum disorders. The ones that have occurred can be characterized as investigating electrophysiology, brain imaging, and neuroendocrinology. The two studies investigating neurophysiology and brain imaging found similarities between patients with MinD and MDD. The one study investigating neuroendocrinology and MinD did not identify differences from normal controls in either the MinD or the MD group. So again there were similar results although this may represent an assay sensitivity problem rather than a distinct biological finding.

One of the difficulties with the study of affective disorders is that there are, at present, no pathognomonic laboratory findings to identify depressive disorders. However, an important study employing polysomnographic data by Akiskal suggested there may be common neurophysiological substrate for subthreshold depression, dysthymia, and MDD [7]. Many characterological depressives were found to have shortened rapid eye movement (REM) latency, increased REM percentage, and redistribution of REM diurnality. REM sleep disturbances were consistently present during consecutive night polysomnography of subthreshold depression groups.

Kumar and colleagues also found common neurobiological data for different forms of depressive disorders. Quantitative magnetic resonance imaging (MRI) was used to investigate the neuroanatomy of patient's late-onset MinD, late-onset MD, and older nondepressed controls. Patients with late-life MinD had smaller prefrontal lobe volumes (0.152) when compared to nondepressed controls (0.167) [25]. Results showed a significant inverse linear gradation between prefrontal lobe volume and severity of clinical depression.

It has been long postulated that increased hypothalamic-pituitary-adrenal axis drive contributes to increased cortisol secretion and dexamethasome nonsuppression in patients with melancholic depression. In a sample of 68 unipolar depression patients (minor, $n = 24$; major, $n = 25$; melancholic, $n = 19$) Maes examined post-Synacthen adrenocorticotropic hormone (ACTH) [ACTH (1–24), 250 mg IV], intact ACTH (1–39), β-endorphin/β-lipotropin, cortisol, androstenedione concentrations, as well as the postdexamethasone (DST) plasma ACTH (1–39), and cortisol values [26]. No significant differences were found between any of the groups in post-Synacthen cortisol or androstenedione secretion or DST nonsuppressors and suppressors.

In summary, there is a paucity of biological studies investigating depressive spectrum disorders. This will be an area of fertile future investigations.

MIND AND THE ELDERLY

Mental disorders in older patients may differ in clinical presentation, pathogenesis, and pathophysiology from mental disorders of younger persons. Diagnosis and treatment is often confounded by coexisting chronic medical illnesses, medications, and cognitive impairment. There is also a lack of consensus about how to define and thus diagnose MinD in older people. Snaith identified anhedonia as the cardinal feature of MinD in later life [27]. Wood emphasized the importance of affective flattening; reporting that 44% of elderly psychogeriatric inpatients displayed unchanging facial expressions, decreased movements, lack of expressive gestures, poor eye contact, emotional nonreactivity, and lack of vocal inflection [28]. Blazer and colleagues identified a unique symptom profile among people aged 60 years and older which was characterized by depressed mood, psychomotor retardation, poor concentration, and constipation [29].

Epidemiological community studies of MinD in older individuals report rates varying between 12.9 and 18.9% [30,31]. However, chronic medical illnesses markedly increase the risk of MinD in older individuals. Oxman and colleagues studied medical clinic outpatients aged 60 years and older and found prevalence rates of 47.4–52.6% for RDC MinD [32]. Rates of MinD depression are also extraordinarily high in nursing home patients with rates reported ranging from 18.1 [33] to 30.5% [34].

The issue of bereavement is especially likely in later life, and as a result many older people are at risk for developing bereavement-related depression. Zisook found subsyndromal symptomatic depression to have a prevalence rate of 27% at 2 months, 19% at 13 months, and 12% at 25 months after the loss of a spouse [35]. Data on the frequency and severity of symptoms in subsyndromal depression and MD in late life spousal bereavement have been reported by Pasternak and colleagues [36]. Patients with depressive spectrum disorder were characterized by the combination of heightened anxiety, early morning awakening, weight loss, and low mood. In the longitudinal portion of the analysis, symptoms of depression, poor sleep, medical burden, functional impairment, perceived social support, and stability of social rhythms over the first 2 years following spousal loss were compared in bereaved subjects presenting with subsyndromal depression (n = 20), nondepressed bereaved subjects (n = 27), and nondepressed, nonbereaved control subjects (n = 20). All subjects were between 60 and 80 years old. Subsyndromal subjects qualified by failing to meet RDC criteria for full syndromal depression but had stable Hamilton Rating Scale for Depression 17 (Ham-D-17) scores, ranging between 11 and 15. Results indicated that subsyndromally depressed subjects had the most elevated HAM-D-17 scores at 6 months (5.7 ± 3.3) and 24 months (5.1 ± 2.5) compared to nondepressed bereaved subjects (4.4 ± 2.4, 3.4 ± 2.5) and nonbereaved controls (1.0 ± 1.5, 1.9 ± 2.0). Functional impairment as measured by the Global Assessment Scale was lower for subsyndromal subjects at 6 months (85.7 ± 4.4) and 24 months (82.3 ± 6.9) than nondepressed bereaved subjects (87.9 ± 6.5, 87.2 ± 5.9) and nonbereaved subjects (95.8 ± 4.5, 98.8 ± 1.9). Pittsburgh Sleep Quality Index scores showed significant disturbance among the subsyndromal subjects at 6 months (5.0 ± 2.0) and 24 months (5.1 ± 2.0) versus nondepressed bereaved subjects (4.4 ± 2.3, 3.8 ± 2.4) and nonbereaved subjects (2.5 ± 1.1, 4.3 ± 2.0). Significant group effects were found in every area except the social rhythm metric. These data suggest that subsyndromally bereaved elders are more impaired than nondepressed bereaved subjects.

Declining physical health is an important risk factor for depression and depressive spectrum disorder in later life. Beekman examined the differences between MinD and MD and poor health in a community-based sample of adults aged 55 years and older [30]. In this sample of 646 individuals, 41.3%

met criteria for MinD and 9.2% for MD. Several health variables were significantly associated with MinD but not MD including chronic disease, heart disease, osteoarthritis, rheumatoid arthritis, and impaired distant vision. Impaired hearing was associated with MD but not MinD. Diabetes mellitus, stroke, and cancer were not significantly associated with either MD or MinD. In this study, results suggest that there is a strikingly high prevalence of MinD among older persons with chronic medical conditions. The relationship between MD and MinD and medical illness in older adults was examined by Koenig in a medical inpatient setting [37]. Significant correlates for MinD included negative life events, hospital stressors, and severity of medical illness. When MinD and MD were compared directly, no significant characteristics between the two were detected. Characteristics of those with MinD versus nondepressed patients included more non–health-related negative life events, diagnosis of immune system disorders, greater complaints of somatic symptoms, and greater severity of medical illness. These data suggest that differences between patients with MD and MinD were minimal.

Older adults are vulnerable to adverse behavioral and cognitive effects of many medications. Medications, especially antihypertensives and cardiac medications, can precipitate a depressive disorder. Bethanidine, clonidine, guanethidine, hydralazone, methyldopa, propranol, and reserpine have all been found to cause either MD or MinD. Some of the factors implicated in the development of medication-related depressive symptoms include age-related changes in drug absorption that increase bioavailability, patient's taking the medication incorrectly and thus overdosing or underdosing of agents, and sensitivity of older patient to medication side effects such as anticholinergic properties.

Depressive spectrum disorders are more common in older individuals. Bereavement, declining physical health, disabilities, chronic illness, and multiple medications may account for some of the increased vulnerability of this group to depressive spectrum disorders. However, more research into the etiology and treatment of depressive spectrum disorders is certainly warranted.

TREATMENT

Psychotherapy

SSD

Barkham conducted the first randomized, controlled trial of very brief psychological intervention in patients with subsyndromal depression [38]. Subjects were split into three levels of severity based on their BDI scores: stressed, subclinical, and low-level depressed. The treatment consisted of two

1-h sessions 1 week apart followed by a third 1-hour session 3 months later. This model was called the two-plus-one (2 + 1) model. The hypothesis was that positive change occurs through highly focused work in the first two sessions, which focused on the successful resolution of problematic situations and experiences. It is postulated that the patient then builds on these corrective experiences during the time before session 3. One hundred and thirty-eight subjects were randomized to receive either CBT or psychodynamic-interpersonal (PI) therapy in one of two time frames: initially or with a 4-week delay. One hundred and sixteen patients completed treatment. BDI scores across treatment for the three severity bands showed the stressed group at a preliminary mean BDI of 7.41 decreasing to a mean 3.96 at assessment four, the subclinical group at a preliminary mean BDI of 12.55 decreasing to a mean 3.87 at assessment four, and the low-level depressed group at a preliminary mean BDI of 18.9 decreasing to a mean 6.0 at assessment four. Overall, patients receiving the 2 + 1 model of treatment improved from baseline screening (M = 13.40, SD = 4.82) to treatment end at assessment 4 (M = 5.24, SD = 6.03). These data suggest that the 2 + 1 model delivering brief CBT or brief PI therapy was a successful treatment intervention for subthreshold depressive symptoms.

MinD

Lynch and colleagues developed a problem-solving telephone treatment protocol for outpatients with MinD identified in a family practice setting [39]. Twenty-nine subjects were randomized to a treatment group or a comparison group. HAM-D scores were equivalent for both groups at baseline. The treatment group received six problem-solving sessions that took subjects through five steps designed to help them develop methods for managing their life problems. The sessions were once a week for 20 min. The HAM-D scores improved from 15.6 to 10.9 for the treatment group and went from 12.4 to 13.3 for the control group. Although these subjects did not reach remission, they seemed to receive some benefit from this telephone intervention.

Miranda and Munoz evaluated the efficacy of a cognitive-behavioral intervention for minor depression in primary care patients [40]. One hundred and fifty subjects were randomly assigned to the intervention (n = 70) or the control condition (n = 78). The 8-week psychoeducational program was designed to teach patients to control negative moods through the use of pleasant activities, constructive thinking, and focus on interpersonal relationships. Patients in the intervention condition had a significant reduction in BDI scores (F = 3.72, df = 3342, P = .01). Reductions in depressive symptoms persisted through the 1-year follow-up for this group. Somatic problems as measured by the Hopkins Symptom Checklist were significantly lower for the treatment group as compared with the control group. This decrease in somatic complaints in the treatment group was maintained at 1-year follow-up.

In summary, the few studies performed investigating the efficacy of psychotherapy suggest that it may be useful in decreasing symptoms of depression in patients with subsyndromal and minor depression. These data suggest that future studies designed to bring patients with SSD and MinD to full remission status are warranted.

Psychopharmacology

SSD

Rapaport and Judd were first to quantify functional impairment and depressive symptomology in a clinical sample of patients with subsyndromal and MinD and to demonstrate that treatment with the selective serotonin reuptake inhibitor, fluvoxamine, was effective in decreasing depressive symptomology and improving psychosocial functioning [41]. Thirty patients, half with MinD and half with SSD, were treated with open-label fluvoxamine 25–100 mg/day for 8 weeks. At baseline, patients were evaluated with a modified Structured Clinical Interview for DSM-IV (SCID), the Global Assessment of Functioning (GAF), the HAM-D, the Inventory of Depressive Symptomatology (IDS-C), the Clinician Global Impression Scale (CGI), the Depression Section of the Diagnostic Interview Schedule, and the Medical Outcome Survey Short Form 36 (SF = 36). During the first week of treatment, patients received fluvoxamine 25 mg daily. Patients who had no significant side effects at the end of week 1 were increased to fluvoxamine 50 mg/day. Patients could be titrated up to 100 mg/day of fluvoxamine based on response and tolerability. The medication could be tapered down to 25 mg/day if side effects were intolerable. The mean dose for the MinD sample was 47 ($\pm$ 28.5) mg and was 48.7 ($\pm$ 29.9) mg for the SSD sample. MinD patients had markedly lower baseline SF-36 scores on measures of physical role functioning, emotional role functioning, emotional well-being, social functioning, and energy/fatigue that remediated to community norms with treatment. SSD patients had distinctly lower baseline SF-36 subscale scores for emotional role functioning, emotional well-being, social functioning, and energy/fatigue; again these scores remediated with treatment. The mean HAM-D-17 for MinD patients was 11.7 at baseline and decreased to a mean of 5.8 at week 8. The mean HAM-D-17 for the SSD cohort was 11.9 at baseline and decreased to a mean of 4.2 by week 8. Treatment improved ratings of severity of illness as assessed by the HAM-D-28, IDS-C, and CGI for both the SSD and MinD groups. GAF scores for both groups improved over the 8-week treatment period. These data suggest that patients with MinD and patients with SSD both responded positively to open-label treatment with fluvoxamine. A remarkable

30% of patients in each group attained complete resolution of depressive symptomology with only 8 weeks of treatment.

MinD

The beneficial effects of paroxetine and maprotiline were compared and contrasted in a randomized double-blind multicenter 6-week study of outpatients with MinD [42]. Patients were initially started on paroxetine 20 mg/day or maprotiline 100 mg/day, and were titrated to paroxetine 40 mg/day and maprotiline 150 mg/day if they failed to show a response by the end of week 3. Patients were assessed at weekly intervals on the HAM-D-17 item, Montgomery-Asberg Depression Rating Scale (MADRS), Bech-Rafaelsen Depression Rating Scale (BRMS), Raskin Depression Rating Scale (RDS), Hamilton Anxiety Rating Scale (HAM-A), and CGI. Both the maprotiline and the paroxetine groups demonstrated improvement on the HAM-D-17 and the MADRS. The HAM-D-17 score for the paroxetine-treated group dropped from 17 to a mean of 4 at week 6; the MADRS score went from a baseline of 17 to a mean 3 at week 6. The HAM-D-17 score for the maprotiline group dropped from 16 at baseline to a mean of 5 at week 6. The MADRS score went from a baseline of 17 to a mean of 5 at week 6. Although not definitive, the investigators suggested that paroxetine treatment may be slightly more efficacious than maprotiline treatment for MinD.

There have been few placebo-controlled trials of mild MD and/or MinD. Stewart and colleagues performed a double-blind efficacy trial of desipramine treatment for MD [43]. Entry criteria required subjects to have a HAM-D score below 19 and meet RDC criteria for MD, MinD, or intermittent depressive disorder. Baseline assessment included HAM-D, CGI, and the Hopkins Symptom Checklist. After a 10-day placebo lead-in, subjects were randomized to double-blind treatment with desipramine or placebo. The clinical status of each patient was assessed weekly for 6 weeks. The initial medication dose was 50 mg daily and was increased by 50 mg every 3 days to a maximum of 300 mg/day. Patients experiencing side effects which prevented maximum titration but tolerating at least 200 mg day were considered to be receiving an adequate trial of desipramine. Unfortunately, the rapid titration and high doses of desipramine caused problems with side effects and dropouts. This meant that the sample size of patients with MinD was too small for any meaningful statistical analysis.

Paykel examined amitriptyline in a 6-week placebo-controlled trial of general practice patients experiencing mild depression [44]. Dosages employed in the first week were 75 mg amitriptyline or placebo, and were titrated in 25-mg increments weekly to a maximum 175 mg/day based on patient response and the research physician's judgment. Approximately two of three of the 178 patients who entered the study completed the entire study. Amitriptyline did not differentiate from placebo in this study; both groups improved over the course of the study.

Hamilton and colleagues randomized 72 mild and moderate depressed patients to flupenthixol or fluvoxamine for 4 weeks in a general practice setting [45]. Thirty-six patients received treatment with flupenthixol dihydrochloride and 36 patients received fluvoxamine. Dosages during the first week were flupenthixol 1 mg or fluvoxamine 100 mg. Patients not responding at the end of week 1 could have their dosages doubled. Assessments included the HAM-D-17, CGI, and a self-assessment visual analogue scale for depression and were conducted on days 1, 8, 15, and 29. Both groups improved from baseline on all measures over the 4-week treatment period.

RBD

Stamenkovic and colleagues are among the few to examine the efficacy of pharmacological treatments in patients with RBD [46]. In two case studies, patients were treated with mirtazapine for 4 months. After 3 days of 15 mg/day mirtazapine, the dosage was increased to 30 mg/day. Assessments used included the CGI, HAM-D, and BDI. Patients were asked to keep a daily diary to document severity, duration, and frequency of their brief depressive episodes. CGI severity scores for both patients were reduced from 6 at baseline to 0 after 4 months of with mirtazapine. These data suggest that mirtazapine may help some patients with RBD.

Corominas reported the case of a 38-year-old man who presented with a history of sudden depressive episodes lasting 2–4 days and recurring monthly [47]. The patient was started with a regimen of clomipramine 75 mg/day, with complete remission after 3 days. However, 1 month later, the patient had a recurrence. Clomipramine was increased to 225 mg/day, but the patient developed suicidal ideation and was hospitalized. Lithium therapy was added and complete resolution of symptoms was seen after 3 days. Lithium treatment was continued at 800–1000 mg/day and clomipramine was gradually tapered. The patient did not have a recurrence during the subsequent months.

Psychotherapy Versus Psychopharmacology

Williams compared the effectiveness of pharmacotherapy and psychotherapy in a randomized, placebo-controlled trial among older patients with minor depression or dysthymia [48]. Four hundred and fifteen primary care patients were randomized to receive paroxetine 10–40 mg a day (n = 137), placebo (n = 140), or receive problem-solving treatment primary care (PST-PC; n = 138). Over 11 weeks, patients randomized to paroxetine or placebo had six visits that included adverse events monitoring and general support.

The PST-PC patients received six sessions of psychotherapy. The primary outcome measures were the Hopkins Symptom Checklist Depression Scale (HSCL-D-20) and the HAM-D-17. Functional status was assessed by the SF-36 physical and mental subscales. Patients treated with paroxetine had moderate improvement in depressive symptoms. Patients treated with PST-PC did not differ significantly from those receiving placebo. These data suggest that paroxetine might improve depressive symptomology in some older patients with MinD. However, unlike the previously described psychotherapy studies, PST-PC did not confer a therapeutic advantage over placebo.

In general, there is a need for more trials investigating the efficacy for depressive spectrum disorders. Preliminary data suggest that pharmacotherapy may be useful for SSD, MinD, and RBD, but large placebo-controlled trials are needed. The preliminary results from the psychotherapy trials are intriguing, but suggest that the development of more specific focused therapies may be required. However, it is clear that depressive spectrum disorders are serious, disabling, and costly. They increase the risk of MD significantly; therefore, further study of their treatment is worthwhile.

CONCLUSION

This chapter should stimulate more questions than answers. The clinical and family history data clearly demonstrate that depressive spectrum disorders are similar to major depressive disorder. The disability and prognostic data suggest that these potential entities certainly seem to be part of the monotonic gradient of dysfunction that extends from euthymia to severe MD. Review of the epidemiological data suggest that (1) for some individuals depressive spectrum disorders may represent the "form furste" presentation of major depression, (2) for some individuals depressive spectrum disorders may be a transitional state as they traverse between MD and euthymia, and (3) for some individuals depressive spectrum disorders may be distinct clinical phenotype of unipolar depressive disorder. These findings are consistent with existing clinical data from longitudinal studies of MD. However, careful review of both epidemiological and clinical data clearly demonstrate that the presence of depressive spectrum states whether as a "form furste" presentation of MD, an entity unto itself, or as a manifestation of residual symptoms of MD is not benign. We need to develop effective treatment strategies for these conditions. Unfortunately, the current treatment literature is limited and fraught with methodological challenges. These problems with the development of consensus about the diagnostic characteristics of the syndromes and questions about the sensitivity of the tools used to measure severity and treatment effects restrict the information we can glean from existing studies. Yet, taken as a whole, the data suggest that the types of treatment interventions we use for MD may be helpful in ameliorating depressive spectrum disorders.

Continued research developing and validating instruments to assess depressive spectrum disorders will be critical to our understanding of these paradigms. These tools will facilitate our understanding of the prevalence of these conditions, their longitudinal course, their relationship to other forms of depressive disorders, and prognosis with treatment.

REFERENCES

1. American Psychiatric Association. Diagnostic and Statistical Manual of Mental Disorders. 3rd ed. Washington, DC: American Psychiatric Association, 1980.
2. KB Wells, A Stewart, RD Hays, MA Burnam, W Rogers, M Daniels, S Berry, S Greenfield, J Ware. The functioning and well-being of depressed patients. Results from the Medical Outcomes Study. JAMA 1989; 262:914–919.
3. CD Sherbourne, KB Wells, RD Hays, W Rogers, MA Burnam, LL Judd. Subthreshold depression and depressive disorder: clinical characteristics of general medical and mental health specialty outpatients. Am J Psychiatry 1994; 151:1777–1784.
4. M Olfson, WE Broadhead, MM Weissman, AC Leon, L Farber, C Hoven, and R Kathol. Subthreshold psychiatric symptoms in a primary care group practice. Arch Gen Psychiatry 1996; 53:880–886.
5. American Psychiatric Association. Diagnostic and Statistical Manual of Mental Disorder. 4th ed. Washington, DC: American Psychiatric Association, 1994.
6. World Health Organization. The ICD-10 Classification of Mental and Behavioural Disorders. Diagnostic Criteria For Research Geneva: World Health Organization, 1993.
7. LL Judd, HS Akiskal, and MP Paulus. The role and clinical significance of subsyndromal depressive symptoms (SSD) in unipolar major depressive disorder. J Affect Disord 1997; 45:5–17.
8. LL Judd, MH Rapaport, MP Paulus, JL Brown. Subsyndromal symptomatic depression: a new mood disorder? J Clin Psychiatry 1994; 55(suppl):18–28.
9. RC Kessler, S Zhao, DG Blazer, M Swartz. Prevalence, correlates, and course of minor depression and major depression in the National Comorbidity Survey. J Affect Disord 1997; 45:19–30.
10. J Angst, B Hochstrasser. Recurrent brief depression: the Zurich Study. J Clin Psychiatry 1994; 55(suppl):3–9 (1994).
11. J Angst. The history and concept of recurrent brief depression. Eur Arch Psychiatry Clin Neurosci 1994; 244:171–173.
12. E Weiller, P Boyer, JP Lepine, Y Lecrubien. Prevalence of recurrent brief depression in primary care. Eur Arch Psychiatry Clin Neurosci 1994; 244:174–181.

13. KS Kendler, CO Gardner Jr. Boundaries of major depression: an evaluation of DSM-IV criteria. Am J Psychiatry 1998; 155:172–177.
14. HW Pretorius, W Bodemer, JL Roos, J Grimbeek, Personality traits, brief recurrent depression and attempted suicide. S Afr Med J 1994; 84;690–694 (1994).
15. J Angst, K Merikangas. The depressive spectrum: diagnostic classification and course. J Affect Disord 1997; 45:31–39.
16. WE Broadhead, DG Blazer, LK George, CK Tse. Depression, disability days, and days lost from work in a prospective epidemiologic survey. JAMA 1990; 264:2524–2528.
17. E Horwath, J Johnson, GL Klerman, MM Weissman. Depressive symptoms as relative and attributable risk factors for first- onset major depression. Arch Gen Psychiatry 1992; 49:817–823.
18. KB Wells, MA Burnam, W Rogers, R Hays, P Camp. The course of depression in adult outpatients. Results from the Medical Outcomes Study. Arch Gen Psychiatry 1992; 49:788–794 (1992).
19. W Maier, M Gansicke, O Weiffenbach. The relationship between major and subthreshold variants of unipolar depression. J Affect Disord 1997; 45:41–51.
20. LL Judd, HS Akiskal, JD Maser, PJ Zeller, J Endicott, W Coryell, MP Paulus, JL Kunovac, AC Leon, TI Mueller, JA Rice, MB Keller. Major depressive disorder: a prospective study of residual subthreshold depressive symptoms as predictor of rapid relapse. J Affect Disord 1998; 50:97–108.
21. ME Thase. Relapse and recurrence in unipolar major depression: short-term and long-term approaches. J Clin Psychiatry 1990; 51(suppl):51–57 (1990).
22. ES Paykel, R Ramana, Z Cooper, H Hayhurst, J Kerr, A Barocka. Residual symptoms after partial remission: an important outcome in depression. Psychol Med 1995; 25:1171–1180.
23. C Faravelli, A Ambonetti, S Pallanti, A Pazzagli. Depressive relapses and incomplete recovery from index episode. Am J Psychiatry 1986; 143:888–891.
24. GA Fava, S Grandi, M Zielezny, R Canestrari, MA Morphy. Cognitive behavioral treatment of residual symptoms in primary major depressive disorder. Am J Psychiatry 1994; 151:1295–1299.
25. A Kumar, Z Jin, W Bilker, J Udupa, and G Gottlieb. Late-onset minor and major depression: early evidence for common neuroanatomical substrates detected by using MRI. Proc Natl Acad Sci USA 1998; 95:7654–7658.
26. M Maes, H Meltzer, P Cosyns, J Calabrese, P D'Hondt, P Blockx, C Vandervorst and J Raus. Pituitary and adrenal hormone responsiveness to Synacthen in melancholic subjects versus subjects with minor depression. Biol Psychiatry 1993; 33:624–629.
27. RP Snaith. The concepts of mild depression. Br J Psychiatry 1987; 150:387–393.
28. KA Wood, H Nissenbaum and M Livingston, Affective flattening in elderly patients. Age Ageing 1990; 19:253–256 (1990).
29. D. Blazer, M Woodbury, DC Hughes, LK George, KG Manton, JR Bachar, N Fowler. A statistical analysis of the classification of depression in a mixed community and clinical sample. J Affect Disord 1989; 16:11–20 (1989).

30. AT Beekman, DJ Deeg, T van Tilburg, JH Smit, C Hooijer and W van Tilbug. Major and minor depression in later life: a study of prevalence and risk factors. J Affect Disord 1995; 36:65–75.
31. A Paivarinta, A Verkkoniemi, L Niinisto, SL Kivela, and R Sulkava. The prevalence and associates of depressive disorders in the oldest-old Finns. Soc Psychiatry Psychiatr Epidemiol 1999; 34:352–359.
32. TE Oxman, JE Barrett, J Barrett, P Gerber. Symptomatology of late-life minor depression among primary care patients. Psychosomatics 1990; 31:174–180.
33. BW Rovner, PS German, LJ Brant, R Clark, L Burton, and MF Folstein. Depression and mortality in nursing homes. JAMA 1991; 265:993–996.
34. PA Parmelee, IR Katz, MP Lawton. Depression among institutionalized aged: assessment and prevalence estimation. J Gerontol 1989; 44:M22–M29.
35. S Zisook, M Paulus, SR Shuchter, and LL Judd. The many faces of depression following spousal bereavement. J Affect Disord 1997; 45:85–94.
36. RE Pasternak, CF Reynolds, III, MD Miller, E Frank, A Fasiczka, H Prigerson, S Mazumdar, DJ Kupfer. The symptom profile and two-year course of subsyndromal depression in spousally bereaved elders. Am J Geriatr Psychiatry 1994; 2:210–219.
37. HG Koenig. Differences in psychosocial and health correlates of major and minor depression in medically ill older adults. J Am Geriatr Soc 1997; 45:1487–1495.
38. M Barkham, DA Shapiro, GE Hardy, A Rees. Psychotherapy in two plus-one sessions: outcomes of a randomized controlled trial of cognitive-behavioral and psychodynamic interpersonal therapy for subsyndromal depression. J Consult Clin Psychol 1999; 67:201–211.
39. DJ Lynch, MB Tamburrino, and R Nagel. Telephone counseling for patients with minor depression: preliminary findings in a family practice setting. J Fam Pract 1997; 44:293–298.
40. J Miranda, R Munoz. Intervention for minor depression in primary care patients. Psychosom Med 1994; 56:136–141.
41. MH Rapaport, LL Judd. Minor depressive disorder and subsyndromal depressive symptoms: functional impairment and response to treatment. J Affect Disord 1998; 48:227–232.
42. A Szegedi, H Wetzel, D Angersbach, M Philipp, O Benkert. Response to treatment in minor and major depression: results of a double-blind comparative study with paroxetine and maprotiline. J Affect Disord 1997; 45:167–178.
43. JW Stewart, FM Quitkin, MR Liebowitz, PJ McGrath, WM Harrison, and DF Klein. Efficacy of desipramine in depressed outpatients. Response according to research diagnosis criteria diagnoses and severity of illness. Arch Gen Psychiatry 1983; 40:202–207.
44. ES Paykel, P Freeling, and JA Hollyman. Are tricyclic antidepressants useful for mild depression? A placebo controlled trial. Pharmacopsychiatry 1988; 21:15–18.

45. BA Hamilton, PG Jones, AN Hoda, PM Keane, I Majid, SI Zaidi. Flupenthixol and fluvoxamine in mild to moderate depression: a comparison in general practice. Pharmatherapeutica 1989; 5:292–297.

46. M Stamenkovic, L Pezawas, M de Zwaan, HN Aschauer, S Kasper. Mirtazapine in recurrent brief depression. Int Clin Psychopharmacol 1998; 13:39–40 (1998).

47. A Corominas, P Bonet, E Nieto. Recurrent brief depression successfully treated with lithium. Biol Psychiatry 1998; 44:927–929 (1998).

48. JW Williams, Jr., J Barrett, T Oxman, E Frank, W Katon, M Sullivan, J Cornell, A Sengupta. Treatment of dysthymia and minor depression in primary care: A randomized controlled trial in older adults. JAMA 2000; 284:1519–1526.

9

Psychotherapeutic Approaches for Prevention and Treatment of Relapse and Recurrence

Edward S. Friedman and Michael E. Thase
Western Psychiatric Institute and Clinic
and University of Pittsburgh Medical Center
Pittsburgh, Pennsylvania, U.S.A.

MAJOR DEPRESSION AND RECURRENCE

Major depressive disorder (MDD) is a recurrent, disabling, and potentially lethal illness with high rates of residual symptoms and persistent psychosocial impairments even among a large percentage of individuals who respond to acute phase therapy. The point prevalence of chronic and recurrent cases of major affective disorder exceeds that for acute, first-episode disorders [1,2]. In the 1970s, Angst and associates [3] and Zis and Goodwin [4] documented the likelihood of relapse and recurrence in the major affective disorders. These findings were prospectively confirmed in a series of studies conducted under the auspices of the National Institute of Mental Health (NIMH) Collaborative Study on the Psychobiology of Depression as summarized by Keller and Hanks [5]. At the least, 50% of those who have experienced one episode of major depression will experience another at some later point. Thus, assuming a lifetime risk for major depression of 5% [6], an individual who has recovered from an initial episode of depression has at least a 10-fold greater risk of having another episode when compared to a person of similar age and sex who has never been clinically depressed. For recurrent (unipolar) major depression and bipolar depression, where recurrence rates of at least 70–90% are expected, the increase in risk for recurrence is 14- to 18-fold when compared with that in the general population [3,5,7–9]. Chronic minor depressions (i.e., dysthymia) have a similarly marked increase in the risk of subsequent major depressive episodes [5].

However, even episodes of depression of such limited duration convey many adverse economic, interpersonal, and medical consequences [5,10–14]. For example, family dysfunction is quite common and may persist after the episode has remitted [12]. Impairment of leisure time and vocational functioning may similarly persist long after resolution of a depressive episode [13,14]. Furthermore, substance abuse, including that of alcohol (ethanol) and hypnosedatives, may develop or worsen during an untreated depressive episode [15,16], and depressed patients are, on average, heavier tobacco users than nondepressed individuals [17]. Thus, for those whose depression remains untreated and who do not remit spontaneously, an ingrained pattern of chronic depression conveys even more negative prognostic implications [5,16].

Consequences of Recurrence

The disability that is associated with suffering from a depressive disorder is well documented. Coryell and colleagues [18] assessed the enduring psychosocial consequences of unipolar depression in 240 patients. These patients were assessed as they sought treatment and across 6 years of follow-up. They reported that at the onset of treatment these patients had deficits in annual income which declined further over the course of follow-up. In addition, over the course of follow-up, these patients experienced declines in job status and other areas of psychosocial functioning. Judd and colleagues [19] subsequently studied psychosocial disability in relation to depressive symptom severity in an expanded study group across 10 years of systematic follow-up. They found that across the decade that the disability associated with unipolar MDD was pervasive and chronic—it affected most areas of everyday function. The investigators also described a continuum of depressive symptom severity ranging from levels of subthreshold depressive symptoms to minor depression or dysthymia to MDD, and that each successive level of greater symptom severity is associated with a significant stepwise increment in psychosocial disability. Keller and Boland [21], also analyzing data from the NIMH Collaborative Depression Study, found that failing to achieve adequate maintenance treatment for unipolar recurrent major depression has psychopathological and psychosocial consequences, decreasing work productivity and the quality of a person's life.

Wells and colleagues [20] examined patients in various types of outpatient treatment as part of the Medical Outcomes Study. This study assessed disability in the areas of physical, social, and role functioning, perceived current health, and bodily pain. They found that the disability associated with the depressive disorders was comparable with or worse than that of eight other major chronic medical illnesses.

The most dire consequence of failing to achieve a sustained remission is suicide. Guze and Robbins [22] estimated the probability of suicide in patients with primary affective disorders at 15%. This finding has been similarly clarified to pertain to the most severe mood disorders [21,23]. Lifetime suicide rates associated with milder depressive episodes are more typically in the 6–8% range. Depression also has been shown to increase the risk of cardiovascular disease and diabetes, as well as to increase the morbidity and mortality associated with a number of illnesses [24–27]. In summary, depressive disorders when incompletely and poorly controlled lead to social and economic disability, morbidity and mortality, and increased biological disturbance. For all these reasons, continuation and maintenance phase treatments are necessary for the completed and successful treatment of depression and the prevention of further episodes of illness.

Psychotherapy and the Treatment and Prevention of Relapse and Recurrence

Current consensus opinion [7,8] on the treatment of depression is represented by the American Psychiatric Association (APA) *Practice Guidelines for the Treatment of Patients with Major Depressive Disorder (Revision)* [7]. These experts have defined the psychiatrist's goal in the treatment of the depressive disorders as effecting improvement of the acute depressive episode and to maintain improvement thereafter. While pharmacotherapy is generally recommended for continuation and maintenance phase treatments, the role of psychotherapy is less clear, but also broadly supported in practice and in contemporary treatment guidelines. The APA Practice Guideline [8] recommends specific and effective psychotherapy alone may be considered as an acute phase treatment modality for patients with mild to moderately severe MDD. This consensus panel also supported the use of psychotherapy during the continuation phase. They recommend that the treatment that was effective in the acute and continuation phase should be used in the maintenance phase as well. This panel highlighted the rarity of studies of combination psychotherapy and pharmacotherapy in the maintenance phase [24–27]; nonetheless, they recommended consideration of such combinations for some patients reflecting the realities of common psychiatric practices [28,29].

Modern, symptom-focused psychotherapies, such as Beck's [30] model of cognitive therapy (CT) and Klerman and Weissman's [31] interpersonal psychotherapy (IPT), have emerged over the past 25 years as alternatives to pharmacotherapy. Although the effectiveness of these time-limited therapies is *generally* comparable to pharmacotherapy after 3–4 months of acute phase treatment [32], the hypothesis that short-term psychotherapy will have a beneficial and enduring impact on the risk of recurrent depression remains largely unproven. Research gathered over the past 20 years, however, has begun to define a role for depression-focused psychotherapy in the treatment and prevention of relapse and recurrence of depression.

Adaptation of the Phases of Treatment Model to the Psychotherapy of Major Depressive Disorder

The conceptualization, rationale, and consensus definitions of terms used to describe the phases in the course of depressive illness were described by Frank and colleagues [33]. This work group examined and operationalized the change points in the course of a depressive episode: response, remission, recovery, relapse, and recurrence. As Figure 1 shows, these definitions correspond to the three phases of treatment. Treatment is defined as consisting of: (1) the *acute phase* during which *remission* of symptoms is induced;

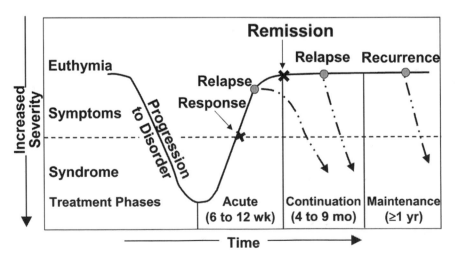

FIGURE 1 Remission is goal of treatment in major depression. (Adapted from Ref. 91, with permission.)

(2) the *continuation phase* during which the state of *remission* is preserved and risk of relapse is minimized; and (3) the *maintenance phase* during which the susceptible patient is treated to prevent a *recurrence* of the depressive disorder. Although these distinctions have not been validated, they represent reasonable working definitions [22]. A clear conceptualization of the course of depressive illness and its treatment provides a framework for a coherent, long-term psychotherapeutic treatment plan [34,35].

Acute Treatment

The acute phase of treatment begins with the selection of a strategy. The treatment modality first chosen for a depressive episode is generally predetermined by the patient's choice of mental health providers. For example, depressed persons treated by family practitioners are likely to receive pharmacotherapy, whereas the clients of psychologists, social workers, and other therapists are almost certain to receive counseling or psychotherapy [36]. At present, most psychiatrists prefer to use a combination of both modalities [29,36,37]. Identifying better means of matching patients with potentially effective treatments would be preferred.

The term *treatment response* is used to categorize the initial therapeutic goal for depressed patients. In addition to the specific effects of an active treatment, response encompasses both spontaneous remissions of symptoms and placebo responses. A response generally corresponds to at least 40–60% reduction of symptoms [38]. This is often achieved within 3–6 weeks after the initiation of antidepressant pharmacotherapy. In controlled studies of mild to moderately depressed outpatients, specified, time-limited psychotherapies [30,31] appear to achieve results comparable with those of tricyclic antidepressants when given over 12–16 weeks [32,39]. With either type of treatment, however, failure to achieve an adequate treatment response after a trial of appropriate duration (e.g., 6–8 weeks for pharmacotherpy and 12–16 weeks for psychotherapy) is considered nonresponse. The Texas Medication Algorithm Project [40], for example, presents evidence-based treatment strategies for the pharmacotherapy of depression at the end of the acute phase and other change points across the phases of treatment. These investigators describe reasonable strategies for the switching or augmentation of medication. No such algorithms exist to recommend the sequencing, intensity, and duration for the psychotherapies.

Continuation Therapy

The acute phase of therapy ends and continuation therapy begins when a patient has achieved a significant response to treatment. Ideally, this should be a full remission of the depressive episode to a level of symptoms so low that the patient would be indistinguishable from someone who had never been depressed. The term *remission* does not (in this instance) convey a resolution of the underlying illness pathophysiology.

During continuation pharmacotherapy, medication dosage typically remains constant and visits to the clinician become less frequent. It is worth noting that the concept and definitions of these change points in the course of treatment of a depressive episode were formulated with regard to pharmacotherapy [41–43]. Later, the concept was expanded by Frank and colleagues [33] to conceptualize psychotherapeutic response across the phases of treatment. Jarrett and Kraft [34] modified cognitive behavior therapy (CBT) to conceptualize and monitor the change points in the course of treatment as fundamental decision points for changes in psychotherapy treatment planning. (We will more fully describe these ideas below.) The goals of continuation phase psychotherapy, which are (1) prevention of relapse and (2) conversion of a response into a remission [10], are equally true for the psychotherapies as for psychopharmacotherapy. Remission is defined by a substantial reduction of symptoms and a return to a level of functioning equal to the patient's premorbid state [10,33]. A patient who achieves a stable remission for at least 4–6 months may be said to have recovered from the index depressive episode [33]. Relapse is defined as an increase of depressive symptoms back to a syndromal level at any point between the initial treatment response and the end of continuation therapy [10,33]. Reviews of empirical studies of pharmacological treatments indicate that the risk of relapse is particularly high if an antidepressant is discontinued within the first 4 months of achieving response, with relapse rates typically ranging from 40 to 60% [10,43,44]. By contrast, relapse rates of only 10–20% are observed during continuation pharmacotherapy [10,43,44]. In our experience at the University of Pittsburgh [10], a relapse rate of only 5% was observed over a 4-month period of continued pharmacotherapy with a maximum dose of antidepressant in combination with IPT [10].

Risk factors for relapse include medication noncompliance and nonadherence; severity of the index depressive episode; the presence of persistent residual (subsyndromal) depressive symptoms; severe personality pathology; older age; high levels of dysfunctional attitudes; poor social support; and ongoing or renewed psychosocial stressors [10,45–48]. Patients who do not achieve stable remissions during continuation treatment represent a particularly high-risk group [10]. The presence of residual symptoms conveys increased risk of relapse despite continuation therapy, suggesting the need for more vigorous treatment and/or the adjunctive use of pharmacotherapy and psychotherapy [49]. Conventionally, continuation therapy ends when the patient meets the criteria for recovery (i.e., after 4–6 months of sustained euthymia) [10,33]. A recovery is presumed to represent a qualitatively distinct state when compared with remission. For example, it is hypothesized that the psychobiological correlates of the acute depressive state become quiescent during recovery [10]. A recurrent or renewed period of depressive symptoms following recovery is thus conceptualized as the onset of a distinctly new episode of affective illness. However, because 10–15% of apparently recovered patients have recurrences within the first 8 weeks of discontinuing antidepressant medication [50], it appears that time alone may not provide an adequate definition of recovery.

Maintenance Therapy

Maintenance pharmacotherapy is recommended [7,8] after continuation therapy for all patients at a high risk of recurrence. The characteristics of such patients include a history of recurrent episodes of depression [35,51]. This is especially true for patients who have experienced multiple episodes of depression within 2 or 3 years prior to the onset of the index episode [50,52]. Other risk factors for recurrent depression include both early and late onset of depression (i.e., before age 25 or after age 60 years), chronicity, gender (i.e., rates may be higher in women), severity of the index episode, a seasonal pattern of mood disturbance, and a family history of affective disorder [35]. The need for maintenance therapy is illustrated by the findings from studies of patients with highly recurrent unipolar depression. In one study, an 85% recurrence rate was observed within 3 years after the withdrawal of imipramine [53]. Conversely, 80% of patients receiving maintenance pharmacotherapy remained well. Most other studies have also documented a superior outcome for patients receiving active maintenance therapy, although the magnitude of the drug-placebo differences is generally smaller [35,51]. The higher recurrence rates observed in earlier studies may have been attributable to the use of lower dosages of maintenance pharmacotherapy. While a modest body of empirical evidence exists to support the popular strategy of combining psychotherapeutic and pharmacological approaches during acute treatment of affective disorders [54], strong empirical justification for the routine combination of these forms of therapy as maintenance treatment strategies is lacking [29]. Similarly, the efficacy of psychotherapy alone as a maintenance treatment has not been definitely established.

REVIEW OF STUDIES OF THE PSYCHOTHERAPEUTIC APPROACHES FOR PREVENTION OF RELAPSE AND RECURRENCE

Interpersonal Psychotherapy

Only three studies have addressed the efficacy of IPT as continuation [55] or maintenance treatments [53,56]. In a study of continuation therapy [55], 150 depressed women who responded to acute phase pharmacotherapy with amitriptyline were subsequently randomized to one of four treatment strategies: (1) individual IPT, (2) placebo pharmacotherapy, (3) maintenance amitriptyline, or (4) a combination of psychotherapy and pharmacotherapy. No additional prophylaxis was conferred by combined psychotherapy and pharmacotherapy when compared with amitriptyline only. Moreover, the relapse risk of those withdrawn from pharmacotherapy and treated only with psychotherapy was not significantly different from that of the group treated with only placebo [55]. There was, however, evidence of improved interpersonal functioning in the women who were treated with psychotherapy and who remained well [57]. In the second study, Frank and associates [53] found that a systematized form of maintenance IPT (IPT-M), provided on a monthly basis following an initial course of weekly sessions (in combination with pharmacotherapy), was significantly more effective than placebo in preventing recurrence. However, IPT-M was significantly less effective than maintenance imipramine pharmacotherapy [53]. Furthermore, patients randomly assigned to receive the combination of IPT-M and imipramine did not show significantly superior prophylaxis when compared with those receiving pharmacotherapy alone (Fig. 2) [53].

In the third study, Reynolds and colleagues [56] found that the combination of nortriptyline and monthly IPT had an additive benefit (relative to the monotherapies) in preventing recurrent depression among an older

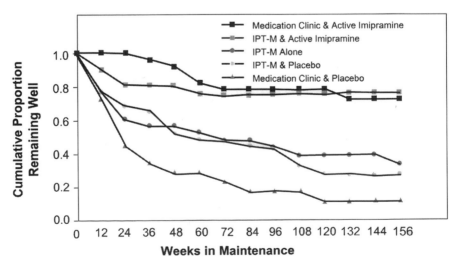

FIGURE 2   Maintenance therapy of recurrent (unipolar) depression. (From Ref. 53.)

sample. Both monotherapies were superior to the placebo control group, and nortriptyline alone and IPT-M alone did not differ significantly. The prophylactic success of IPT-M was found to be linked to the quality of the therapeutic relationship [58,59]. Specifically, those patients who participated in high-quality therapy (i.e., defined by above-average scores on a measure that assessed the quality of therapy) were at significantly lower risk of relapse than patients whose therapy scores were below the mean on this measure. In fact, recurrence rates for those patients undergoing high-quality therapy did not differ from those who received pharmacotherapy until the third year of the study. In contrast, the fate of the patients in the low-quality therapy group was virtually identical to that of patients treated with placebo alone. In a subsequent report, Spaner and associates [59] found that higher quality IPT actually partially offset the increased recurrence risk associated with electroencephalographic (EEG) sleep disturbance. Thus, IPT-M was either a potent prophylactic therapy or was ineffective, depending on the fidelity of the therapy. It remains to be seen if more frequent psychotherapeutic contact enhances the efficacy of IPT-M. A study by Frank and colleagues is currently underway at the University of Pittsburgh to determine if continued weekly or twice-monthly psychotherapeutic contact is superior to monthly sessions of therapy.

Cognitive Therapy and the Treatment and Prevention of Relapse and Recurrence

Cognitive therapy (CT) [30] has received the most extensive empirical evaluation of the newer psychotherapies, and overall, the efficacy of CT in acute phase treatment is comparable to pharmacotherapy [60,61]. Although CT has demonstrated a poorer response in severe depression in some studies [62,63], that finding has not been observed by others [64,65]. CT treats depression through a combination of symptom reduction and the learning of new and better adaptive strategies. The patient is taught to overcome behavioral inactivation, to identify and alter their negative automatic thoughts, and in so doing gain greater emotional stability. As a result, the individual learns to monitor their perceptions about their interactions and behaviors. Thus, some have speculated that CT could have a prophylactic effect on relapse and recurrence [30,66]. Some studies support this supposition. Kovacs and associates [67] reported a 1-year naturalistic follow-up of patients who responded to acute phase CT or imipramine. The CT patients had lower levels of self-rated depression at the end of 1 year.

There are several studies that have compared the long-term outcome of patients who have responded to acute phase CT with the outcome of patients who responded to acute phase pharmacotherapy and whose antidepressant medications were withdrawn at the end of the acute phase. Shea and colleagues [68] presented findings from the NIMH Treatment of Depression Collaborative Research Program on the course of depressive symptoms during an 18-month naturalistic follow-up period. In this study, patients with MDD were treated in a 16-week acute phase with one of four treatments: CT, IPT, imipramine hydrochloride (IMI) plus clinical management (CM), or placebo and CM. Follow-up assessments were conducted at 6, 12, and 18 months of treatment. Of all the patients who entered treatment and who participated in the follow-up phase, the percentage who recovered (defined by the investigators as 8 weeks of minimal or no symptoms following the end of acute phase treatment) and remained well during the follow-up phase did not differ significantly among the four treatments: 20% for the CT group; 26% for the IPT group; 19% in the IMI + CM group; and 20% for the placebo + CM group. Shea et al. also reported the rates of relapse among patients who had recovered: 36% for the CT group; 33% for the IPT group; 50% for the IMI + CM group; and 33% in the CM group. Their overall conclusion was that 16 weeks of any of these specific forms of therapy were insufficient for most patients to achieve a full recovery and a lasting remission. They also argue for improving strategies for continuation and maintenance treatments.

Our group [52] studied 50 patients with major depression who responded during a 16- to 20-week course of CT for a 1-year prospective follow-up. We defined relapse as, at minimum, a 2-week period in which the subject met the Diagnostic and Statistical Manual of Mental Illness, Revised (DMS-III-R) criteria for MDD and a Hamilton depression scale score of 15 more. We found that 32% of patients relapsed during the 1-year follow-up phase. Correlates of relapse included a history of depressive episodes (recurrence), higher levels of depressive symptoms and dysfunctional attitudes, slower response to therapy, and unmarried status. We found that patients who had a full recovery during the acute phase treatment (a Hamilton depression score of 6 or less for 8 weeks or more) were at significantly lower risk for relapse than those patients who were partially recovered (9 and 52%, respectively) (Fig. 3). The factors of being slower to respond, unmarried status, and high residual scores on the Dysfunctional Attitudes Scale were independently and additively related to increased risk of relapse. We concluded that there is a relation between the persistence of residual symptoms and the risk of relapse after the cessation of active treatment. This evidence lead us to recommend that models of longer term psychotherapy need to be developed for depressed patients who do not fully recover during time-limited, acute phase, CT.

Evans and associates [69] attempted to determine whether CT prevents relapse after successful acute phase treatment. Patients were randomly assigned to 12 weeks of treatment with an experienced cognitive therapist

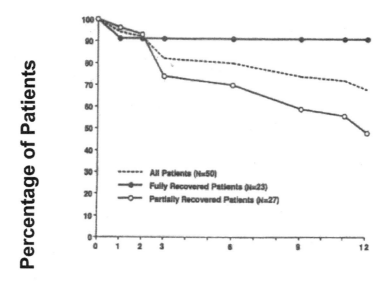

Months of Follow-up

FIGURE 3   Survival curves of time to relapse after termination of cognitive be-havior therapy for depressed patient. Significant difference between fully recov-ered and partially recovered patients (Wilcoxon $x' = 10.63$, $df = 1$, $p = 0.004$).

and/or pharmacotherapist. Treatment conditions included imipramine phar-macotherapy, with posttreatment continuation; imipramine pharmacother-apy without posttreatment continuation; CBT; and combined CBT and pharmacotherapy. Medications were tapered and discontinued in the medi-cation–no continuation condition and in the combined treatment condition at the end of the 12-week acute treatment phase. CT was terminated at the end of the acute treatment phase (i.e., after 12 weeks) for all responders in the CBT condition and in the combined treatment condition. After 12 months of follow-up, the medication of those in the medication continuation group was tapered and discontinued. In reporting on the acute phase of the protocol [70], Evans et al. concluded that CT and pharmacotherapy did not differ in terms of their effect on symptomatic response; initial severity did predict response with pharmacotherapy alone but not with CBT; and combination therapy did not markedly improve response over that observed for monotherapy alone. During the 2 years of posttreatment follow-up phase, monthly contacts were maintained and patients were reevaluated every 6 months or at the time relapse occurred (as measured by two consecutive BDI scores of ≥16 over a

2-week period). Because Evans et al. were unable to discern a difference between the two CT conditions, they were combined in the analyses. They concluded that CBT, alone or in combination with medication, appears to prevent relapse after treatment termination. They report that CBT was at least as effective in preventing relapse as continuation medication, the current standard of care. The combination of CBT and pharmacotherapy was not superior to CBT alone. Evans et al. interpret this as suggesting that adding pharmacotherapy to CBT does not interfere with its preventive effects and that combined therapy may maximize both acute response and relapse prevention. However, the investigators do note that the duration of their study may have been too brief to determine if this preventive effect also applies to the prevention of recurrence of major depression.

Blackburn and colleagues [66] naturalistically followed a group of inpatients and outpatients with major unipolar depression who responded to acute phase CT, pharmacotherapy, or combination treatment. This study showed a clear advantage in favor of the prophylactic effect of CT. At 6 months, significantly more patients in the drug group relapsed versus the CT group and the combination group. This pattern was consistent throughout the 2 years of follow-up. Blackburn and Moore [64] performed a randomized, controlled trial of CT and antidepressants in acute and maintenance treatment. Seventy-five outpatients with major unipolar depression were randomized to 16 weeks of acute treatment with (1) antidepressants and maintenance antidepressants, (2) CT and maintenance CT, and (3) antidepressants and maintenance CT (which consisted of three weekly sessions in the first month, two sessions in the second month, and once a month thereafter). In the acute phase of treatment, all patients improved significantly, and there was no difference among treatments or in the pattern of improvement over time. In the maintenance phase, patients kept improving over time in all three groups, and there was no significant difference among treatments. Blackburn et al. concluded that maintenance CT has a similar prophylactic effect to maintenance medication.

Fava and colleagues [49] present another strategy for addressing the risk of relapse and recurrence following successful treatment of MDD. Unlike the acute-continuation-maintenance model, they have adopted a two-stage, sequential, intensive approach focusing on residual symptoms of MDD. Fava and Kellner [71] suggest that residual symptoms of MDD may progress to become prodromal symptoms of relapse. This group studied [49,72] 40 patients with MDD who had been successfully treated with antidepressant drugs. Patients were randomized to CBT focused on residual symptoms and healthy lifestyle or standard CM for an additional 10 biweekly sessions. In both cells, the antidepressant drugs were gradually tapered and discontinued. The CBT group had a significantly lower level of residual symptoms after discontinuation of medication therapy than did the CM group. CT treatment also resulted in a significantly lower rate of relapse (35%) at 4-year follow-up than did CM (70%). After 6 years, Fava et al. [72] found that the protective effects of CT that were evident at the 4-year follow-up faded. In another population of recurrent MDD patients, however, Fava and associates [74] similarly found that 20 weeks of continuation phase CT, focusing on residual symptoms, resulted in a lower relapse rate (25%) than did CM (80%) at the end of 2-year follow-up. They challenge the assumption that long-term drug treatment is the only tool to prevent relapse in patients with recurrent depression. CT modified for continuation and maintenance treatment may offer an alternative to pharmacotherapy for some patients. As Teasdale and associates [77] noted, the the possibility of (1) capitalizing on the cost efficiency of antidepressant medication to reduce acute symptomology while (2) avoiding the need for patients to remain indefinitely on maintenance medication to reduce future relapse and recurrence. This group [77] similarly found that a modified form of CT, provided in eight group sessions, significantly reduced the risk of recurrent depression from 66 to 40% in a 60-month follow-up study of 145 pharmacotherapy responders who had already discontinued medication. Therefore, it appears that a relatively short course of focused CT provides a useful way to offset the risk of recurrent illness following medication withdrawal.

Blackburn and Moore [64] and Paykel and associates [75] largely replicated these finding using Beck's model of CT. In the study of Paykel and associates [75], 18 sessions of CT reduced the risk of relapse from 36 to 22% in a group of 158 partially remitted patients receiving maintenance pharmacotherapy. Jarrett and colleagues [76] also report findings consistent with the hypothesis that continuation phase CT helps patients achieve and maintain long-term remission of depressive symptoms. The rate of relapse or recurrence was determined in two sequential pilot studies of MDD patients treated with CT in the acute phase (A-CT). Seventy-six percent of 49 patients responded to acute CT and were eligible for follow-up. Thirty patients completed the continuation-CT (C-CT) phase, which consisted of four sessions over the first 2 months and 6 monthly sessions thereafter. The relapse rate in patients who responded to A-CT was 40% at 6 months, 45% at 8 months, 50% at 12 months, and 74% at 24 months. The relapse rate in patients who completed C-CT was 20% at 6 months, 27% at 12 months, and 36% at 18 months and 24 months after A-CT. The investigators suggest that C-CT can reduce depressive relapse or recurrence.

Approaching the problem of who really needs continuation and maintenance treatment our group has focused on patients who responded to acute CT. We have found that most patients who remit fully during the acute phase do not require further treatment. Such patients have only a 10–20% risk of relapse/recurrence in the year following therapy. This effect is comparable to the benefit of continuation phase pharmacotherapy for antidepressant responders [43]. We have found that patients who obtain slower or less complete remissions during acute phase CT have a 40–60% risk of relapse within 12 months of terminating therapy. Such patients are at about the same risk of relapse as patients abruptly withdrawn from medication after acute phase therapy [43]. This high risk of relapse is reduced significantly by providing 10 sessions of continuous phase CT. Continuous phase CT lowers the risk of relapse to a level comparable to that of patients who achieved a full and complete remission within the first 8 weeks of acute phase CT.

MODEL OF CT ADAPTED FOR THE TREATMENT AND PREVENTION OF RELAPSE AND RECURRENCE

Cognitive and behavioral models of relapse prevention are based on the premise that patients can learn new ways of coping in response to various challenges [34,78,79]. During A-CT, patients learn certain skills (e.g., self-monitoring, logical analysis, and hypothesis testing) to restructure attitudes about self, world, and future and to shift attributional styles toward more flexible and specific explanations. The theoretical foundation of CT draws heavily on learning theory by emphasizing behavioral strategies to promote acquiring, generalizing, and maintaining coping responses [80]. CT also incorporates social learning theory [81] by using in vivo strategies such as behavior rehearsal and guided practice, aiming for subjective mastery of coping responses (i.e., self-efficacy). From these perspectives, an incomplete remission may simply reflect an idiosyncratic difference in the higher risk patient's learning curve, which can be remedied by a longer course of therapy.

Cognitive theories of depressive vulnerability also posit that dysfunctional core beliefs or schema in critical areas pertaining to approval, achievement, loss, and romantic attachment mediate the risk of symptom exacerbation in response to relevant or matching stressors. Such cognitive diatheses may be "silent" during better times, but can be deduced from the themes reflected in the person's thoughts and statements during times of affective distress. From this perspective, an incomplete remission may reflect persistent cognitive vulnerability. The therapeutic implication is that additional sessions of therapy would provide the opportunity to reduce long-term risk by focusing on revising depressogenic attributional styles or dysfunctional attitudes. Pharmacotherapy, on the other hand, would reduce the vulnerability by dampening excessive emotional responses to negative cognitions within limbic-cortical circuits [82]. Consistent with this view, Segal and associates [83] found that patients who responded to CT experienced fewer negative cognitions during dysphoric mood induction when compared to patients who responded to antidepressants. This supports the hypothesis that C-CT specifically reduces the risk of recurrent depression by targeting dysfunctional attitudes and beliefs and cognitive-affective reactivity.

It is also possible that C-CT has a symptom-suppressing effect akin to pharmacotherapy but no long-term benefit. This view posits that depressed patients at high risk for recurrent episodes have more persistent and dys-regulated affective responses that are either inherited or acquired via sensitization of neurohormonal responses to stress (e.g., "kindling") [84]. If true, C-CT and medication may both have protective effects when treatment is being received, but the risk of relapse will not be reduced after treatment is withdrawn. Our group [85,86] has found some evidence of persistent risk in a study of 90 patients treated with 16 weeks of CT. We found that post-treatment sleep profiles of nearly 50% of CT responders remained abnormal and, even among patients who fully recovered, an abnormal sleep profile was associated with an increased risk of recurrent depression during a 24-month controlled follow-up period.

Jarrett and Kraft [34] have defined theoretical principles to guide practice during continuation and maintenance CT (C/M-CT). *Cognitive therapists treat and teach* is the first principle. This underscores the dual goals of CT: symptom reduction and symptom prevention. The focus of acute phase CT is to reduce depressive symptom severity. This focus is continued and amplified in C/M-CT with the further goal of symptom elimination and the prevention of the return of symptoms. The means of accomplishing prevention is teaching of critical skills to reduce and prevent depressive symptoms or decrease the conditions that foster recurrence. The second principle is that *C/M-CT is not simply the acute phase made longer*: The goal is to promote and maintain complete recovery. The basic theories of CT guide the therapist in identifying the patient's cognitive and emotional vulnerabilities and learning theory guides the therapist in teaching the patient new behaviors and skills. The teaching is directed at the patient's identified vulnerabilities and at the vulnerabilities that are a consequence of living with a recurrent and sometimes chronic, illness. CT theory recommends that patients explore and analyze their view of themselves, the world, and their future; this is equally important in C/M-CT. The major teaching goal of C/M-CT is to generalize the skills the patient acquired during acute phase CT. The goal is to identify and match the critical skills the patient must learn with characteristics of the patient and their environment that promote or impede learning or the generalization of skills. The desired consequence of the generalization of skills is evidence that the patient is successfully using these skills in highly emotionally laden situations that previously lead to depressive episodes. Over time, continued evidence that the acquired skills are being used and that the patient independently applies them to novel circumstances constitutes relapse prevention. Further, it is assumed that the likelihood of relapse and recurrence is increased when the patient (1) incompletely learns critical CT skills, (2) ceases to use learned skills, and/ or (3) confronts situations which activate depressive assumptions that have not been adequately restructured. The clinical goal of acute phase CT is to achieve a remission of symptoms, which is the foundation for a complete and sustained recovery—the goal of C/M-CT.

The third principle states that *CT therapists use data to make clinical decisions*. The psychoeducation of the patient on the characteristics of continuation and maintenance phases of depressive illnesses and the use of self-rating instruments help the therapist and patient to monitor symptomatic recurrence. The ongoing assessment process guides the content of therapy and the application of therapeutic strategies. C/M-CT builds upon the CT skills learned in acute phase CT: (1) understanding the relationship between cognitions, moods, and behavior; (2) observing and identifying the interplay of these factors in episodes derived from their day-to-day lives; and (3) challenging the accuracy of distorted thoughts and the benefit of dysfunctional attitudes. C/M-CT, in addition, focuses on (1) identifying the patient's schemas that underly and organize their distorted, often negative, thoughts; (2) restructuring schema through logical analysis; (3) using experimentation and empiricism to test alternative rules, beliefs, and schemas; (4) using these skills to make behavioral changes associated with long-term positive outcomes; and (5) teaching of remedial skills not mastered during the acute phase.

The fourth principle states that *the use of* coping skills must be clearly demonstrated before encouraging the patient to use them in novel ways or situations. Patients can demonstrate their mastery of these skills by demonstrating comprehension, role playing with the therapist, successful homework completion, and using the skills in everyday situations. This leads to the fifth principle, which states during C/M-CT that *the therapist encourages the generalization of critical cognitive therapy skills*. This is accomplished through the reduction in the frequency of sessions, causing the patients to rely on themselves to utilize their skills in between sessions. The therapist gradually turns the control of the session over to the patient, uses fewer prompts, has the patient set the agenda, and uses Socratic questioning to guide discovery of unresolved issues. Using the "collaborative empiricism" model, the therapist and patient identify any factors (biological, cognitive, behavioral, interpersonal, or situational) that would promote or impede the use of critical skills. The therapist helps patients identify their therapeutic strengths and weaknesses. If symptoms return, the therapist and patient review the patient's personal risk factors for relapse and address the identified vulnerabilities. Brief episodes of subsyndromal symptoms—"blips"—are distinguished from actual recurrences of MDD, and patients learn to endure such episodes with less hopelessness, anxiety, and dread.

The sixth principle is *stress inoculation is a primary intervention used to maintain therapeutic gains and to prevent relapse/recurrence*. Through "stress inoculation," the therapist challenges the patient's reactions to premorbid stressors through the use of imaginal techniques, bibliotherapy, role play, and homework assignments. The patient rehearses different possible reactions to these stressors choosing a strategy that they have logically identified, reviewed the utility and possible outcomes of, and are willing to accept as "good enough" out of the available options. Those cognitions, behaviors, and situations that were associated with the onset of the depressive episode highlight areas of future vulnerability, and hence the content of stress inoculation.

Finally, Jarrett and Kraft [34] reinforce a core CT technique; principle seven reminds the therapist that *termination begins at the first acute phase session and is emphasized throughout C/M-CT*. Termination is the logical end of the generalization of skills process, the final transfer of the therapeutic locus of control to the patient, and an endpoint to the learning phase, the patient's graduation to autonomy.

Our group, in conjunction with Jarrett's group in Texas, have incorporated these principles into a self-rated therapist checklist that we are employing in our current study of relapse prevention using C/M-CT. The checklist is entitled "Generalizing Skills to Prevent Recurrent Depression" (Table 1). This checklist helps the therapist attend to the core techniques of C/M-CT as demonstrated in or reported during a C/M-CT session.

TABLE 1 Generalizing Skills to Prevent Recurrent Depression

Check off each of the following as they are reported or demonstrated in a session:
____ Early warning signs identified and discussed?
____ Adaptive skills identified and being used?
____ Depressive beliefs being spotted?
____ Depressive beliefs being tested?
____ Thought logs being used for mood shifts an recording facts reviewed?
____ Risks ahead to stability of mood being spotted and discussed?
____ Tracking what promotes positive mood shifts?

Source: UPMC: Relapse Prevention Study; Continuation Phase Checklist. Kornblith, Friedman, Jarrett, and Thase.

MAJOR METHODOLOGICAL ISSUES IN
PSYCHOTHERAPY STUDIES

There are a dozen or so studies that comprise the literature on the psycho-therapeutic treatment and prevention of relapse and recurrence. The phases of treatment (acute-continuation-maintenance phases) and the sequential treatment of residual symptom models present strategies for defining and conceptualizing relapse, recurrence, and health maintenance for patients suffering from MDD. And taking these studies in sum, many methodological issues make it difficult to draw definitive conclusions about the utility of continuation and maintenance psychotherapies.

Many basic issues are not controlled in these studies, such as the adequacy of sample sizes; cohort differences such as gender, socioeconomic, and racial representation in these samples; diagnostic reliability and validity between different study cohorts; and varying inclusion and exclusion criteria. Psychotherapy studies can be biased by investigator affiliation [87], lack of the equivalent of a pill/placebo control [88], and the interaction between patient characteristics and therapist characteristics [89,90], including the lack of control of therapist competence. Despite the stated allegiance to a therapeutic model in these studies, issues of treatment integrity and treatment drift from the manualized therapy remains problematic. Furthermore, the larger issue of whether it is the stated active factors of the depression specific psychotherapies or nonspecific factors common to the psychotherapeutic process (such as the strength and efficacy of the patient-therapist dyad) [89,90] that effect change is poorly understood. Further study is needed to determine which components of the depression-specific psychotherapies are responsible for efficacy of these treatments.

Other areas for further study include the indications for various forms of therapy—can we adapt the depression-specific psychotherapies to appropriate depressive subtypes or associated risk factors. It remains to be determined what are the optimal parameters for psychotherapeutic treatment, for example, the optimal frequencies of contacts in the acute, continuation, and maintenance phases of treatment. We can only speculate on the proper duration of maintenance phase treatment, and follow-up studies are needed to clarify long-term effects of treatment.

ACKNOWLEDGMENTS

This research was supported by grants MHIRC MH30915, MH-41884, and MH-58356 from the National Institute of Mental Health. We wish to thank Janice Jozefov and Christine Johnson for their assistance in preparation of this manuscript.

REFERENCES

1. Weissman MM, Leaf PJ, Tischler GL, Blazer DG, Karno M, Bruce ML, Florio LP. Affective disorders in five United States communities. Psychol Med 1983; 18:141–153.
2. Weissman MM, Leaf PJ, Bruce ML, Florio L. The epidemiology of dysthymia in five communities: rates, risks, comorbidity, and treatment. Am J Psychiatry 1988; 145:815–819.
3. Angst J, Baastrup P, Grof P, Hippius H, Poldinger W, Weis P. The course of monopolar depression and bipolar psychoses. Psychiatr Neurol Neurochirurgia 1973; 76:489–500.
4. Zis AP, Goodwin FK. Major affective disorder as a recurrent illness: A critical review. Arch Gen Psychiatry 1979; 36:835–839.
5. Keller MB, Hanks DL. The natural history and heterogeneity of depressive disorders: Implications for rational antidepressant therapy. J Clin Psychiatry 1994; 55(suppl 9):25–31.
6. Robins LN, Holzer JE, Weissman MM, Orvaschel H. Lifetime prevalence of specific psychiatric disorders in 3 sites. Arch Gen Psychiatry 1984; 41:949–958.
7. Consensus Development Panel. Mood disorders: pharmacologic prevention of recurrences [NIMH/NIH Consensus Development Conference Statement]. Am J Psychiatry 1985; 142:469–476.
8. Consensus statement: WHO mental health collaborating centers. J Affect Disord 1989; 17:197–198.
9. Goodwin KF, Jamison KR. Manic-Depressive Illness. New York. Oxford University Press, 1990.
10. Thase ME. Relapse and recurrence in unipolar major depression: short-term and long-term approaches. J Clin Psychiatry 1990; 51(suppl 6):51–57.
11. Barnett PA, Gotlib IA. Psychosocial functioning and depression: Distinguishing among antecedents, concomitants, and consequences. Psychol Bull 1988; 104:97–126.
12. Keitner GI, Miller IW. Family functioning and major depression: an overview. Am J Psychiatry 1990; 147:1128–1137.
13. Bauwens F, Tracy A, Pardoen D, Elst MV, Mendlewicz J. Social adjustment of remitted bipolar and unipolar outpatients: A comparison with age- and sex-matched controls. Br J Psychiatry 1991; 159:239–244.
14. Perugi G, Maremmani I, McNair D, Cassano GB, Akiskal HS. Differential changes in areas of social adjustment from depressive episodes through recovery. J Affect Disord 1988; 15:39–43.
15. Buydens-Branchey L, Branchey MG, Noumair D. Age of alcoholism onset. I: Relationship to psychopathology. Arch Gen Psychiatry 1989; 46:225–230.
16. Akiskal HS. Factors associated with incomplete recovery in primary depressive illness. J Clin Psychiatry 1982; 43:266–271.
17. Bresalau N, Kilbey MM, Andreski P. Nicotine dependence, major depression, and anxiety in young adults. Arch Gen Psychiatry 1991; 48:1069–1074.
18. Coryell W, Scheftner W, Keller M, Endicott J, Masur J, Klerman GL. The enduring psychosocial consequences of mania and depression. Am J Psychiatry 1993; 150:720–727.

19. Judd LL, Akiskal HS, Zeller PJ, Paulus M, Leon AC, Mase JD, Endicott J, Coryell W, Kunovac JL, Mueller TI, Rice JP, Keller M. Psychosocial disability during the long-term course of unipolar major depressive disorder. Arch Gen Psychiatry 2000; 57:375–380.

20. Wells KB, Steward A, Hays RD, Berman A, Rogers W, Daniels M, Berry S, Greenfield S, Ware J. The functioning and well-being of depressed patients: Results of the medical outcomes study. JAMA 1989; 262:914–919.

21. Keller MB, Boland RJ. Implications of failing to achieve long-term maintenance treatment of recurrent unipolar major depression. Biol Psychiatry 1998; 44(suppl 5):348–360.

22. Guze SB, Robins E. Suicide and primary affective disorders. Br J Psychiatry 1970; 117:437–438.

23. Robins LN, Kulbok PA. Epidemiologic studies in suicide. In: Frances AJ, Hales RE, ed. Review of Psychiatry. Vol 7. Washington, DC: American Psychiatric Press, 1988:289–306.

24. Frank E, Anderson B, Reynolds CF, Ritenour A, Kupfer DJ. Life events and the research diagnostic criteria endogenous subtype: a confirmation of the distinction using the Bedford College methods. Arch Gen Psychiatry 1994; 51: 519–524.

25. Meedor-Woodruff JH, Gurguis G, Grunhaus L, Haskett RF, Greden JF. Multiple episodes and plasma postdexamethasone cortisol levels. Biol Psychiatry 1987; 22:583–592.

26. Thase ME, Kupfer DJ, Buysse DJ, Frank E, Simons AD, McEachran AB, Rashid KF, Grochocinski VJ. Electroencephalographic sleep profiles in single-episode and recurrent unipolar forms of major depression: 1. Comparison during acute depressive states. Biol Psychiatry 1995; 38:506–515.

27. Thase ME, Kupfer DJ. Recent developments in the pharmacotherapy of mood disorders. J Consult Clin Psychol 1996; 64(suppl 4):1–14.

28. Karasu TB. Psychotherapy and Pharmacotherapy: toward an integrative model. Am J Psychiatry 1982; 139:1102–1113.

29. Friedman ES. Combined therapy for depression. J Pract Psychiatry Behav Health July 1997; 3:211–222.

30. Beck AT, Rush AJ, Shaw BG, Emery G. Cognitive Therapy of Depression. New York: Guilford Press, 1979.

31. Klerman GL, Weissman MM, Rounsaville BJ, Chevron ES. Interpersonal Psychotherapy of Depression. New York: Basic Books, 1984.

32. Dobson KS. A meta-analysis of the efficacy of cognitive therapy for depression. J Consult Clin Psychol 1989; 57:414–419.

33. Frank E, Prien RF, Jarrett RB, Keller MB, Kupfer DJ, Lavori P, Rush AJ, Weissman MM. Conceptualization and rationale for consensus definitions of terms in major depressive disorder: Remission, recovery, relapse, and recurrence. Arch Gen Psychiatry 1991; 48:851–855.

34. Jarrett RB, Kraft D. Prophylactic cognitive therapy for major depressive disorder. In Session: Psychotherapy in Practice 1997; 3:65–79.

35. Thase ME. Long-term treatments of recurrent depressive disorders. J Clin Psychiatry 1992; 53(suppl):33–44.

36. Orleans CT, George LK, Houpt JH, Brodie HKH. How primary care physicians treat psychiatric disorders: A national survey of family practitioners. Am J Psychiatry 1985; 142:52–57.
37. Karasu TB. Psychotherapy and pharmacotherapy: toward an integrative model. Am J Psychiatry 1982; 139:1102–1113.
38. Prien RF, Carpenter LL, Kupfer DJ. The definition and operational criteria for treatment outcome of major depressive disorder: a review of the current research literature. Arch Gen Psychiatry 1991; 48:796–800.
39. Robinson LA, Berman JS, Neimer RA. Psychotherapy for treatment of depression: A review of the controlled outcome research. Psychol Bull 1990; 108:30–49.
40. Crismon ML, Trivedi M, Pigott TA, Rush JA, Hirschfeld RMA, Kahn DA, DeBattista C, Nelson JC, Nierenberg AA, Sackeim HA, Thase ME, The Texas Consensus Conference Panel on Medication Treatment of Major Depressive Disorder. The Texas medication algorithm project: Report of the Texas consensus conference panel on medication treatment of major depressive disorder. J Clin Psychiatry 1999; 60(suppl 3):142–156.
41. Quitkin FM, Rabkin JG, Stewart JW, McGarth PJ, Harrison W. Study duration in antidepressant research: Advantage of a 12-week trial. J Psychiatr Res 1986; 20:211–216.
42. Prien RF, Kupfer DJ, Mansky PA, Small JG, Tuason VB, Voss CB, Johnson WE. Research and methodological issues for evaluating the therapeutic effectiveness of antidepressant drugs. Psychopharmacol Bull 1984; 20:250–257.
43. Prien RF, Kupfer DJ. Continuation drug therapy for major depressive episodes: How long should it be maintained? Am J Psychiatry 1986; 143:18–23.
44. Montgomery SA, Doogan DP, Burnside R. The influence of different relapse criteria on the assessment of long-term efficacy of sertraline. Int Clin Psychopharmacol Dec 1991; 6(suppl 2):37–46.
45. Belsher G, Costello CG. Relapse after recovery from unipolar depression: A critical review. Psychol Bull 1988; 104:84–96.
46. Faravelli C, Ambonetti A, Pallanti S, Pazzagli A. Depressive relapses and incomplete recovery from index episode. Am J Psychiatry 1986; 143:888–891.
47. Hammen C, Ellicott A, Gitlin M, Jamison KR. Sociotropy-autonomy and vulnerability to specific life events in patients with unipolar depression and bipolar disorders. J Abnorm Psychol 1989; 98:154–160.
48. Hooley JM, Teasdale JD. Predictors of relapse in unipolar depressives: Expressed emotion, marital distress, and perceived criticism. J Abnorm Psychol 1989; 98:229–235.
49. Fava GA, Grandi S, Zielezny M, Canestrari R, Morphy MA. Cognitive behavioral treatment of residual symptoms in primary major depressive disorder. Am J Psychiatry 1994; 151:1295–1299.
50. Frank E, Kupfer DJ, Perel JM. Early recurrence in unipolar depression. Arch Gen Psychiatry 1989; 46:397–400.
51. Prien RF. Long-term treatment of affective disorders. In: Meltzer HY, ed. Psychopharmacology: The Third Generation of progress. New York: Raven Press, 1987:1051–1058.

52. Thase ME, Simons AD, McGeary J, Cahalane JF, Hughes C, Harden T, Friedman ES. Relapse following cognitive behavior therapy of depression: Potential implications for longer-term forms of treatment? Am J Psychiatry 1992; 149:1046–1052.

53. Frank E, Kupfer DJ, Perel JM, Cornes CL, Jarrett P, Mallinger A, Thase ME, McEachran AB, Grochocinski VJ. Three-year outcomes for maintenance therapies in recurrent depression. Arch Gen Psychiatry 1990; 47:1093–1099.

54. Conte HR, Plutchik R, Wild KV, Karasu TB. Combined psychotherapy and pharmacotherapy for depression. Arch Gen Psychiatry 1986; 43:471–479.

55. Klerman GL, DiMascio A, Weissman M, Prusoff B, Paykel E. Treatment of depression by drugs and psychotherapy. Am J Psychiatry 1974; 131:186–191.

56. Reynolds CF III, Frank E, Perel JM, Imber SD, Cornes C, Miller MD, Mazumdar S, Houck PR, Dew MA, Stack JA, Pollock BG, Kupfer DJ. Nortriptyline and interpersonal psychotherapy as maintenance therapies for recurrent major depression. A randomized controlled trial in patients older than 59 years. JAMA 1999; 281:39–45.

57. Weissman MM, Klerman GL, Paykel ES, Prusoff BA, Hanson B. Treatment effects on the social adjustment of depressed patients. Arch Gen Psychiatry 1974; 30:771–778.

58. Frank E, Kupfer DJ, Wagner EF, McEachran AB, Cornes C. Efficacy of interpersonal psychotherapy as a maintenance treatment of recurrent depression: contributing factors. Arch Gen Psychiatry 1991; 48:1053–1059.

59. Spanier, Frank E, McEachran AB, Grochocinski VJ, Kupfer DJ. The prophylaxis of depressive episodes in recurrent depression following discontinuation of drug therapy: Integrating psychological and biological factors. Psychol Med 1996; 26:461–475.

60. Roth A, Fonagy P. What Works for Whom? A Critical Review of Psychotherapy Research. New York: The Guilford Press, 1996.

61. Rush AJ, Thase ME. Indications and planning of psychotherapies. In: Maj M, Sartorius N, eds. World Psychiatric Association Series on Evidence and Experience in Psychiatry. Vol 1. Winchester, UK: J Wiley, 1999.

62. Elkin I, Shea MT, Walkins JT, Imber SD, Sotsky SM, Collins JF, Glass DR, Pilkonis PA, Leber WR, Docherty JP, Fiester SJ, Parloff MB. National Institute of Mental Health Treatment of Depression Collaborative Research Program General effectiveness of treatments. Arch Gen Psychiatry 1989; 46: 971–993.

63. Thase ME, Simons AD, Cahalane J, McGeary J, Harden T. Severity of depression and response to cognitive behavior therapy. Am J Psychiatry 1991; 148: 784–789.

64. Blackburn IM, Moore RG. Controlled acute and follow-up trial of cognitive therapy and pharmacotherapy in out-patients with recurrent depression. Br J Psychiatry 1997; 171:328–334.

65. DeRubeis RJ, Gelfand LA, Tang TZ, Simmons AD. Medication versus cognitive behavior therapy for severely depressed outpatients: mega-analysis of four randomized comparisons. Am J Psychiatry 1999; 156(suppl 7):1007–1013.

66. Blackburn IM, Eunson KM, Bishop S. A two-year naturalistic follow-up of depressed patients treated with cognitive therapy, pharmacotherapy and a combination of both. J Affect Disord 1986; 10:67–75.

67. Kovacs M, Rush AJ, Beck AT, Hollon SD. Depressed out-patients treated with cognitive therapy or pharmacotherapy. A one-year follow-up. Arch Gen Psychiatry 1981; 38:33–39.

68. Shea MT, Elkin I, Imbeer SD, Sotsky SM, Watkins JT, Collins JF, Pilkonis PA, Beckham E, Glass DR, Dolan RT, Parloff MB. Course of depressive symptoms over follow-up. Findings from the National Institute of Mental Health treatment of depression collaborative research program. Arch Gen Psychiatry 1992; 49: 782–787.

69. Evans MD, Hollon SD, DeRubeis RJ, Piasecki JM, Grove WM, Garvey MJ, Tuason VB. Differential relapse following cognitive therapy and pharmacotherapy for depression. Arch Gen Psychiatry 1992; 49:802–808.

70. Hollon SD, DeRubeis RJ, Evans MD, Wiemer MJ, Garvey MJ, Grove WM, Tuason VB. Cognitive therapy and pharmacotherapy for depression: singly and in combination. Arch Gen Psychiatry 1992; 49:774–781.

71. Fava GA, Kellner R. Prodromal symptoms in affective disorders. Am J Psychiatry 1991; 148:823–830.

72. Fava GA, Grandi S, Zielezny M, Rafanelli C, Canestrari R. Four-year outcome for cognitive behavioral treatment of residual symptoms in major depression. Am J Psychiatry 1996; 153(7):945–947.

73. Fava GA, Rafanelli C, Grandi S, Canestrari R, Morphy MA. Six-year outcome for cognitive behavioral treatment of residual symptoms in major depression. Am J Psychiatry 1998a; 155(10):1443–1445.

74. Fava GA, Rafanelli C, Grandi S, Conti S, Belluardo P. Prevention of recurrent depression with cognitive behavioral therapy. Arch Gen Psychiatry 1998b; 55: 816–820.

75. Paykel ES, Scott J, Teasdale JD, Johnson AL, Garland A, Moore R, Jenaway A, Cornwall PL, Hayhurst H, Abbott R, Pope M. Prevention of relapse in residual depression by cognitive therapy. Arch Gen Psychiatry 1999; 56:829–835.

76. Jarrett RB, Bosco MR, Risser R, Ramanan J, Marwill M, Kraft D, Rush AJ. Is there a role for continuation phase cognitive therapy for depressed outpatients. J Consult Clin Psychol 1999; 66(suppl 6):1036–1040.

77. Teasdale JD, Segal ZV, Williams JMG, Ridgeway VA, Soulsby JM, Lou MA. Prevention of relapse/recurrence in major depression by mindfulness-based cognitive therapy. J Consult Clin Psychol 2000; 64(suppl 4):615–623.

78. Marlatt GA, Barrett K. Relapse prevention. In: Galanter M, Kleber HD, eds. The Textbook of Substance Abuse Treatment. Washington, DC: American Psychiatric Press, 1994:285–299.

79. Segal ZV. Summary of relapse and recurrence from a cognitive perspective. Depressive disorders: Index and reviews 1996; 1:3–17.

80. Ferster CB. A functional analysis of depression. Am Psychol 1973; 856–870A.

81. Bandura. Principles of Behavior Modification. New York: Holt, Reinhardt Winston, 1969.

82. Drevets WC, Frank E, Price JC, Kupfer DJ, Holt D, Greer PJ, Huang Y, Gautier C, Mathis C. PET imaging of serotonin 1A receptor binding in depression. Biol Psychiatry 1999; 46:1375–1387.

83. Segal ZV, Gemar M, Williams S. Differential cognitive response to a mood challenge following successful cognitive therapy or pharmacotherapy for unipolar depression. J Abnorm Psychol 1999; 108(suppl 1):3–10.

84. Post RM. Transduction of psychosocial stress into the neurobiology of recurrent affective disorder. Am J Psychiatry 1992; 149:999–1010.

85. Thase ME, Simons AD, Reynolds CF. Abnormal electroencephalographic sleep profiles in major depression. Association with response to cognitive behavior therapy. Arch Gen Psychiatry 1996; 53:99–108.

86. Thase ME, Fasiczka AL, Berman SR, Simons AD, Reynolds CF. Electroencephalographic sleep profiles before and after cognitive behavior therapy of depression. Arch Gen Psychiatry 1998; 55:144.

87. Robinson LA, Berman JS, Neimeyer RA. Psychotherapy treatment for the treatment of depression: a comprehensive review of controlled outcome research. Psychol Bull 1990; 108:30–49.

88. Hollon SD, Shelton RC, Loosen PT. Cognitive therapy and pharmacotherapy for depression. J Consult Clin Psychol 1991; 59:88–99.

89. AD Horvath. There are no main effects; only interaction. Paper presented at the international meeting of the Society for Psychotherapy Research, Toronto, Ontario, Canada, June 1989.

90. Jarrett RB, Rush AJ. Short term psychotherapy of depressive disorders: current status and future directions. Psychiatry 1994; 57:115–132.

10

Psychopharmacological Approaches to Prevention and Treatment of Relapse and Recurrence

Timothy J. Petersen, Andrew A. Nierenberg, Julie L. Ryan, and Jonathan E. Alpert
Massachusetts General Hospital
and Harvard Medical School
Boston, Massachusetts, U.S.A.

INTRODUCTION

Preventing a reemergence of depressive symptoms is the primary goal in the long-term pharmacotherapy of chronic depression. Nevertheless, return of clinically significant depression occurs all too commonly both during and following treatment. Depressive episodes that reappear within 6 months of acute response are called relapses and those that occur after 6 months are called recurrences [1]. Theoretically, relapses are considered a return of the original episode, whereas recurrences represent a new episode. Although these distinctions are based on limited data, the phases of treatment to prevent relapse and recurrence have been differentiated correspondingly into continuation and maintenance phases, respectively. Without long-term antidepressant treatment, depressive relapses or recurrences occur in 50–80% of patients [1–6]. Double-blind discontinuation studies reveal that antidepressants lower the risk of relapse and recurrence, and they have repeatedly been shown to be superior to placebo substitution [2,7–10]. Nonetheless, even while taking long-term antidepressants for prophylaxis, observational studies have shown that within 1–5 years after an acute response, 20–80% of patients develop another depressive episode [6,8,11–19]. Estimated rates of relapse and recurrence vary because of factors related to study design (controlled vs observational; flexible vs fixed dosing; duration of follow-up; definitions of relapse/recurrence) and patient samples (degree of recurrence/chronicity; outpatient vs inpatient; primary vs specialty care settings; demographic/clinical factors). A succinct term for relapse or recurrence during long-term antidepressant treatment is depressive breakthrough. In this chapter, we review existing guidelines for longer term treatment of depression for prevention of relapse and recurrence, current knowledge concerning the use of contemporary agents for continuation and maintenance treatment, the evolving appreciation for the clinical phenomenon of depressive breakthrough, and psychopharmacological strategies for treatment of breakthrough.

CURRENT PRACTICE GUIDELINES

Over the past decade, several guidelines have helped provide an outline for long-term depression treatment in primary and specialty care. The Agency for Health Care Policy and Research (AHCPR) produced a book entitled, *Depression in Primary Care: Treatment of Major Depression* [20] that recommends an initial 4–9 months of continuation antidepressant treatment following acute phase response (continuation dosage should equal acute phase dosage) for all patients with unipolar depression. However, the guideline stipulates that patients with the following clinical factors should be provided longer term maintenance treatment following sustained response during continuation treatment. The factors are ranked as either leading to recommending maintenance treatment "very strongly" or "strongly."

- Three or more lifetime depressive episodes—Very strongly recommended
- Two or more depressive episodes within a 5-year time frame and (1) family history of bipolar disorder, (2) previous recurrence within 1 year of medication discontinuation, (3) family history of recurrent a major depressive disorder (MDD), (4) early-onset depression (< 20 years old), or (5) both episodes severe, sudden, or life threatening—Strongly recommended

In addition, the guideline recommends consideration of other factors in determining the need for maintenance treatment: time between prior episodes, severity of episodes, previous suicide risk, acuteness of onset, patient preference, and practitioner comfort in management of maintenance medications. Finally, the guideline highlights the need to determine if patients can forego maintenance treatment after a certain period of time.

The American Psychiatric Association (APA) Work Group on Major Depressive Disorders subsequently developed the *Practice Guideline for the Treatment of Patients with Major Depressive Disorder* [21]. Although it recommended 16–20 weeks on full doses of antidepressants following acute phase remission, the guideline recommended that the following factors be considered when making the decision to provide maintenance treatment: (1) risk of recurrence (number of prior episodes, presence of comorbid conditions, and residual symptoms between episodes); (2) severity of episodes (suicidality, psychotic features, severe functional impairments); (3) side effects experienced with continuous treatment; and (4) patient preferences. The same factors considered in the decision to initiate maintenance treatment should be used in the decision to discontinue treatment. If maintenance treatment is provided, antidepressant dosing should be equivalent to the acute and continuation phase treatments.

The APA guideline also highlights the need for more research on the timing and nature of psychotherapeutic interventions in long-term treatment for depression, for the role of electroconvulsive therapy (ECT) in continuation and maintenance treatment, and the role of combined treatments involving more than one modality and/or a combination of medications.

Two additional clinical guidelines [22,23]—the United Kingdom Defeat Depression Consensus Statement and guidelines published by the British Association for Psychopharmacology—also make formal recommendations for the duration of continuation antidepressant treatment (after acute phase response) and for which patients longer "maintenance" treatment is appropriate. The UK Consensus Statement recommends 4–6 months of continuation treatment, whereas the British Association for Psychopharmacology recommends six months of continuation treatment. The first guideline recommends longer, maintenance treatment in the case of a patient who has experienced two or more prior depressive episodes. The latter guideline recommends maintenance treatment for patients with three or more depressive episodes in the prior 5 years or six or more lifetime episodes.

Although the optimal length of maintenance treatment, once initiated, is unknown, it is clear that many individuals with chronic depressions do not receive even minimally adequate durations and dosing for long-term prophylaxis [24,25]. In contemporary practice, the decision of whether and when to discontinue treatment after a period of 1 or more years of maintenance pharmacotherapy involves weighing putative risk factors for recurrence (including number of previous episodes and completeness of interepisode recovery), severity of the index episode (e.g., disability, suicidality, psychosis), appreciation of anticipated stressors (e.g., starting a new job), and supports (e.g., family, friends, religious, and other group affiliations), feasibility of treatment (e.g., ability to tolerate and afford medications and monitoring), and patient preference for medications and other forms of treatment, particularly psychotherapy. When a decision is made to embark upon treatment discontinuation, a plan needs to be in place for a gradual taper with adequate monitoring for depressive reemergence. Psychoeducation to the patient and, where relevant, an involved family member, concerning warning signs of depressive recurrence (vs more temporary "roughenings" in response to stressors) is often helpful in ensuring that recurrences, if they develop, will be diagnosed and treated without delay.

STUDIES OF LONG-TERM PHARMACOTHERAPY

Long-Term Course of Depression: Observational Studies

Observational studies generally reveal a worse long-term prognosis for depressed patients than controlled trials. As part of the National Institute of Mental Health (NIMH) Collaborative Program on the Psychobiology of Depression, Lavori and colleagues [12] followed 359 patients. These patients had recovered from their index episode of depression for at least 8 weeks and were then followed for up to 5 years. Of those patients who continued to take high levels of somatic treatment, over 20% became depressed again within the first 6 months. Thereafter, patients who had continued to feel well up until that time relapsed at the same rate regardless of treatment status. Overall, 88% of the entire cohort had a relapse or recurrence by the end of 5 years. The clinical implications of these findings are profound: When followed naturalistically, many patients become depressed again despite putatively adequate long-term pharmacotherapy and the advantages of maintenance antidepressant treatment may diminish after 6 months of wellness. It is unclear whether depressive relapse and recurrence rates may be even higher in purely clinical populations who are not enrolled in follow-up studies.

Mueller and colleagues [26], in another analysis of the NIMH Collaborative Program database, examined 15 years of naturalistic follow-up data for 380 patients who recovered from the index episode of major depression. In addition, they identified 105 of these patients who had remained well for at least 5 years after recovery. Baseline demographic and clinical characteristics were also examined as predictors of recurrence. A cumulative proportion of 85% of the 380 recovered patients experienced a recurrence, as did 58% of those who remained well for at least 5 years. Female sex, a longer index episode, more prior episodes, and never marrying were significant predictors of recurrence in the larger group but not for the patients who remained well for at least 5 years. Naturalistic treatment was characterized as lower than recommended doses for all phases of treatment. Similar to the findings of Lavori and colleagues the level of treatment reportedly received by patients did not significantly differ between those who did and did not experience a recurrence [12]. In addition, even in patients who sustained a long period of recovery, recurrence rates were high and no significant predictors of recurrence were identified.

In another observational study, Ramana and colleagues [16] followed 70 patients (53 inpatients and 17 outpatients) for up to 15 months: 80% remitted by 15 months; of those who remitted, Kaplan-Meier survival analysis [27] showed that 40% experienced at least one depressive relapse within 10 months of remission. Relapsers and nonrelapsers had the same levels of long-term antidepressant treatment, again consistent with Lavori and colleagues' [12] findings.

Montgomery et al. [28] followed a group of 217 patients who had remitted to three different 6-week acute phase treatments— mirtazapine, amitriptyline, or placebo—and then continued on the same treatments during a 2-year follow-up phase. Dosing during follow-up was flexible, but maximum permitted dosages were mirtazapine 35 mg/day, amitriptyline 280 mg/day, and placebo 7 capsules/day. Survival analysis indicated that patients treated with mirtazapine had a significantly longer time to relapse than recipients of amitriptyline or placebo, and amitriptyline-treated patients showed a significantly longer time to relapse than recipients of placebo. At study endpoint, survival analysis indicated that patients treated with mirtazapine or amitriptyline had a significantly longer time to relapse than recipients of placebo did. Relapse rates during the first 20 weeks of follow-up were 4.1, 7.0, and 28.0% for the mirtazapine, amitriptyline, and placebo groups, respectively. At study endpoint, relapse rates were 4.1, 11.6, and 28.1%. Tolerability was lower to amitriptyline than to mirtazapine or placebo.

Claxton and colleagues [29] utilized the UK Primary Care Database to identify 7293 patients treated for depression with a selective serotonin reuptake inhibitor (SSRI). They then examined rates of relapse and recurrence during an 18-month follow-up period. Four cohorts were identified: patients who had < 120 days of any antidepressant treatment (73% of sample); patients who had at least 120 days of treatment, but who switched agents or added a second antidepressant (4% of sample); patients who maintained treatment on the original SSRI for at least 120 days, but had thier dosage titrated upward during the 6-month treatment period (2% of sample); and patients who used the index SSRI at a stable dosage throughout the treatment period (21% of sample). The investigators found that the stable-use cohort experienced a somewhat lower rate of relapse or recurrence (20%) than the other three groups: 23, 29, and 24%. Younger age, increased psychiatric comorbidity, and anxiolytic use during the index episode were associated with higher rates of relapse and recurrence. Primary limitations of this study were a small effect size for risk between groups and heterogeneity within definitions of relapse and recurrence. Moreover, inferences regarding causality are limited by the nonrandomized design.

Controlled Studies Of Continuation Treatment

In the last 5 years, there has been a proliferation of studies that evaluate continuation and maintenance phase treatments for patients responding to acute phase antidepressant treatments. Most of these trials have involved comparing active medication versus placebo, but some have compared two or more active medication groups without a placebo control. In addition, there is some degree of heterogeneity in patient samples used for these studies. The most notable variation is in degree of previous recurrence and/or resistance. It is important to keep this in mind when examining relapse and recurrence rates; those patients with a more recurrent and/or resistant illness history have been shown to have higher rates of relapse and recurrence irrespective of treatments administered. Owing to the size of this recent literature, we will only review in detail the key representative studies.

Sackheim et al. [30] randomized 84 patients (stratified by medication resistance) who had remitted to acute phase ECT to three continuation treatment groups: nortriptyline, nortriptyline and lithium, or placebo. By the end of this 24-week continuation phase, relapse rates were 60, 39, and 84% for the nortriptyline, nortriptyline + lithium, and placebo groups, respectively. Nortriptyline-lithium combination therapy had a marked advantage in time to relapse, which was superior to both placebo and nortriptyline alone. All but one instance of relapse with nortriptyline-lithium occurred within 5 weeks of ECT termination, whereas relapse continued throughout treatment with placebo or nortriptyline alone. Medication-resistant patients, female patients, and those with more severe depressive symptoms following ECT had more rapid relapse.

Versiani [31] treated 283 patients with recurrent depression during a 6-week open trial of reboxetine. Responders went on to be randomized to continuation reboxetine versus placebo for a 46-week period. During this time period, 22% of patients receiving reboxetine and 56% of patients receiving placebo relapsed. Confirming previous work that indicates the importance of treating patients acutely to full remission, Versiani and colleagues found that patients in full remission at the end of acute treatment had even lower relapse rates: 16 and 48% for the reboxetine and placebo groups, respectively.

Feiger et al. [17] conducted a trial in which patients were treated acutely with open nefazodone. One hundred and thirty-one remitters were then randomized to continuation nefazodone versus placebo. Rates of relapse during the 36-week continuation treatment phase were 1.8 and 18.3% for the nefazodone and placebo groups, respectively. Rates of discontinuation because of lack of efficacy were 17.3 and 32.8% for the same two groups.

Several other studies have examined effectiveness of continuation active treatments versus placebo in patients having demonstrated partial and/or full acute phase response. In a pooled analysis from four randomized controlled trials, Entsuah [18] found that relapse rates (after 6 months of continuation treatment) between acute phase responders treated with continuation placebo versus venlafaxine were 23 and 11%, respectively. Thase et al. [32] treated 410 patients diagnosed with moderate to severely recurrent or chronic major depression with open mirtazapine. One hundred and fifty-six fully remitted patients were randomized to mirtazapine or placebo for a 40-week continuation phase. Relapse rates during continuation treatment were 19.7% for the mirtazapine group and 43.8% for the placebo group. Discontinuation rates due to adverse events were 11.8 and 2.5% for these same groups. Ferreri et al. [33] used 200 mg of open-label amineptine to treat 458 patients with depression during a 3-month acute trial. They reported an acute phase response rate of 66%. These responders (n = 284) were then randomized to continuation amineptine or placebo during a 9-month continuation phase. Relapse rates were found to be 6.6% for the medication group and 18.7% for the placebo group. Of note is that patients in this protocol met criteria for MDD or dysthymia.

Some more recent work has evaluated a switch to weekly fluoxetine for those patients who responded acutely to an SSRI. Miner et al. [34] found that responders to paroxetine, citalopram, or sertraline demonstrated a 9.3% relapse/discontinuation rate over a 12-week continuation treatment phase. Schmidt and colleagues [35] randomized acute phase fluoxetine responders to fluoxetine 20 mg/day, 90 mg fluoxetine weekly, and placebo, and found no difference in efficacy between the two active drug groups. Doogan and Caillard [7] followed depressed patients who responded to an 8-week trial of sertraline. After patients responded, they were randomized to either continue on the sertraline (N = 184) or be switched to placebo (N = 105). Thirteen percent of the sertraline patients and over 45% of the placebo-substituted patients had another episode of major depression within 44 weeks. Note that if a depression reappeared, the dose of sertraline could be increased to up to 200 mg daily (mean daily dose ranged between 69.3 and 82.1 mg daily). The investigators did not specify if patients who had another depressive episode and then responded to an increase in dose were considered to have a relapse or recurrence. No mention was made of how many patients first required and then responded to an increase in dose. Furthermore, although about 75% of the original group had recurrent depression, there was no information about the number of prior episodes. For these reasons, the

investigators' finding that 13% of patients relapsed during long-term sertraline treatment may be an underestimate of the true relapse rate.

Montgomery and Dunbar [13] treated 172 depressed patients who had a
history of recurrences with open paroxetine (20–40 mg/day) for 8 weeks.
Patients who responded were randomized to either continue on paroxetine
(20–30 mg/day; N = 68) or placebo (N = 67) for the next 52 weeks. Three
percent of the patients who took paroxetine had depressive relapses as
compared to 19% of the placebo group. Similarly, Claghorn and Feighner
[11] followed patients for 52 weeks and found relapse rates of 25% among 32
patients who had responded to placebo initially, 15% among 60 paroxetine-
treated patients, and 4% among imipramine-treated patients. The dose of
long-term medication used in Montgomery and Dunbar's study could be
maintained, decreased, or increased at the discretion of the physician. The
mean dose of paroxetine that patients responded to was 40 mg during the
acute trial and 38 mg during the extension phase. The dose of the SSRI in this
study, therefore, was stable during continuation and maintenance treatment.
As with the studies noted above, no information was provided about
subsequent treatment of those patients who had breakthrough depressions
while on active medications.

Quitkin and colleagues [15] have proposed that the loss of efficacy
within 6 weeks after an acute response may reflect the loss of an initial placebo
response to an antidepressant rather than a true drug effect. They reported the
results of a 12-week double-blind trial of imipramine (N = 174), phenelzine
(N = 169), and placebo (N = 164) for patients with atypical depression. Of
the group that responded by 6 weeks, the proportions of patients who had a
relapse were 11.8% (imipramine), 8.8% (phenelzine), and 31.3% (placebo).
The authors' hypothesis is that between 36 and 100% of relapsers initially
had a placebo response to medication and then lost it. Given the parallel
design used in this study, such inference may be tentative as, after all, the
majority of the placebo responders still remained well during continuation
treatment. Nevertheless, it is not an uncommon clinical observation that early
responses to antidepressants which then waiver during acute treatment often
do not hold well in the long term; the ebbing of these responses with time may
be due in part to loss of a placebo response. In the individual patient, other
hypotheses need to be explored, including the possibility of mood cycling due
to undiagnosed bipolar disorder.

Uncontrolled Studies of Maintenance Antidepressant Treatment

Peselow and colleagues [14] studied 217 patients with unipolar depression
who responded to tricyclic antidepressants (mean imipramine equivalence
dose 159.6 mg daily), were stable for at least 6 months, and then followed for

up to 5 years. They compared patients who stayed on medication to a group of 28 patients who were stable for 6 months and then discontinued medication. Relapse rates were 30%, 50%, and 60%, at 1, 2, and 3 years, respectively, while on active drug versus 51, 74, and 83% on no treatment. Overall 87 of 217 patients on active drug (40.1%) were observed to have suffered a depressive relapse over the 5-year course.

Controlled Studies of Maintenance Antidepressant Treatment

Controlled studies suggest that imipramine therapy, either alone or with lithium, is ore effective in preventing recurrence than lithium alone. Prien and coworkers [38] compared strategies for maintenance treatment for 150 unipolar depressed patients. These patients were treated initially for their index depressive episode with a variety of antidepressants (usually imipramine), antidepressants plus lithium, lithium alone, neuroleptics, or ECT and then stabilized for 2 months with a combination of imipramine plus lithium. After stabilization, patients were randomized to take imipramine alone (mean daily dose 137 mg), lithium alone (mean blood level 0.66 ng/mL), the combination of imipramine plus lithium, or placebo. Over the next 27 months, 33% of the imipramine group, 26% of the combination group, 57% of the lithium group, and 65% of the placebo group had a recurrence. Although imipramine prevented recurrences in a substantially higher proportion of patients than either placebo or lithium alone, a third of these patients experienced a depressive recurrence while taking maintenance imipramine. Greenhouse et al. [36] suggests that the reappearance of the depressive syndrome in patients on lithium alone may have been due to discontinuation of the imipramine rather than to a loss of efficacy of this agent. This explanation, however, does not apply to those who became depressed again while they continued on the imipramine.

Frank and colleagues [2] demonstrated the advantages of taking full doses of imipramine for 3 years after an acute response to imipramine plus interpersonal therapy in those patients who had at least their third episode of depression; only about 20% of patients had a recurrence while taking imipramine at the acute effective dose (with and without interpersonal psychotherapy) as compared to about 80% of those who were switched over to placebo alone. Prior studies that examined the usefulness of lower doses of maintenance antidepressants tend to have recurrence rates of about 50–70% [5]. Even though Frank and colleagues' [2] data are encouraging when compared to previous reports, note that [1] these patients had been treated with interpersonal psychotherapy during the acute treatment phase and might have been more able to cope with stressors and less likely to suffer from recurrences, and [2] 20% of the patients who took full antidepressant doses for maintenance became depressed again. No mention is made of how these patients were subsequently treated.

In a follow-up study of those patients who experienced a recurrence treated with interpersonal psychotherapy, Frank et al. [37] restabilized these patients on a full dose of imipramine plus interpersonal therapy. They were then randomized to continue on full or half-dose imipramine (N = 10 each group). Thirty percent of the full-dose group and 70% of the half-dose group had a recurrence. Note that although the full-dose group had a lower recurrence rate as compared to the half-dose group, the 30% recurrence rate of the full-dose group is substantial.

Rouillon et al. [38] examined patients who had remitted to acute phase milnacipran treatment and maintained remission throughout the 18-week continuation treatment phase. These patients were randomized to maintenance phase milnacipran versus placebo. Recurrence rates were significantly different between groups: 23.6% for placebo and 16.3% for active drug. Gilberte et al. [39], in another placebo-controlled maintenance phase trial, randomized patients who had maintained a total of 32 weeks of response to fluoxetine to the same dose of fluoxetine or placebo. They found recurrence rates (20% fluoxetine and 40% placebo) as well as time to recurrence to differ significantly between groups. Adverse events did not significantly differ between groups.

In a study of geriatric patients, Klysner et al. [40] randomized 121 patients (who had maintained response to 20–40 mg of citalopram throughout acute and continuation treatment phases) to the same dose of citalopram or placebo. He found recurrence rates of 32% for citalopram and 66% for placebo. Using a similar study design, Terra and colleagues [41] followed 204 patients who maintained response to fluvoxamine for both 6 weeks of acute treatment and 18 weeks of continuation treatment. These patients were randomized to continuing on active drug or placebo. Significantly fewer recurrences were observed in the active drug group when compared with the placebo group. Robinson and colleagues [9] studied the long-term efficacy of maintenance phenelzine in 47 depressed patients. Patients were first treated with phenelzine at a dose of 1 mg/kg for 6–13 weeks. Responders were stabilized for 16 weeks after acute recovery and then randomized to phenelzine 60 mg daily (N = 19), phenelzine 45 mg daily (N = 12), or placebo (N = 16) for 2 years. Although maintenance phenelzine at both doses was superior to placebo, after 12 months, a substantial proportion of patients relapsed while taking the active drug (total proportions of patients who either had a relapse or recurrence were phenelzine 60 mg = 26%; phenelzine 45 mg = 33%; and placebo = 81%). One problem with these data is that only eight patients were able to complete the entire 2-year maintenance phase.

Montgomery et al. [8] compared fluoxetine (N = 88) with placebo (N = 94) to prevent recurrences in unipolar depressed patients who had responded to an open trial of fluoxetine (40–80 mg daily). Subjects were stable for 6 months on fluoxetine 40 mg/day prior to randomization to either staying on the same dose of fluoxetine 40 mg or switching to placebo. At the end of 1 year, 26% of subjects who took prophylactic fluoxetine and 57% who took placebo had a recurrence. As with the Frank [1] and Kupfer [4] studies, Montgomery et al. [8] demonstrated that active antidepressant maintenance therapy is superior to placebo, but that a substantial proportion (26%) of patients experience a depressive recurrence despite active treatment.

Stewart et al. [42] applied pattern analysis to distinguish between "true drug response," which was delayed and sustained, and "placebo response," which was early or nonpersistent, among 428 responders to 12 weeks of open treatment with fluoxetine 20 mg/day. Among the 392 subjects willing to be randomized to fluoxetine versus placebo over the next 12 months, those identified as true drug responders showed a significant drug-placebo difference in relapse/recurrence rates during continuation/maintenance, whereas those with an initial placebo response pattern had an equivalent outcome whether maintained on fluoxetine or not. In addition, placebo pattern responders were significantly more likely to experience depressive breakthrough on drug compared with those who had shown a true drug response.

One study of the long-term treatment of depression with paroxetine differentiated continuation and maintenance prophylaxis [13]. Paroxetine was superior to placebo, but 14% of patients experienced a recurrence during active long-term paroxetine treatment. Montgomery et al. [43] randomized 147 patients who had responded to either citalopram 20 mg (n = 68) or 40 mg (n = 79) during a 6-week acute treatment trial to receive the same dose or placebo over a 24-week period. Relapse rates were significantly lower on citalopram (8% on 20 mg, 12% on 40 mg) than placebo (31%). In a similar study, 226 responders to citalopram flexibly dosed between 20 and 60 mg over 8 weeks were randomized 2:1 to citalopram or placebo [44]. Citalopram-treated subjects continued on the dose to which they had responded acutely. Relapse rates were 13.8% on citalopram compared with 24.3% on placebo. In an active comparator study among 297 depressed patients treated in general practice, there was no significant difference in depression severity at 22 weeks between patients randomized to one of two levels of citalopram (10–30 mg or 20–60 mg) versus imipramine (50–150 mg), although relapse rates were not reported [45].

Franchini et al. [46] reported a high recurrence rate (50%) among 32 patients with recurrent major depression who had maintained response to citalopram 40 mg/day over a 4-month period and were then treated with 20 mg/day over 24 months. Although the absence of a comparison group treated with 40 mg/day hinders any definitive conclusions, the high rate of depressive breakthrough on the lower dose would tend to support the premise that full-dose maintenance treatment of this SSRI is required for adequate prophylaxis among patients at risk for recurrence. In an extension of this work, Franchini et al. [47] examined 32 patients who had maintained response through acute and continuation phases of treatment at citalopram 40 mg/day and continued on the same dosage during maintenance phase treatment. They reported a 34% recurrent rate for patients on the maintenance citalopram dose of 40 mg/day. Hochstrasser et al. [48] also examined citalopram as a maintenance phase treatment but in a placebo-controlled manner. Time to recurrence was found to be significantly longer in the maintenance phase citalopram-treated group versus placebo. All of these patients (n = 269) had demonstrated response to flexible citalopram dosing (20–60 mg) throughout the acute and continuation phases of treatment.

Overall *controlled trials* show that within 1–3 years of long-term antidepressant treatment after an acute response, at least 14–30% of patients have a reappearance of depression. In contrast to controlled trials, *observational studies* show that within 5 years of acute response, 40–80% of patients have depressive breakthrough.

Meta-analyses of Long-Term Pharmacotherapy

Geddes and colleagues [49] recently published a comprehensive meta-analysis of randomized trials of continuing treatment with antidepressants in patients with depressive disorders who had responded to acute treatment. They pooled data from 31 randomized trials (a total of 4410 patients) and found that continued antidepressant treatment (following acute phase response) reduced the odds of relapse and recurrence by 70% compared with treatment discontinuation (placebo). The average rate of relapse on placebo was 41% compared with 18% on active treatment. The modal length of follow-up after randomization for these trials was 12 months with a range of 6–36 months. Rates of relapse did not seem to differ between the type of antidepressant or treatment duration before randomization. In addition, the proportional risk reduction was found to be similar in patients with short (6 months) and long (36 months) follow-up periods, which suggests no increased or decreased risk with increasing time since response. These observations, as suggested by the Geddes et al., challenges the validity of clear demarcation of continuation and maintenance treatment phases. In addition, they were unable to discern an obvious difference in prevention of relapse and recurrence across patient subpopulations, although the study was not designed for a systematic analysis of predictive clinical and demographic factors. As acknowledged by these researchers, one limitation of this meta-analysis is that patients were mainly drawn from secondary care settings, where patients may have a higher risk for relapse. Nevertheless, these findings confirm the clear benefit of continued antidepressant treatment in terms of reduction of the risk of relapse and recurrence.

MANAGEMENT OF DEPRESSIVE BREAKTHROUGH

Although the preponderance of evidence clearly supports the efficacy of long-term pharmacotherapy to prevent relapse and recurrence, depressive breakthroughs are nevertheless an all too common and seriously understudied clinical problem. When they occur, they tend to be dispiriting for patients who had reason to hope that faithfulness to recommended treatment would keep their depression under good control. Depressive breakthrough is estimated to occur in 14–80% of patients taking adequate continuation and maintenance doses of medication. The average antidepressant breakthrough rate cited in the meta-analysis by Geddes et al. [49] was 18%. According to Byrne and Rothschild [50], breakthrough is more likely to occur with monoamine oxidase inhibitors (MAOIs) and SSRIs. However, this is based on very limited data. Some investigators have referred to breakthrough as "antidepressant tachyphylaxis" or "drug tolerance." However, such terms tend to imply a particular pharmacological mechanism for relapse/recurrence, and in the majority of patients, the basis for the depressive breakthrough remains speculative. Several factors have been suggested as contributing to depressive breakthrough, including pharmacological factors (receptor tolerance; inadequate levels; changes in drugmetabolite ratio; reduced delivery across membranes related to drug transport proteins; drug interactions; drug side effects such as fatigue or "apathy"; intermittent withdrawal symptoms related to missed doses) [51–56]; loss of an initial placebo effect [15,57,58]; undetected mood cycling within a bipolar spectrum illness or psychotic depression [51,52,53]; increase in disease severity [52]; stressful life events [56]; residual depressive symptoms [56]; and other psychiatric or medical comorbidities complicating long-term course (56) (e.g., anxiety disorders or substance abuse).

Although case series and some controlled studies have described the return of major depression during long-term antidepressant treatment, very few studies have examined the management of those patients who have depressive breakthrough.

Case Reports and Uncontrolled Trials for Depressive Breakthrough

The phenomenon of depressive breakthrough has been noted more widely over the past decade. However, even within an older literature, treatments that worked initially and then lost efficacy over weeks to months included MAOIs [52,59,60], tricyclic antidepressants [51,59], and amoxapine [61]. Following loss of efficacy, a variety of somatic therapies helped patients, with some patients receiving multiple subsequent treatments. These therapies included increasing the dose of the medication that had stopped working, changing the medication to another antidepressant, switching to ECT, and adding either lithium or thyroxin. Overall, 34 cases were reported, and of these, only 6 (17.6%) responded to the next treatment. Subsequently, however, in a series of 18 outpatients with major depression who had relapsed on fluoxetine 20 mg/day, we found that 15 (83%) had a full or partial acute response to raising the dose of the SSRI to 40 mg/day [58]. Eleven of the 15 patients who responded (73%) maintained their response during follow-up (up to 12 months), and two patients who experienced a subsequent break-through on 40 mg/day remitted again on 80 mg/day. In a more recent case series [62], Sharma followed 15 treatment resistant patients who were diagnosed with either unipolar or bipolar depression (11 unipolar/4 bipolar II). All patients had experienced a loss of antidepressant response to adequate doses of at least two antidepressants, resulting in relapses following a complete remission of at least 2 weeks but not more than 6 months in duration. Each patient had experienced a loss of response to at least one antidepressant prior to assessment, and in 11 patients, the loss of antidepressant response was also observed prospectively at least once. Although not entirely clear, it appears that Sharma found all 15 of these patients responded to antidepressant discontinuation and the addition of a mood stabilizer (in most cases lithium). Sharma asserts that these results suggest careful consideration of bipolar diathesis in depressed patients with a history of loss of antidepressant efficacy and/or treatment resistance. However, the trial is clearly limited in that patients were highly recurrent and/or resistant, the treatment for breakthrough was not standardized, and several of the patients had been diagnosed with or had a positive family history of bipolar disorder.

McGrath et al. [63] studied 12 patients who had experienced a stable remission for at least 1 month on an SSRI and then relapsed. They treated these patients by adding the ergot derivative dopamine agonist, bromocriptine mesylate (2.5–10.0 mg daily) for 4 weeks to the SSRI. The rationale derived from previous evidence that fluoxetine can diminish dopamine levels in the nucleus accumbens and nucleus striatum [64]. Six of the 12 patients experienced a response, which was sustained for at least 2 months. Response was achieved within 14 days of initiation of treatment. One of the six re-sponders lost the benefit of bromocriptine and changed treatments after 2 months. Three patients were considered nonresponders, and three were intolerant of side effects. Two limitations of this study are that the patient sample included those with both unipolar and bipolar depression and the inability to determine if the bromocriptine-treatment response was achieved simply by the activating properties of the medication.

In another recent trial [65], the first systematically to compare active treatments for depressive breakthrough, Schmidt and colleagues examined patients who had responded to a 13-week open-label, acute treatment with fluoxetine 20 mg daily. These patients were randomized to a double-blind continuation treatment with either 90 mg enteric-coated fluoxetine once weekly, fluoxetine 20 mg once daily, or placebo. Of the 125 patients who relapsed during the continuation treatment phase, 123 elected to be treated within a rescue protocol as follows. Patients who had been taking fluoxetine 20 mg daily had their dose increased to 40 mg daily, and those taking fluoxetine 90 mg weekly had their dose increased to 90 mg twice weekly. Results indicate no significant differences between groups in the percentage of patients who responded and maintained response (for up to 6 months after relapse; 57% in patients receiving 40 mg of fluoxetine and 72% in patients receiving 90 mg fluoxetine). There was also no significant difference in the degree of change in the Hamilton Rating Scale for Depression 17 (Ham-D-17) [66] and CGI-S scores between the treatment groups. Although the comparability of daily and weekly fluoxetine for addressing relapse is not necessarily surprising, the results of this study generally support increasing dose as a reasonable first-line treatment strategy for patients who relapse while taking a previously effective dose of an antidepressant.

Overall the published literature is surprisingly limited given the apparent prevalence of breakthrough in clinical settings, and, as yet, there exist no randomized, placebo-controlled, double-blind studies which compare different treatments for depressive breakthrough.

Options to Treat Depressive Breakthrough

Although we lack controlled trials to guide treatment of depressive breakthrough, clinicians broadly have four options for its pharmacological management [67]: (1) maximizing the dose of the maintenance antidepressant [68–70], (2) lowering the antidepressant dose, (3) adding another agent, or (4) switching to another antidepressant.

When presented with hypothetical cases of breakthrough depression, the most popular choice for first-step treatment among 145 Massachusetts' psychopharmacologists surveyed was to increase dose [71]. Augmentation or combination with other agents was the next favored approach, followed by switching to another antidepressant. Dose increase to address depressive relapse was also the first-choice strategy among over 75% of the 432 clinicians from across the United States in a subsequent survey [67].

Maximizing Dose

Several studies have shown that fluoxetine at 20 mg daily is as effective as fluoxetine 60 mg daily for the acute treatment of depression [72–74]. However, among those patients who are nonresponsive to lower doses (20 mg), a considerable proportion nevertheless do respond to a dose increase. This finding during acute treatment appears to translate to management of depressive breakthrough as well. As described previously, 83% of 18 patients who relapsed following remission on 20 mg/day responded to a dose increase to 40 mg, many sustaining the response for up to 12 months and two responding to a further dose increase to 80 mg when depression returned [58]. The advantages of using higher doses of the maintenance antidepressant are that it is parsimonious and generally well accepted, as the patient is already familiar with the drug and its associated side effects. The potential disadvantage of this approach is that increasing the dose may cause more side effects. Because of its simplicity and acceptability to patients, it appears to make sense to consider a dose increase as a first step for those who have depressive breakthrough and then test further strategies for those who fail to respond.

The importance of subsyndromal symptoms as a risk factor for major depressive breakthrough [75] begs the question of what level of depression severity and duration should prompt intervention. Should a change in treatment to address breakthrough be triggered by a subsyndromal depressive reemergence or only a clearly defined syndromal return of major depression? In the absence of studies examining this question, the decision often reflects a best judgement balancing the aim of reducing risk of a full depressive breakthrough with that of minimizing a patient's long-term side effect burden and costs. In practice, we often do recommend a change in treatment (often starting with dose increase) in response to the subsyndromal return of depressive symptoms among previously remitted individuals with chronic depression. This is particularly when we anticipate that the breakthrough is not simply a transient response to an identifiable stressor and is already causing distress and/or impairment.

Lowering Dose

Although no studies have examined the strategy of dose lowering, Byrne and Rothschild [50] suggest that its potential advantages are reduction of side effects that overlap with depressive symptoms and an alteration of drug: metabolite ratios in favor of active forms. An obvious disadvantage of this strategy is the potential exacerbation of breakthrough due to subtherapeutic dosing. Nevertheless, under circumstances in which antidepressant side effects are suspected to be contributing to apparent depressive breakthrough, a closely monitored dose reduction may help clarify if this is the case.

Adding Another Agent

A third approach is to combine two antidepressants. Among the agents that appear to be most popular for combination with SSRIs during acute treatment is buproprion [67] despite remarkably limited published data [76]. The efficacy of bupropion for SSRI breakthrough remains unknown. More generally, the current clinical approach to adding another agent for depressive breakthrough parallels that to resistant depression by featuring antidepressant combinations that are thought to have complementary mechanisms (e.g., venlafaxine and mirtazapine) and, when possible, that have the added advantage of addressing troublesome chronic side effects (e.g., nefazodone may reduce sexual dysfunction on an SSRI).

Another option to regain an antidepressant response is to add an augmenting agent that by itself may have limited antidepressant potential. This is also a widely used strategy to manage treatment-resistant depression [77,78]. Lithium augmentation has been the most widely studied and used treatment [79,80], but it has not been tested in the context of recurrent depression that occurs while patients take continuation/maintenance antidepressants.

Lithium augmentation has been shown in a case series to be effective for patients who do not respond to fluoxetine [81]. Another study showed, however, that although lithium augmentation was effective for about 60% of patients who failed to respond to either fluoxetine or desipramine, about a third of the responders to lithium augmentation of fluoxetine had a depressive relapse at 14 weeks of follow-up. In contrast, none of the responders to lithium augmentation of desipramine had a relapse [82]. In a more recent trial that examined lithium versus placebo augmentation of nortriptyline for patients with highly refractory depression [83], response rate for the lithium augmentation group was only 12.5% and for placebo 20.0%. However, the likelihood of response to any treatment in this population is very low. Another lithium versus placebo continuation phase augmentation trial found a 0% relapse rate for the lithium group versus 47% for the placebo group [84]. However, all of these patients had received lithium augmentation of an antidepressant during the acute phase of treatment. In addition, antidepressant choice was not fixed but seminaturalistic. Patients received either a tricyclic or tetracyclic (150 mg/day), an SSRI (paroxetine, 20 mg/day), or trazodone or venlafaxine (150 mg/day) for more than 2 weeks. Despite these studies, we do not know if lithium augmentation is effective, both acutely and for the long-term, for patients who have breakthrough depressive episodes and are maintained on fluoxetine or any other SSRI.

Augmentation of antidepressants in response to breakthrough depression also draws heavily upon the options marshaled for treatment-resistant depression [85]. These include adding to the initial antidepressant the dopamine agonists (e.g., pramipexole,), psychostimulants, modafanil, atypical antipsychotics such as olanzapine or ziprasidone, anticonvulsants (e.g., lamotrigene), triiodothyronine, or buspirone.

The advantages of an augmentation or combination strategy are several and include the ability to recruit an additional psychopharmacological mechanism without sacrificing the first, a potential for synergistic effect, the possibility of targeting side effects (e.g., insomnia) and comorbid conditions (e.g., attention deficit–hyperactivity disorder [ADHD]), and opportunity to address putative changes in companion systems (e.g., mesocorticolimbic dopamine underactivity due to an SSRI) [63,86,87]. The disadvantages of such strategies are the regimen becomes more complicated and potentially reduces patient adherence, the possible introduction of new side effects, and greater potential for drug-drug interactions.

Switching Antidepressants

A fourth alternative is to switch to another antidepressant. The greatest advantages of switching are that the patient can remain on monotherapy, hence lowering risks of drug interactions and lowered treatment adherence, and may also achieve relief from side effects associated with the previous agent. If switching from one antidepressant to another involves changing to another class of antidepressant then the different mechanism of action may also be beneficial, although this theory has not been proven. However, evidence from studies on SSRI to SSRI switches suggest that even switching from one SSRI to another may be effective in up to 60% of patients who fail to respond to the first SSRI [88–90]. Other information about switching can be inferred from the literature on treatment-resistant depression. Nierenberg and colleagues [91] found that venlafaxine was effective for about a third of patients who had failed a minimum of three other antidepressants plus at least one attempt at augmentation [91]. In follow-up, however, about half of the responders to venlafaxine relapsed within 3 months. More recently, DeMontigny et al. [92] reported that switching to venlafaxine after patients fail up to three other antidepressants can result in over 70% responding. In a more recent report, Faya and colleagues [93] examined 29 patients who had not responded to an 8- to 12-week trial of fluoxetine and were then switched to bupropion SR. Sixty-five of patients exhibited a response, and 23% fully remitted. In a double-blind crossover study, subjects with chronic depression who had failed to respond to 12 weeks of sertraline or imipramine were switched over to the alternate medication [94]. Over 50% of antidepressant nonresponders benefited from the crossover, although the SSRI was somewhat better tolerated than the tricyclic antidepressant. Overall, then, both switching across and within a class of antidepressants offer a reasonable possibility of benefit following an insufficient response to an antidepressant. For present purposes, of course, our question is whether this holds for treatment of breakthrough depression in which an individual had been an initial responder to a treatment that subsequently fails. This question has not yet been systematically addressed.

The disadvantage of switching to another antidepressant is that it involves abandoning a previously effective and tolerated treatment for an unfamiliar medication; the switchover may still be complicated by drug interactions, particularly if the original antidepressant has a long half-life (e.g., fluoxentine), and careful consideration needs to be given to the possibility of discontinuation of emergent symptoms when deciding when and how rapidly to taper the initial antidepressant. Another potential disadvantage is that although there was breakthrough, the initial antidepressant may be providing some benefit which will be lost on taper, and it may take as long as 6–8 weeks to determine whether a patient will respond to the new antidepressant.

A recent open-label trial evaluated a switch versus augmentation strategy for a heterogeneous group of patients (n = 74) [95] who had experienced nonresponse, partial response, or depressive breakthrough (34% of the sample). Treatment decisions were left entirely to the clinician in a nonrandomized manner. The main result of this study was that no statistically significant differences were found between the treatment groups; there was a trend favoring augmentation for acute response. More than 2 months after initiating the switch or augmentation strategy, some patients exhibited a delayed response. In this respect, the switch strategy showed a trend toward greater efficacy in the long run. This study was informative although limited by a small and diverse sample, nonrandomized treatment, the use of several treatments, and nonblinding of clinicians. Systematic comparisons of augmentation and switching strategies are much needed in devising optimal strategies in the treatment of depressive breakthrough.

CONCLUSION

Controlled studies of continuation and maintenance pharmacotherapy have consistently shown the advantage of drug over placebo for prevention of relapse and recurrences, particularly when antidepressant medications are maintained at the full dose required initially to establish remission. Although the evolving literature has generally supported the longer term use of antidepressants for individuals with chronic or particularly severe depression, the question of whether and when to consider tapering treatment after a long-term course is still largely unaddressed. Furthermore, both controlled and observational studies have found substantial rates of relapse and recurrence even among individuals who are maintained on antidepressant treatment.

Although it is a common clinical challenge, there are few uncontrolled studies and no controlled trials on management of depressive breakthrough. Four principal pharmacological strategies, similar to those for addressing acutely resistant depression, appear to be increasing dose, lowering dose, adding another agent, and switching antidepressants within or across classes. Although resourceful clinicians will continue to devise tactics for reestablishing antidepressant response in those patients who have lost it, controlled studies of long-term treatment are needed to identify the optimal nature and sequence of approaches for reemergent depression and to determine what symptom severity and duration should prompt a change in treatment when the current long-term regimen is no longer working well enough.

REFERENCES

1. Frank E, Prien RF, Jarrett RB, et al. Conceptualization and rationale for consensus definitions of terms in major depressive disorder: remission, recovery, relapse, and recurrence. Arch Gen Psychiatry 1991; 48:851–855.
2. Frank E, Kupfer DJ, Perel JM. Three-year outcomes for maintenance therapies in recurrent depression. Arch Gen Psychiatry 1990; 47:1093–1099.
3. Keller M, Klerman G, Lavori D. Long-term outcome of episodes of major depression. JAMA 1984; 252:788–792.
4. Kupfer DJ, Frank E, Perel JM, et al. Five year outcome for maintenance therapies in recurrent depression. Arch Gen Psychiatry 1992; 49:769–773.
5. Prien RF, Kupfer DJ, Mansky PA. Drug therapy in the prevention of recurrences in unipolar and bipolar affective disorders: a report of the NIMH Collaborative Study Group comparing lithium carbonate, imipramine, and a lithium carbonate-imipramine combination. Arch Gen Psychiatry 1984; 41:1096–1104.
6. Hirschfeld RM. Clinical importance of long-term antidepressant treatment. Br J Psychiatry 2001; 42(suppl):S4–S8.
7. Doogan DP, Caillard V. Sertraline in the prevention of depression. Br J Psychiatry 1992; 160:217–222.
8. Montgomery SA, Dufour H, Brion S. The prophylactic efficacy of fluoxetine in unipolar depression. Br J Psychiatry 1988; 153(suppl 3):69–73.
9. Robinson DS, Lerfald SC, Bennett B, et al. Continuation and maintenance treatment of major depression with the monoamine oxidase inhibitor phenelzine: a double-blind placebo-controlled discontinuation study. Psychopharmacol Bull 1991; 27:31–39.
10. Wade AG, Hochstrasser B, Isakson PM, et-al. A double-blind, placebo controlled study of citalopram for depressive recurrence. ACNP abstract. San Juan, Puerto Rico, 1999
11. Claghorn JL, Feighner JP. A double-blind comparison of paroxetine with imipramine in the long term treatment of depression. J Clin Psychopharm 1993; 13(6 suppl 2):23s–27s.
12. Lavori PW, Keller MB, Scheftner W, et al. Recurrence after recovery in unipolar MDD: an observational follow-up study of clinical predictors and somatic treatment as a mediating factor. Int J Methods Psychiatr Res 1994; 4:211–220.
13. Montgomery SA, Dunbar G. Paroxetine is better than placebo in relapse prevention and prophylaxis of recurrent depression. Int Clin Psychopharmacol 1993; 8:189–195.
14. Peselow ED, Dunner DL, Fieve RR, et al. The prophylactic efficacy of tricyclic

antidepressants—a five year followup. Prog Neuropsychopharmacol Biol Psychiatry 1991; 15:71–82.

15. Quitkin FM, Stewart JW, McGrath PJ. Loss of drug effects during continuation therapy. Am J Psychiatry 1993; 150:562–565.

16. Ramana R, Paykel E, Cooper Z. Remission and relapse in major depression: a two-year prospective follow-up study. Psychol Med 1995; 25:1161–1170.

17. Feiger AD, Bielski RJ, Bremner J, Heiser JF, Trivedi M, Wilcox CS, Roberts DL, Kensler TT, McQuade RD, Kaplita SB, Archibald DG. Double-blind, placebo-substitution study of nefazodone in the prevention of relapse during continuation treatment of outpatients with major depression. Int Clin Psychopharmol 1999; 14(1):19–28.

18. Entsuah AR, Rudolph RL, Hackett D, Miska S. Efficacy of venlafaxine and placebo during long-term treatment of depression: a pooled analysis of relapse rates. Int Clin Psychopharmacol 1996; 11(2):137–147.

19. Anton SF, Robinson DS, Roberts DL, Kensler TT, English PA, Archibald DG. Long-term treatment of depression with nefazodone. Psychopharmacol Bull 1994; 30(2):165–169.

20. U.S. Department of Health and Human Services: Depression in Primary Care. Vol. 2. Treatment of Major Depression. Washington, DC: U.S. Government Printing Office (AHCPR 930551), 1993.

21. American Psychiatric Association. Practice Guideline for the Treatment of Patients with Major Depressive Disorder (revision) [review]. Am J Psychiatry 2000; 157(suppl 4):1–45.

22. Paykel ES, Priest RG. Recognition and management of depression in general practice: consensus statement. BMJ 1992; 305:1198–1202.

23. Anderson IM, Nutt DJ, Deakin JF. Evidence-based guidelines for treating depressive disorders with antidepressants: a revision of the 1993 British Association for Psychopharmacology Guidelines. J Psychopharmacol 2000; 14:3–20.

24. Keller MB. Long-term treatment of recurrent and chronic depression. J Clin Psychiatry 2001; 62(suppl 24):3–5.

25. Dunner DL. Acute and maintenance treatment of chronic depression. J Clin Psychiatry 2001; 62(suppl 6):10–16.

26. Mueller TI, Leon AC, Keller MB, Martin B, Solomon DA, Endicott J, Coryell W, Warshaw M, Maser JD. Recurrence after recovery from major depressive disorder during 15 years of observational follow-up. Am J Psychiatry 1999; 156(7):1000–1006.

27. Kaplan E, Meier P. Nonparametric estimation from incomplete observations. J Am Stat Assoc 1958; 58:690–700.

28. Montgomery SA, Reimitz PE, Zivkov M. Mirtazapine versus amitriptyline in the long-term treatment of depression: a double-blind placebo-controlled study. Int Clin Psychopharmacol 1998; 13(2):63–73.

29. Claxton AJ, Li Z, McKendrick J. Selective serotonin reuptake inhibitor treatment in the UK: risk of relapse or recurrence of depression. Br J Psychiatry 2000; 177:163–168.

30. Sackeim HA, Haskett RE, Mulsant BH, Thase ME, Mann JJ, Pettinati HM,

Greenberg RM, Crowe RR, Cooper TB, Prudic J. Continuation pharmacotheraphy in the prevention of relapse following electroconvulsive therapy: a randomized controlled trial. JAMA 2001; 285(10):1299–1307.

31. Vesiani M, Mehilane L, Gaszner P, Arnaud-Castiglioni R. Reboxetine, a unique selective NRI, prevents relapse and recurrence in long-term treatment of major depressive disorder. J Clin Psychiatry 1999; 60(6):400–406.

32. Thase ME, Nierenberg AA, Keller MB, Panagides J. The relapse prevention study group. Efficacy of mirtazapine for prevention of depressive relapse: a placebo controlled double-blind trial of recently remitted high-risk patients. J Clin Psychiatry 2001; 62(10):782–788.

33. Ferreri M, Colonna L, Leger JM. Efficacy of amineptine in the prevention of relapse in unipolar depression. Int Clin Psychopharmacol 1997; 12(suppl 3):S39–S45.

34. Miner CM, Brown EB, Gonzales JS, Munir R. Switching patients from daily citalopram, paroxetine, or sertraline to once-weekly fluoxetine in the maintenance of response for depression. J Clin Psychiatry 2002; 63(3):232–240.

35. Schmidt ME, Fava M, Robinson JM, Judge R. The efficacy and safety of a new enteric-coated formulation of fluoxetine given once weekly during the continuation treatment of major depressive disorder. J Clin Psychiatry 2000; 61(11):851–857.

36. Greenhouse JB, Stangl D, Kupfer DJ, et al. Methodologic issues in maintenance therapy clinical trials. Arch Gen Psychiatry 1991; 48:313–318.

37. Frank E, Kupfer DJ, Perel JM. Comparison of full-dose versus half-dose pharmacotherapy in the maintenance treatment of recurrent depression. J Affect Disord 1993; 27:139–145.

38. Rouillon F, Warner B, Pezous N, Bisserbe JC. Milnacipran efficacy in the prevention of recurrent depression: a 12-month placebo-controlled study. Int Clin Psychopharmacol 2000; 15(3):133–140.

39. Gilaberte I, Montejo AL, de la Gandara J, Perez-Sola V, Bernardo M, Massana J, Martin-Santos R, Santiso A, Noguera R, Casais L, Perez-Camo V, Arias M, Judge R. Fluoxetine in the prevention of depressive recurrences: a double-blind study. J Clin Psychopharmacol 2001; 21(4):417–424.

40. Klysner R, Bent-Hansen J, Hansen HL, Lunde M, Pleidrup E, Poulsen DL, Andersen M, Petersen HE. Efficacy of citalopram in the prevention of recurrent depression in elderly patients: placebo-controlled study of maintenance therapy. Br J Psychiatry 2002; 181:29–35.

41. Terra JL, Montgomery SA. Fluvoxamine prevents recurrence of depression: results of long-term, double-blind, placebo-controlled study. Int Clin Psychopharmacol 1998; 13(2):55–62.

42. Stewart J, Quitkin F, McGrath PJ, et al. Use of pattern analysis to predict differential relapse of remitted patients with major depression during 1 year of treatment with fluoxetine or placebo. Arch Gen Psychiatry 1998; 55:334–343.

43. Montgomery SA, Rasmussen JGC, Tanghoj P. A 24-week study of 20 mg citalopram, 40 mg citalopram, and placebo in the prevention of relapse of major depression. Int Clin Psychopharmacol 1993; 8:181–188.

44. Robert PH, Montgomery SA. Citalopram in doses of 20–60 mg is effective in depression relapse prevention: a placebo-controlled 6 month study. Int Clin Psychopharmacol 1995; 10(suppl 1):29–35.
45. Rosenberg et al., 1994.
46. Franchini L, Zanardi R, Gasperini M, et al. Two-year maintenance treatment with citalopram, 20 mg, in unipolar subjects with high recurrence rate. J Clin Psychiatry 1999; 60:861–865.
47. Franchini L, Spagnolo C, Rampoldi R, Zanardi R, Smeraldi E. Long-term treatment with citalopram in patients with highly recurrent forms of unipolar depression. Psychiatry Res 2001; 105(1–2):129–133.
48. Hochstrasser B, Isaksen PM, Koponen H, Lauritzen L, Mahnert FA, Rouillon F, Wade AG, Andersen M, Pedersen SF, Swart JC, Nil R. Prophylactic effect of citalopram in unipolar, recurrent depression: placebo-controlled study of maintenance therapy. Br J Psychiatry 2001; 178:304–310.
49. Geddes JR, Carney SM, Davies C, Furukawa TA, Kupfer DJ, Frank E, Goodwin GM. Relapse prevention with antidepressant drug treatment in depressive disorders: a systematic review. Lancet 2003; 361(9358):653–661.
50. Byrne S, Rothschild AJ. Loss of antidepressant efficacy during maintenance therapy: possible mechanisms and treatments. J Clin Psychiatry 1998; 59:279–288.
51. Cohen BM, Baldessarini RJ. Tolerance to therapeutic effects of antidepressants. Am J Psychiatry 1985; 142:489–490.
52. Donaldson SR. Tolerance to phenelzine and subsequent refractory depression: three cases. J Clin Psychiatry 1989; 50:33–35.
53. Cohen BM, Baldessarini RJ. Tolerance to therapeutic effects of antidepressants. Am J Psychiatry 1985; 142(4):489–490.
54. Cain JW. Poor response to fluoxetine: underlying depression, serotonergic overstimulation or a "therapeutic window"? J Clin Psychiatry 1992; 53:272–277.
55. Chisholm DD. Change in serum antidepressant level at a constant dose of medication. Am J Psychiatry 1986; 143:388.
56. Alpert JE. Management of depressive breakthrough during long term treatment. 154th Annual Meeting of the American Psychiatric Association, New Orleans, 2001.
57. Quitkin FM, Stewart JW, McGrath PJ, Nunes E, Ocepek-Welikson K, Tricamo E, Rabkin JG, Klein DF. Further evidence that a placebo response to antidepressants can be identified. Am J Psychiatry 1993; 150:566–570.
58. Fava M, Rappe SM, Pava JA, et al. Relapse in patients on long-term fluoxetine treatment: Response to increased fluoxetine dose. J Clin Psychiatry 1995; 56:52–55.
59. Leib J, Balter A. Antidepressant tachyphylaxis. Med Hypotheses 1984; 15:279–291.
60. Mann JJ. Loss of antidepressant effect with long-term monoamine oxidase inhibition. J Clin Psychopharmacol 1983; 3:363–366.
61. Zetin M, Aden G, Moldawsky R. Tolerance to amoxapine antidepressant effects. Clin Ther 1983; 5:638–643.

62. Sharma V. Loss of response to antidepressants and subsequent refractoriness: diagnostic issues in a retrospective case series. J Affect Disord 2001; 64:99–106.
63. McGrath PJ, Quitkin FM, Klein DF. Bromocriptine treatment of relapses seen during selective serotonin re-uptake inhibitor treatment of depression. J Clin Psychopharmacol 1995; 15(4):289–291.
64. Gardier AM, Lepoul E, Trouvin JH, Chanut E, Dessalles DC, Jacquot C. Changes in dopamine metabolism in rat forebrain regions after cessation of long-term fluoxetine treatment: relationship with brain concentrations of fluoxetine and norfluoxetine. Life Sci 1994; 54:51–56.
65. Schmidt ME, Fava M, Zhang S, Gonzales J, Raute NJ, Judge R. Treatment approaches to major depressive disorder relapse. Psychother Psychosom 2002; 71:190–194.
66. Hamilton M. A rating scale for depression. J Neurol Neurosurg Psychiatry 1960; 23:56–62.
67. Fredman SJ, Fava M, White CN, et al. Partial response, non-response and relapse on SSRIs in major depression: a survey of current "next-step" practices. Am J Psychiatry. In press.
68. Amsterdam J, Brunswick DJ, Mendels J. High dose desipramine plasma drug levels and clinical response. J Clin Psychiatry 1979; 40:141–143.
69. Schuckit MA. Safety of high-dose tricyclic antidepressant therapy. Am J Psychiatry 1972; 128:1456–1459.
70. Simpson GM, Lee UH, Cucuilc Z, Kellner R. Two doses of imipramine in hospitalized depressives. Arch Gen Psychiatry 1976; 33:1093–1102.
71. Rothschild AJ, Byrne S. Psychiatrists' responses to failure of maintenance therapy with antidepressants. Psychiatr Serv 1997; 48:835–837.
72. Altamura AC, Montgomery SA, Wernicke JF. The evidence of 20 mg a day of fluoxetine as the optimal dose in the treatment of depression. Br J Psychiatry 1988; 153(suppl 3):109–112.
73. Dornseif BE, Dunlop SR, Potvin JH, Wernicke JF. Effect of dose escalation after low-dose fluoxetine therapy. Psychopharmacol Bull 1989; 25:71–79.
74. Schweitzer E, Rickels K, Amsterdam JD. What constitutes and adequate antidepressant trial for fluoxetine? J Clin Psychiatry 1990; 51:8–11.
75. Judd et al.
76. Bodkin JA, Lasser RA, Wines JD Jr, et al. Combining serotonin reuptake inhibitors and bupropion in partial responders to antidepressant monotherapy. J Clin Psychiatry 1997; 58:137–145.
77. Fava M, Rosenbaum JF, McGrath PJ, et al. A double-blind, controlled study of lithium and tricyclic augmentation of fluoxetine in treatment resistant depression. Am J Psychiatry 1994; 151:1372–1374.
78. Nierenberg AA, Cole JO. One antidepressant fails: what next? A survey of northeastern psychiatrists. J Clin Psychiatry 1991; 52:383–385.
79. de Montigny C, Grunberg F, Mayer A. Lithium induces rapid relief of depression in tricyclic antidepressant drug nonresponders. Br J Psychiatry 1981; 138:252–256.
80. Kramlinger KG, Post RM. The addition of lithium to carbamazepine: anti-

depressant efficacy in treatment-resistant depression. Arch Gen Psychiatry 1989; 46:794–800.

81. Pope HG, McElroy SL, Nixon RA. Possible synergism between fluoxetine and lithium in refractory depression. Am J Psychiatry 1988; 145:1292–1294.

82. Ontiveros A, Fontaine R, Elie R. Refractory depression: the addition of lithium to fluoxetine or desipramine. Acta Psychiatr Scand 1991; 83:188–192.

83. Nierenberg AA, Iacoviello BM, Worthington JJ, Tedlow J, Alpert JE, Fava M. Lithium augmentation of nortriptyline for subjects resistant to multiple antidepressants. J Clin Psychopharmacol 2003; 23(1):92–95.

84. Bauer M, Bschor T, Kunz D, Berghofer A, Strohle A, Muller-Oerlinghausen B. Double-blind, placebo-controlled trial of the use of lithium to augment antidepressant medication in continuation treatment of unipolar major depression. Am J Psychiatry 2000; 157(9):1429–1435.

85. Fava M. Augmentation and combination strategies in treatment-resistant depression. J Clin Psychiatry 2001; 62(suppl 18):4–11.

86. Dording CM, Mischoulon D, Petersen TJ, Kornbluh R, Gordon JA, Nierenberg AA, Rosenbaum JF, Fava M. The pharmacologic management of SSRI-induced side effects: a survey of psychiatrists. Ann Clin Psychiatry. In press.

87. Nelson JC. Augmentation strategies in depression 2000. J Clin Psychiatry 2000; 61(suppl 2):13–19.

88. Apter JT, Birkett M.Fluoxetine treatment in depressed patients who failed treatment with sertraline. Presented at the 34th annual meeting of the American College of Neuropsychopharmacology, San Juan, Puerto Rico, December 11–15, 1995.

89. Brown WA, Harrison W. Are patients who are intolerant to one serotonin selective reuptake inhibitor intolerant to another? J Clin Psychiatry 1995; 56:30–34.

90. Kreider MS, Bushnell WD, Oakes R, et al. A double-blind, randomized study to provide safety information on switching fluoxetine-treated patients to paroxetine without an intervening washout period. J Clin Psychiatry 1994; 56:142–145.

91. Nierenberg A, Feighner JP, Rudolph R. Venlafaxine for treatment-resistant depression. J Clin Psychopharmacol 1994; 14:419–423.

92. de Montigny C, Debonnel G, Bergeron R, St-André E, Blier P. Venlafaxine in treatment-resistant depression: an open-label multicenter study. Poster presented at the 34th Annual Meeting of the American College of Neuropsychopharmacology, San Juan, Puerto Rico, 1995.

93. Fava M, Papakostas GI, Petersen T, Mahal Y, Quitkin F, Stewart J, McGrath P. Switching to buproprion in fluoxetine-refractory depression. Ann Clin Psychiatry. In press.

94. Thase M, Rush AJ, Howland RH, et al. Double-blind switch study of imipramine or sertraline treatment of antidepressant-resistant chronic depression. Arch Gen Psychiatry 2002; 59:233–239.

95. Posternak MA, Zimmerman M. Switching versus augmentation: a prospective, naturalistic comparison in depressed, treatment-resistant patients. J Clin Psychiatry 2001; 62(2):135–142.

11

Psychopharmacological Management of Residual Symptoms and Treatment Resistance in Major Depressive Disorder

Maurizio Fava

Massachusetts General Hospital
and Harvard Medical School
Boston, Massachusetts, U.S.A.

INTRODUCTION

Treatment-resistant depression typically refers to the occurrence of an inadequate response following adequate antidepressant therapy among patients suffering from major depressive disorder (MDD). What constitutes an inadequate response has been the object of considerable debate in the field, and most experts nowadays probably would argue that an inadequate response is the failure to achieve remission. Although the more traditional view of treatment resistance has focused on nonresponse (e.g., patients who have reported minimal or no improvement with drug therapy), from the perspective of clinicians and patients/consumers, not achieving remission despite adequate treatment represents a significant challenge [1]. There is substantial evidence that a significant proportion of patients suffering from MDD fail to achieve full remission despite adequate treatment and significant symptom improvement [2]. These patients, including those who respond (e.g., experience a ≥50%

reduction of symptoms), may continue to be affected by residual symptoms. Residual symptoms can be psychological, behavioral, and/or physical in nature [3], and include depressed mood, lack of interest, excessive guilt, fatigue, sleep disturbances, changes in appetite, and pain. For example, a study from our group [3] showed that approximately one-third of patients who had responded to fluoxetine treatment (with a Hamilton Rating Scale for Depression [HAM-D] score <8) reported fatigue as a subthreshold or threshold residual symptom of their MDD.

Relapse and recurrence after successful treatment of MDD is a common and debilitating outcome [4], and patients with MDD who do not achieve complete remission of their symptoms are particularly vulnerable to relapse [5–7]. For example, in a 15-month study of the long-term outcome of treatment of depression, Paykel et al. [5] followed 60 patients diagnosed with unipolar major depression [Research Diagnostic Criteria (RDC)] to relapse or remission. Thirty-two percent (19 of 60) of the patients reported residual symptoms at remission. Although improvement occurred moderately rapidly, relapse was common. In fact, relapses occurred within the first 10 months of follow-up in 76% (13 of 17) of patients with residual symptoms but in only 25% (10 of 40) of patients without residual symptoms.

All these data strongly urge the need for improved methods of treating depression that will result in remission without residual symptoms.

ASSESSING RESIDUAL SYMPTOMS

In order to target residual symptoms in depression, it is important to be able to assess such symptoms adequately. There are several well-established clinician-rated instruments, such as the HAM-D [8], the Montgomery-Asberg Depression Rating Scale (MADRS) [9], and the Inventory of Depressive Symptomatology—Clinician-Rated (IDS-C) [10], which have shown good sensitivity to detect changes among patients with depressive disorders. Although the use of clinician-rated instruments is preferred, it is more common for clinicians to use clinician or patient global assessment measures, often combined with self-rated instruments, such as the Inventory of Depressive Symptomatology—Self-Rated (IDS-SR) [10], the Beck Depression Inventory (BDI) in its original and revised version [11], the Symptom Questionnaire (SQ) [12], or the Harvard National Depression Screening Day Scale (HANDS) [13].

Given the fact that physical and somatic residual symptoms are highly prevalent in MDD, the use of sensitive scales in clinical practice to assess such symptoms is uncommon, as conventional scales used to measure depression in clinical trials rarely include significant numbers of physical symptoms. For example, the MADRS is a 10-item clinician-rated scale that includes only three physical symptoms (decreased appetite, insomnia, and fatigue) [9]. Most depression scales tend to concentrate on psychological symptoms, with the exception of the Symptom Questionnaire (SQ) [12], which includes a somatic symptom subscale and has shown excellent sensitivity to detect change in physical symptoms following antidepressant treatment [14]. The importance of assessing physical residual symptoms is underscored by a recent study from our group showing that patients who remitted following 8 weeks of antidepressant therapy (HAM-D-17 score $\leq$5) had significantly (P < .03) lower SQ somatic symptom scores at endpoint compared with patients who responded (50% or greater reduction in HAM-D score from baseline to endpoint) but did not achieve remission [15].

TREATMENT TACTICS

Clinicians can employ a number of basic treatment tactics to increase the chance of a patient achieving full remission, including psychoeducation, enhancing treatment adherence, ensuring adequacy of dose, ensuring adequacy of treatment duration, choosing antidepressant treatments with relatively greater efficacy in specific subtypes or populations and adding psychotherapy.

> *Psychoeducation.* It is considered quite helpful to explain to patients that depression is a medical illness that is associated with changes in brain functioning and that antidepressants are used to help the brain function better. Psychoeducational materials and an emphasis on the importance of communication and collaboration may help set the stage for meaningful dialogue. Psychoeducation may therefore increase the degree of collaboration between the patient and the treating clinician and may enhance the acceptability of any subsequent proposed treatment approach.
>
> *Enhancing treatment adherence.* Adequate follow-up with patients (office visits or phone contacts) is known to lead to better adherence to treatment. Also, the use of antidepressants that have relatively greater tolerability and fewer side effects also affects adherence in a positive way, although it is important to discuss side effects that may occur during antidepressant treatment and approaches to their management in the event of their occurrence.
>
> *Ensuring adequacy of dose.* Although antidepressant medication is typically administered at doses within the recommended therapeutic range, some patients may require doses well above the therapeutic

range in order to respond. Monitoring antidepressant blood levels may be useful for patients who are not responding and do not report side effects even with the newer antidepressants for which there is no clear blood level–response relationship.

Ensuring adequacy of treatment duration. Most patients require 6–12 weeks of treatment to achieve an adequate response [16]. On the other hand, studies [16,17] have shown that minimal improvement by week 4 or 5 leads to a very small chance of response. In fact, a study from our group has demonstrated [17] that nonresponse as early as week 4 or 6 predicted poor outcome at week 8. These findings suggest that, in general, clinicians must consider taking action if symptom improvement is not significant by week 5 or 6. In addition, an improved long-term outcome for patients may be achieved by the use of longer courses of treatment, which may ultimately enable recovery from depressive symptoms.

Choosing antidepressant treatments with relatively greater efficacy in specific subtypes or populations. Although remission rates tend to be comparable across antidepressant drugs and antidepressant classes, the chances of remission may be enhanced by choosing agents with relatively greater efficacy in a specific depressive subtype. For example, dual-action antidepressants, acting to inhibit the reuptake of both serotonin and norepinephrine, have performed better than certain single-action selective serotonin reuptake inhibitors (SSRIs) in evoking remission among patients with melancholic/endogenous depression [18,19].

Adding psychotherapy. Recent evidence indicates that for those who respond but do not remit to a medication, cognitive therapy not only removes the residual symptoms but is associated with an improved prognosis [20].

All these treatment tactics may increase the chance of a depressed patient achieving full remission, although it is not clear whether there is synergy across them or whether each tactic affects treatment outcome independently. Future studies are needed to investigate in a systematic fashion the effectiveness of these tactics in managing treatment resistance and eliminating residual symptoms in MDD.

TREATMENT STRATEGIES

The pharmacological strategies used in the management of residual symptoms and treatment resistance in MDD typically derive from those employed for patients who are resistant to antidepressant treatment. However, the assumption that pharmacological strategies proven to be effective in the management of patients with little or no response to standard treatments would work as well in the management of residual symptoms in MDD has never been empirically tested. The actual acceptability, clinical benefit, and side effect burden of these treatments in MDD populations with partial response or response with residual symptoms is also not well known. In the literature, there are only two double-controlled studies of MDD patients with partial response, and they are both from our group [21,22]. This suggests that this is an area of great need for systematic studies to guide clinicians in their therapeutic decisions.

Four typical strategies are used in treatment-resistant depression and, subsequently, in the management of residual symptoms in MDD: (1) dose increase, (2) augmentation, (3) combination, and (4) switching. Although the first option has been shown to be the most common approach to the management of residual symptoms and partial response in a survey of approximately 400 psychiatrists [23], switching is an option that is considered when side effects may be significant. In fact, when depressed patients respond to treatment with an antidepressant but they are still symptomatic and experience troublesome side effects, clinicians may choose to switch them to another antidepressant (switching strategy). On the other hand, if the side effects are tolerable or absent, clinicians may decide to keep the patient on same antidepressant and to add another "augmenting" compound. Such augmentation strategy involves the use of a pharmacological agent that is not considered to be a standard antidepressant but may boost or enhance the effect of an antidepressant. Alternatively, clinicians may choose to combine the antidepressant that did not produce adequate response with another antidepressant, typically of a different class. The latter approach is called combination strategy, and its popularity has increased over time, with the introduction of newer antidepressants with a fairly benign side effect profile and with fewer concerns about drug-drug interactions. In the following four sections of this chapter, we are going to review the studies concerning the efficacy of dose increase, augmentation, combination, and switching strategies.

Dose Increase

From a pharmacological standpoint, raising the dose of the antidepressant is a commonly used strategy in the management of treatment-resistant depression. Raising the dose of an antidepressant is a strategy of dose escalation usually within the recommended therapeutic dose range, although, in some cases, the dose increase may exceed such a range, particularly in the absence of side effects. In a recent survey of 412 psychiatrists from across the United States [23], respondents indicated their preferred strategies when a patient failed to respond to 8 weeks or more of an adequate dose of a SSRI; interestingly, in the case of partial response, raising the dose was the first choice for 82% of the respondents, whereas raising the dose was endorsed only by 27% of the respondents in the case of nonresponse, with the remainder of the respondents selecting either switching or augmentation/combination strategies. Dose increase with the newer antidepressants was first studied in an open trial on 15 depressed outpatients [24] who had failed to respond to 8–12 weeks of open treatment with fluoxetine 20 mg/day and was found to be associated with a significant improvement in depressive symptomatology. In a subsequent double-blind study (Fig. 1) [22] among 41 MDD patients who had not responded to fluoxetine 20 mg/day, 53% of 15 patients treated with high-dose fluoxetine (40–60 mg/day) responded (i.e., their HAM-D-17 score was ≤7) versus 29% of 14 patients treated with fluoxetine plus lithium (300–600 mg/day) and 25% of 12 patients treated with fluoxetine plus desipramine (25–50 mg/day). Although high-dose fluoxetine was the most effective treatment among partial responders (response rate: 83%), fluoxetine 20 mg/day plus lithium 300–600 mg/day (response rate: 50%) was nonsignificantly more effective than the other two strategies among nonresponders. A larger study from our group [21] among 101 MDD patients nonresponding to fluoxetine 20 mg/day for 8 weeks found that there was a nonsignificant superiority in response rates of dose increase compared to the other two treatment groups (high-dose fluoxetine: 42.4%; fluoxetine plus desipramine: 29.4%; fluoxetine plus lithium: 23.5%). There were also nonsignificant differences in response

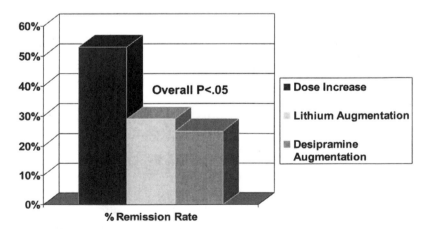

FIGURE 1   Double-blind study in 41 nonresponders and partial responders to an 8-week fluoxetine trial. (From Ref. 22.)

rates across the three treatment groups among partial responders (high-dose fluoxetine: 50.0%; fluoxetine plus desipramine: 33.3%; fluoxetine plus lithium: 33.3%) and nonresponders (high-dose fluoxetine: 35.3%; fluoxetine plus desipramine: 26.3%; fluoxetine plus lithium: 12.5%). These studies suggest that, particularly among partial responders, raising the dose may indeed be a helpful strategy.

Augmentation Studies

Over the past few decades, numerous compounds have been used as augmenting agents of antidepressants. Although the majority of the studies of this therapeutic approach are open label, many investigations are also double blind and often placebo controlled. This certainly allows us to draw relatively firm conclusions about the efficacy of some of the augmenting agents, such as lithium and thyroid hormones. It appears that the improvement following antidepressant augmentation tends to occur within 3–4 weeks, so it may be too premature to decide in first few days or couple of weeks whether or not an augmentation strategy is working. Almost all the studies on the efficacy of these augmentation strategies have focused on the short-term outcome, and very little is known about the minimum duration of the augmentation trial in responders to such strategy. Although there are many augmentation strategies that have been studied or reported in the literature [25], the best-studied augmentation strategies in resistant depression are lithium, thyroid hormone, and buspirone.

Lithium

Lithium augmentation is not as popular currently as it was in the 1980s, although there are a lot of studies that have clearly shown that the addition of a dose of 600 mg or more a day of lithium, typically in divided doses, and with reasonably good blood levels, leads to a robust increase in the chances of a response in patients who have not responded to tricyclic antidepressants (TCAs), monoamine oxidase inhibitors (MAOIs), and SSRIs. Eleven double-blind controlled trials of lithium augmentation in depression have been published; of those, 12 actually reported the observed response rate, which averaged 42% for a total of 187 lithium-treated patients [21,22,26–37]. On the other hand, in several studies, lithium did not do particularly well when added to SSRIs [21,22,32]. Similarly, the efficacy of lithium augmentation in the only two double-blind studies in partial responders to SSRIs in the literature is rather modest, with an overall response rate of 27% (7 of 26 patients) [21,22]. Therefore, despite the relative robust findings concerning lithium augmentation of TCAs in the literature, the role of lithium in managing residual symptoms among MDD patients treated with the newer antidepressants remains to be established.

Thyroid Hormone

In treatment-resistant depression studies, L-triiodothyronine (T3) has been used in preference to and has been shown to be superior to thyroxine (T4) [38]. Among four randomized double-blind studies of T3 augmentation of antidepressants, pooled effects were not significant (relative response: 1.53; 95% CI, 0.70 to 3.35; $P = .29$), but one study with negative results accounted for most of the intertrial heterogeneity in results [39]. Since all the published studies of T3 augmentation involved the use of TCAs, the efficacy of this strategy in SSRI-resistant patients is not known yet. Similarly, there is no published study that has examined specifically the role of T3 augmentation in the management of residual symptoms in MDD.

Buspirone

Buspirone is typically a well-tolerated antianxiety drug, with serotonin (5-HT1A) partial agonist properties. Studies using buspirone 5–15 mg twice a day have shown significant improvement in refractory patients [30,40–42]. Although the first placebo-controlled study in refractory depression comparing buspirone to placebo augmentation did not find any statistically significant difference in response rates between these two treatment (51% vs 47%, respectively) [43], a more recent double-blind study showed that, among the SSRI-resistant patients with severe depression, buspirone was more effective than placebo augmentation [44]. Again, there is no published study that has examined specifically the role of buspirone augmentation in the management of residual symptoms in MDD.

Pindolol

Pindolol augmentation is rarely used in clinical practice in the United States, but it is relatively more popular in Europe and Canada in the management of resistant depression. Pindolol is a beta-blocker and a serotonin 5-HT1A antagonist. A dose of pindolol 2.5 mg three times a day has been used in most depression studies. This agent has generated a lot of interest, because it has been shown to accelerate an antidepressant response when combined with SSRIs in some [45–49], but not all [50], the studies. A study by Moreno and colleagues [51] found no response among 10 refractory depressed patients, and a study by Perez and colleagues [52] showed no difference from placebo in a very short (10-day) trial of augmentation in a refractory depressed population.

Dopaminergic Drugs

Augmentation with dopaminergic drugs is an interesting strategy. In an open trial, Bouckoms and Mangini [53] used with some success the antiparkinsonian drug pergolide 0.25–2.0 mg/day in resistant depression. Similarly, there have been reports of the usefulness of antidepressant augmentation with the dopaminergic drugs amantadine (100–200 mg twice a day) [54], pramipexole (0.125–0.50 mg three times a day) [55,56], and ropinirole (0.5–1.5 mg three times a day) [57]. Unfortunately, these studies concerning the augmentation of antidepressants with dopaminergic agents were uncontrolled and had relatively small sample sizes. Therefore, the effectiveness of these augmenting agents, particularly in the management of residual symptoms in MDD, remains to be established.

Psychostimulants

In line with the potential role of dopaminergic agents as augmentors of antidepressants, psychostimulants, which have significant effects on dopamine neurotransmission, have been used to augment TCAs, MAOIs, SSRIs, and serotonin norepinephrine reuptake inhibitors (SNRIs) [25]. Clinicians typically use methylphenidate 20–80 mg/day or dextroamphetamine 10–40 mg/day in divided doses. In addition to the lack of controlled studies, the main issues concerning the use of psychostimulant augmentation are the potential for abuse in some patients with history of substance abuse, the possible emergence of anxiety and irritability, and their relatively short half-life.

Modafinil

Modafinil is a novel psychostimulant with pharmacological actions somewhat different from those of the amphetamines. In a retrospective case series, Menza et al. [58] reported the usefulness of modafinil (in doses up to 200 mg/day) as an adjunct to antidepressants in resistant depression. A recent report by DeBattista et al. [59] showed that 57% of 14 patients not responding to SSRIs or venlafaxine regarded themselves as being much improved following augmentation with up to 400 mg/day of modafinil. The effectiveness of modafinil as an augmenting agent remains to be established, since these studies concerning its use were uncontrolled and had relatively small sample sizes. However, the relatively greater user friendliness of this agent, compared to the psychostimulants, has made it a relative popular augmentor of antidepressants for the management of residual symptoms in MDD. In particular, the presence of residual symptoms such as fatigue, sleepiness, and lethargy may guide clinicians to use an augmenting agent such as modafinil [59].

Atypical Antipsychotics

Risperidone [60], olanzapine [61], and ziprasidone [63] have all shown good responses in some small trials in SSRI nonresponders. The typical doses in augmentation of antidepressants are 0.5–2.0 mg/day for risperidone, 5–20 mg/day for olanzapine, and 40–160 mg/day for ziprasidone. The rapid onset of the effect of this strategy [61] has made it relatively popular among clinicians in the treatment of resistant depressed patients, although very little is known about its efficacy in the management of residual symptoms in MDD.

Inositol

Despite initial anecdotal positive reports of the usefulness of augmentation of antidepressants with doses of inositol up to 12 g/day, a recent controlled, double-blind augmentation trial did not support its use in SSRI treatment nonresponders [62], and a study by Levine et al. [64] showed no difference in outcome between patients treated with SSRIs and placebo versus those treated with SSRIs and inositol.

Opiates

There is very modest evidence, mostly based on case reports and case series, of the usefulness of augmentation of antidepressants with opiates, such as oxycodone, oxymorphone [65], and buprenorphine [66]. The lack of adequate studies and the potential risk for abuse markedly limit the use of these augmenting agents.

Estrogen

Estrogen exerts profound effects on behavior by interacting with neuronal estrogen receptors [67]. There is mostly anecdotal evidence for the efficacy of estrogen augmentation of antidepressants in resistant depression among postmenopausal women. In addition, as pointed out by Stahl [68] in his review of the literature, there are no guidelines on how to optimize antidepressant administration with estrogen, especially in women insufficiently responsive to antidepressants.

Dehydroepiandrosterone and Testosterone

Dehydroepiandrosterone (DHEA), a major circulating corticosteroid in humans, has an unclear physiological role. In addition to serving as a precursor to testosterone and estrogen, DHEA and its sulfated metabolite, DHEA-S, most likely have important biological roles, and have been hypothesized to be involved in regulating mood and a sense of well-being [69]. A very small, preliminary, double-blind study suggests its usefulness up to 90 mg/day as an adjunct to antidepressants in refractory depression [69]. Further studies are clearly necessary given the small number of patients studied. Similarly, an 8-week randomized, placebo-controlled trial of testosterone transdermal gel among 23 men aged 30–65 years who had resistant depression and low or borderline testosterone levels, testosterone was significantly better than placebo in treating depressive symptoms [70]. However, there are no published studies that have examined specifically the role of DHEA or testosterone augmentation in the management of residual symptoms in MDD.

Folate and S-Adenosyl-Methionine (SAMe)

Folate, in particular its active form methyltetrahydrofolate (MTHF), and S-adenosyl-methionine (SAMe) are compounds closely involved in the one-carbon cycle and in methylation processes of the brain. These compounds have been studied extensively in depression, and the literature suggests that they may have antidepressant properties [71,72]. An open trial of methylfolate (up to 30 mg/day) in SSRI-refractory patients suggested its usefulness as an adjunct [73], and a recent open study with SAMe from our group (J.E. Alpert, personal communication) has also shown the usefulness of this augmenting agent in SSRI nonresponders. The availability of SAMe over-the-counter has made this agent a relatively popular augmentation agent among MDD patients with residual symptoms. Our group hopefully will have a chance in the future to study in a placebo-controlled fashion the effect of SAMe augmentation for the treatment of partial responders and nonresponders to SSRIs.

Combination Studies

Although there are numerous double-blind studies of augmentation strategies, there are less than five double-blind studies of combination strategies, reflecting the need for further studies in this area. It appears that the improvement following the combination of antidepressants tends to occur within 4–6 weeks, so it may be too premature to decide in the first few days or couple of weeks whether or not a combination strategy is working. Almost all the studies on the efficacy of these strategies have focused on the short-term outcome, and very little is known about the minimum duration of the combination trial in responders to such strategy. A typical approach is to maintain the combination for 6–9 months after obtaining remission and then to attempt a gradual discontinuation of one of the two antidepressants. One of the issues concerning combination strategies in resistant depression is that, in the case of a therapeutic response, it is not possible to dissect what is due to the combination (and perhaps the synergy between the two antidepressants) and what is due to the simple exposure to another antidepressant. In fact, most combination strategies employ full doses of both antidepressant agents.

Bupropion Plus SSRIs

Bupropion sustained release (SR) (100–150 mg once or twice a day) combined with SSRIs was the first strategy chosen by 400 psychiatrists surveyed by Fredman et al. [23]. On the other hand, the evidence for this combination is primarily based on anecdotal reports, case series, or small open trials [25]. Future studies need to assess in a systematic fashion the effectiveness of this combination among MDD patients with residual symptoms.

Mirtazapine Plus SSRIs

Mirtazapine is a dual-action antidepressant that (1) increases both serotonergic and noradrenergic activity by blocking the α_2-adrenergic auto- and heteroreceptors and (2) blocks the serotonergic 5-HT$_2$ and 5-HT$_3$ receptors. Mirtazapine (15–30 mg qhs) combined with SSRIs has been reported to be helpful in an open study of nonresponders to SSRIs [74] and to be more effective than placebo plus SSRIs in a subsequent double-blind study among 20 SSRI-resistant depressed patients [75]. A recent study by Debonnel et al. [76] showed a significantly higher response rate to the combination of paroxetine and mirtazapine than monotherapy with either drug alone and a 64% response rate to the switch to combination therapy for patients not responding to monotherapy. All these studies suggest the potential usefulness of combining mirtazapine with SSRIs in MDD with residual symptoms, particularly perhaps among those with insomnia and weight loss as residual symptoms.

Desipramine or Other TCAs Plus SSRIs

An early study by Nelson et al. [77] showed that the TCA plus SSRI combination may produce a more rapid onset of action. A more recent study by Nelson [78] has shown that remission rates are significantly higher in patients on desipramine plus fluoxetine than in those on either drug alone. This is consistent with the reports that desipramine and other TCAs were effective in combination with SSRIs in small cohorts of patients [79,80]. The main issue related to combining TCAs with SSRIs is that TCAs are substrates of cytochrome P450 2D6, so there may be accumulation when coadministered with SSRIs inhibiting this pathway, leading potentially to cardiac toxicity. Low doses of TCAs (25–75 mg/day) are therefore typically used, and monitoring of the TCA blood levels is necessary. The efficacy of the combination of

TCAs with SSRIs has been put in question by two studies that showed that adding low-dose desipramine to fluoxetine was less effective than raising the dose of fluoxetine in patients who had not responded to 8 weeks of treatment with fluoxetine 20 mg/day [21,22].

Reboxetine/Atomoxetine Plus SSRIs

After an initial anecdotal report from our group that the addition of reboxetine, a relatively selective norepinephrine reuptake inhibitor (NRI), was helpful in patients refractory to SSRI treatment [81], three open trials, using doses up to 8 mg/day, have suggested the usefulness of this agent combined with SSRIs in resistant depression [82–84]. Given the fact that reboxetine is not available in the United States, a number of clinicians have been using in combination with SSRIs the newly marketed atomoxetine, a relatively selective NRI that has been approved in the United States for the treatment of attention deficit disorder. Future studies are needed to support this off-label use of this compound.

Nefazodone/Venlafaxine Plus SSRIs

There have been only anecdotal reports suggesting the efficacy of combining SSRIs with nefazodone or venlafaxine. One possible issue concerning this strategy is related to some reports of a serotonin syndrome [85,86]. In addition, venlafaxine is a substrate of the cytochrome P450 2D6, and there have been reports of accumulation of venlafaxine when coadministered with some SSRIs inhibiting the 2D6 pathway, leading to marked blood pressure elevation and severe anticholinergic side effects [87].

Switching Studies

Several "theoretical" principles commonly guide antidepressant pharmacotherapy choices with respect to switching strategies in resistant depression:

1. A switch from one agent that affects one neurotransmitter system (e.g., from a serotonin reuptake blocker) to one that affects another (e.g., selective norepinephrine reuptake blocker) will be more effective than a switch to another agent affecting the same system. This rationale has become a common basis of clinical practice, although its validity has not been studied in double-blind, controlled clinical trials.

2. Agents that affect more than one neurotransmitter system (e.g., serotonin and norepinephrine) will be more effective than more selective agents (e.g., a selective serotonin reuptake inhibitor agent) in those who have failed a more selective agent initially. This hypo-

thesis has been indirectly supported by the Danish University Anti-depressant Group (DUAG) study [19], but it needs empirical evaluation.

3. A switch to an agent that produces changes in neuronal systems by different mechanisms of action (e.g., norepinephrine and serotonin reuptake inhibition plus postsynaptic receptor antagonism vs monoamine oxidase inhibition) than the previously failed agent will be more effective than switches to agents with similar mechanisms of action as the failed prior agent (e.g., switching from a TCA to a TCA will be less effective than switching from a TCA to an MAOI). This hypothesis has been supported by several studies with TCAs and MAOIs [88,89], but it has not been investigated in a systematic fashion with the newer agents.

Switching from One SSRI to Another

Three uncontrolled studies [90–92] found that participants who did not respond to one SSRI had a 50–65% response rate to another SSRI. However, it has been suggested [93] that markedly lower response rates to a switch within SSRIs would be observed when the failure to respond is documented prospectively, when medication doses are adjusted upward for the initial SSRI, and when only those who do not respond to (as opposed to those who were intolerant to) the first SSRI are included. For this reason, it is not surprising that a recent double-blind study [94] showed that, among MDD patients with a history of resistance to two previous antidepressant treatments (mostly SSRIs) and a CGI improvement score of 3 at the beginning of treatment, the response rate was significantly greater for the SNRI venlafaxine than for the SSRI paroxetine.

Switching to Venlafaxine

Nierenberg et al. [95] found a 30–33% response to the serotonin norepinephrine reuptake inhibitor (SNRI) venlafaxine among 84 consecutive treatment-resistant depressed patients (who had failed at least three trials). Another open study found that, among 152 patients with MDD and a documented history of unsatisfactory improvement after a minimum of 8 weeks of treatment with an adequate dose of an antidepressant, treatment with venlafaxine was followed by a response (50% improvement from baseline) in 58% of the patients [96]. These studies do support the hypothesis that dual-action agents (e.g., agents that affect both the serotonin and norepinephrine systems) may be more effective than more selective agents (e.g., a selective serotonin reuptake inhibitor agent) in those who have failed a more selective agent initially.

Switching to Duloxetine

Duloxetine is another dual-action SNRI which has shown greater efficacy than an SSRI comparator in the treatment of MDD [97]. For this reason, an open-label study on the efficacy of the SNRI duloxetine among SSRI non-responders is currently ongoing.

Switching to Mirtazapine

A recent multicenter study [14] has shown a 48% response rate to mirtazapine switch (15–45 mg/day) among 69 SSRI nonresponders whose treatment with the SSRI did not exceed 6 months. A recent study by Thase [98] has shown no significant difference in outcome between mirtazapine and the SSRI sertraline in patients who had not responded to other SSRIs. It should be noted, however, that the latter study enrolled solely patients with a retrospective history of nonresponse to SSRI treatment and that there was no upper limit in the duration of the failed SSRI trial, creating the bases for significant recall biases and for relapses being misclassified as nonresponses.

Switching from SSRIs to TCAs

The switch to TCAs has also been shown to be effective among SSRI nonresponders in a large randomized and controlled study (n = 117) of a switch from sertraline to imipramine (response rate: 44%) [99]. Approximately 40% of 92 patients with treatment-resistant DSM-III-R (Diagnostic and Statistical Manual of Mental Disorders, 3rd., revised) major depression, with resistance defined by at least one, but no more than five, well-documented adequate trials of antidepressants during the current episode, responded to open treatment with nortriptyline for 6 weeks [100].

Switching to Bupropion

Even though switching to bupropion appears to be a very popular strategy among psychiatrists [23], as pointed out in a recent review [93], only small, uncontrolled studies have reported significant improvement upon switching SSRI-treated patients to bupropion. We have recently reported the results of an open trial where a group of fluoxetine nonresponders showed a good response to a switch to bupropion [101]. Future studies should investigate the usefulness of switching MDD with residual symptoms to bupropion.

Switching to Reboxetine

In a recent study of 128 adult outpatients with MDD who had not responded to at least 6–12 weeks of fluoxetine treatment, and with at least 3 weeks of treatment on a minimum dose of 40 mg/day of fluoxetine, a statistically significant ($P < .001$) improvement in the mean total HAM-D-17 score was seen from baseline to endpoint following a switch to open treatment with the selective norepinephrine reuptake inhibitor reboxetine [102].

Switching to MAOIs

Switching to MAOIs, a very effective strategy for resistant depression, was relatively popular in the 1970s and 1980s, but is now typically considered at the end of a treatment algorithm, primarily because of the dietary restrictions and the risk of spontaneous and nonspontaneous hypertensive crises. Several studies have examined the efficacy of MAOIs in the treatment of patients who had failed to respond to TCAs [93]. In a crossover study of patients with mood-reactive, nonmelancholic depression of 46 patients previously unresponsive to imipramine who completed phenelzine treatment, 31 (67%) responded to phenelzine, whereas of 22 patients previously unresponsive to phenelzine who completed imipramine treatment, 9 (41%) responded to imipramine [103].

CONCLUSIONS

Several pharmacological approaches have been developed in the management of MDD patients with residual symptoms and/or treatment resistance. Further studies are needed to investigate the effects of those pharmacological treatments specifically in MDD patients with residual symptoms. Clinicians must marshal the different treatment options to increase their patients' chances of achieving sustained remission from depression and resolution of residual symptoms. The ongoing Sequenced Treatment Alternatives to Relieve Depression (STAR*D) study [104], funded by the National Institute of Mental Health, is determining which treatment options are most effective for patients who fail to benefit adequately after initial treatment with antidepressant therapy. The results of this study will hopefully inform and guide future treatment options for psychiatrists and primary care physicians alike in the pharmacological management of residual symptoms and treatment resistance in MDD.

REFERENCES

1. Fava M. Diagnosis and definition of treatment-resistant depression. Biol Psychiatry 2003; 53:649–659.
2. Fava M, Davidson KG. Definition and epidemiology of treatment-resistant depression. Psychiatr Clin North Am 1996; 19:179–200.

3. Nierenberg AA, Keefe BR, Leslie VC, Alpert JE, Pava JA, Worthington JJ III, Rosenbaum JF, Fava M. Residual symptoms in depressed patients who respond acutely to fluoxetine. J Clin Psychiatry 1999; 60(4):221–225.
4. Fava M, Kaji J. Continuation and maintenance treatments of major depressive disorder. Psychiatr Ann 1994; 24:281–290.
5. Paykel ES, Ramana R, Cooper Z, et al. Residual symptoms after partial remission: an important outcome in depression. Psychol Med 1995; 25:1171–1180.
6. Ramana R, Paykel ES, Cooper Z, et al. Remission and relapse in major depression: a two-year prospective follow-up study. Psychol Med 1995; 25:1161–1170.
7. Judd LL, Paulus MJ, Schettler PJ, et al. Does incomplete recovery from first lifetime major depressive episode herald a chronic course of illness? Am J Psychiatry 2000; 157:1501–1504.
8. Hamilton M. A rating scale for depression. J Neurol Neurosurg Psychiatry 1960; 23:56–62.
9. Montgomery SA, Asberg M. A new depression scale designed to be sensitive to change. Br J Psychiatry 1979; 134:382–389.
10. Rush AJ, Gullion CM, Basco MR, Jarrett RB, Trivedi MH. The Inventory of Depressive Symptomatology (IDS): psychometric properties. Psychol Med 1996; 26:477–486.
11. Beck AT, Steer RA. Internal consistencies of the original and revised Beck Depression Inventory. J Clin Psychol 1984; 40:1365–1367.
12. Kellner R. A symptom questionnaire. J Clin Psychiatry 1987; 48:268–274.
13. Baer L, Jacobs DG, Meszler-Reizes J, Blais M, Fava M, Kessler R, et al. Development of a brief screening instrument: The HANDS. Psychother Psychosom 2000; 69:35–41.
14. Fava M, Dunner DL, Greist JH, Preskorn SH, Trivedi MH, Zajecka J, Cohen M. Efficacy and safety of mirtazapine in major depressive disorder patients after SSRI treatment failure: an open-label trial. J Clin Psychiatry 2001; 62(6):413–420.
15. Denninger JW, Mahal Y, Merens W, et al. The relationship between somatic symptoms and depression. In: New Research Abstracts of the 155th Annual Meeting of the American Psychiatric Association, May 21. Philadelphia: P Abstract NR251, 2002:68–69.
16. Quitkin FM, McGrath PJ, Stewart JW, et al. Chronological milestones to guide drug change: when should clinicians switch antidepressants? Arch Gen Psychiatry 1996; 53:785–792.
17. Nierenberg AA, McLean NE, Alpert JE, et al. Early nonresponse to fluoxetine as a predictor of poor 8-week outcome. Am J Psychiatry 1995; 152:1500–1503.
18. Thase ME, Entsuah AR, Rudolph RL. Remission rates during treatment with venlafaxine or selective serotonin reuptake inhibitors. Br J Psychiatr 2001; 178:234–241.
19. Danish University Antidepressant Group. Paroxetine: a selective serotonin reuptake inhibitor showing better tolerance, but weaker antidepressant effect

than clomipramine in a controlled multicenter study. J Affect Disord 1990; 18: 289–299.

20. Fava GA, Rafanelli C, Grandi S, et al. Prevention of recurrent depression with cognitive therapy: preliminary findings. Arch Gen Psychiatry 1998; 55:816–820.

21. Fava M, Alpert J, Nierenberg A, Lagomasino I, Sonawalla S, Tedlow J, Worthington J, Baer L, Rosenbaum JF. Double-blind study of high-dose fluoxetine versus lithium or desipramine augmentation of fluoxetine in partial responders and nonresponders to fluoxetine. J Clin Psychopharmacol 2002; 22(4): 379–387.

22. Fava M, Rosenbaum JF, McGrath PJ, Stewart JW, Amsterdam JD, Quitkin FM. Lithium and tricyclic augmentation of fluoxetine treatment for resistant major depression: a double-blind, controlled study. Am J Psychiatry 1994; 151(9):1372–1374.

23. Fredman SJ, Fava M, Kienke AS, et al. Partial response, non-response, and relapse on SSRIs in major depression: a survey of current "next-step" practices. J Clin Psychiatry 2000; 61:403–407.

24. Fava M, Rosenbaum JF, Cohen L, Reiter S, McCarthy M, Steingard R, Clancy K. High-dose fluoxetine in the treatment of depressed patients not responsive to a standard dose of fluoxetine. J Affect Dis 1992; 25:229–234.

25. Fava M. Augmentation and combination strategies in treatment-resistant depression. J Clin Psychiatry 2001; 62(suppl 18):4–11.

26. Baumann P, Souche A, Montaldi S, et al. A double-blind, placebo-controlled study of citalopram with and without lithium in the treatment of therapy-resistant depressive patients: a clinical, pharmacokinetic, and pharmacogenetic investigation. J Clin Psychopharmacol 1996; 16:307–314.

27. Cournoyer G, de Montigny C, Oulette J, et al. Lithium addition in tricyclic-resistant unipolar depression: a placebo-controlled study. Presented at the XIVth Congress of the Collegium Internationale Neuropsychopharmacologicum (CINP), Florence, Italy, June 19–23, 1984.

28. de Montigny C, Cournoyer G, Morissette R, et al. Lithium carbonate addition in tricyclic antidepressant-resistant unipolar depression. Correlations with the neurobiologic actions of tricyclic antidepressant drugs and lithium ion on the serotonin system. Arch Gen Psychiatry 1983; 40:1327–1334.

29. Heninger GR, Charney DS, Sternberg DE. Lithium carbonate augmentation of antidepressant action: an effective prescription for treatment refractory depression. Arch Gen Psychiatry 1983; 40:1335–1342.

30. Joffe RT, Singer W, Levitt AJ, MacDonald C. A placebo-controlled comparison of lithium and triiodothyronine augmentation of tricyclic antidepressants in unipolar refractory depression. Arch Gen Psychiatry 1993; 50:387–393.

31. Kantor D, McNeven S, Leichner P, et al. The benefit of lithium carbonate adjunct in refractory depression: fact or fiction? Can J Psychiatry 1986; 31:416–418.

32. Katona CL, Abou-Saleh M, Harrison DA, et al. Placebo-controlled trial of lithium augmentation of fluoxetine and lofepramine. Br J Psychiatry 1995; 166:80–86.

33. Schopf J, Baumann P, Lemarchand T, Rey M. Treatment of endogenous de-

pressions resistant to tricyclic antidepressants or related drugs by lithium addition. Pharmacopsychiatry 1989; 22:183–187.

34. Stein G, Bernadt M. Double-blind trial of lithium carbonate in tricyclic resistant depression. In: Birch NJ, ed. Lithium: Inorganic Pharmacology and Psychiatric Use. Oxford, UK: IRL Press, 1988:35.

35. Stein G, Bernadt M. Lithium augmentation therapy in tricyclic-resistant depression: a controlled trial using lithium in low and normal doses. Br J Psychiatry 1993; 162:634–640.

36. Zusky PM, Biederman J, Rosenbaum JF, et al. Adjunct low dose lithium carbonate in treatment-resistant depression: a placebo-controlled study. J Clin Psychopharmacol 1988; 8:120–124.

37. Nierenberg AA, Papakostas GI, Petersen T, Montoya HD, Worthington JJ, Tedlow J, Alpert JE, Fava M. Lithium augmentation of nortriptyline for subjects resistant to multiple antidepressants. J Clin Psychopharmacol 2003; 23(1): 92–95.

38. Joffe RT, Singer W. A comparison of triiodothyronine and thyroxine in the potentiation of tricyclic antidepressants. Psychiatry Res 1990; 32(3):241–251.

39. Aronson R, Offman HJ, Joffe T, Naylor CD. Triiodothyronine augmentation in the treatment of refractory depression: a meta-analysis. Arch Gen Psychiatry 1996; 53:842–848.

40. Bouwer C, Stein DJ. Buspirone is an effective augmenting agent of serotonin selective reuptake inhibitors in severe treatment-refractory depression. South Afr Med J 1997; 87(suppl 4):534–537, 540.

41. Dimitriou EC, Dimitriou CE. Buspirone augmentation of antidepressant therapy. J Clin Psychopharmacol 1998; 18:465–469.

42. Jacobsen FM. A possible augmentation of antidepressant response by buspirone. J Clin Psychiatry 1991; 52:217–220.

43. Landen M, Bjorling G, Agren H, Fahlen T. A randomized, double-blind, placebo-controlled trial of buspirone in combination with an SSRI in patients with treatment-refractory depression. J Clin Psychiatry 1998; 59:664–668.

44. Appelberg BG, Syvalahti EK, Koskinen TE, et al. Patients with severe depression may benefit from buspirone augmentation of selective serotonin reuptake inhibitors: results from a placebo-controlled, randomized, double-blind, placebo wash-in study. J Clin Psychiatry 2001; 62:448–452.

45. Perez V, Gilaberte I, Faries D, et al. Randomized, double-blind, placebo-controlled trial of pindolol in combination with fluoxetine antidepressant treatment. Lancet 1997; 349:1594–1597.

46. Tome MB, Isaac MT, Harte R, et al. Paroxetine and pindolol: a randomized trial of serotoninergic autoreceptor blockade in the reduction of antidepressant latency. Int Clin Psychopharmacol 1997; 12:81–89.

47. Zanardi R, Artigas F, Franchini L, et al. How long should pindolol be associated with paroxetine to improve the antidepressant response? J Clin Psychopharmacol 1997; 17:446–450.

48. Bordet R, Thomas P, Dupuis B. Effect of pindolol on onset of action of paroxetine in the treatment of major depression: intermediate analysis of a double-blind, placebo-controlled trial. Am J Psychiatry 1998; 155:1346–1351.

49. Blier P, Bergeron R. The use of pindolol to potentiate antidepressant medication. J Clin Psychiatry 1998; 59(suppl 5):16–23.
50. Berman RM, Anand A, Cappiello A, et al. The use of pindolol with fluoxetine in the treatment of major depression: final results from a double-blind, placebo-controlled trial. Biol Psychiatry 1999; 45:1170–1177.
51. Moreno F, Gelenberg AJ, Bachar K, et al. Pindolol augmentation of treatment-resistant depressed patients. J Clin Psychiatry 1997; 58:437–439.
52. Perez V, Soler J, Puigdemont D, et al. A double-blind, randomized, placebo-controlled trial of pindolol augmentation in depressive patients resistant to serotonin reuptake inhibitors. Arch Gen Psychiatry 1999; 56:375–379.
53. Bouckoms A, Mangini LP. An antidepressant adjuvant for mood disorders? Psychopharmacol Bull 1993; 29:207–211.
54. Michelson D, Bancroft J, Targum S, et al. Female sexual dysfunction associated with antidepressant administration: a randomized, placebo-controlled study of pharmacologic intervention. Am J Psychiatry 2000; 157:239–243.
55. Sporn J, Ghaemi SN, Sambur MR, et al. Pramipexole augmentation in the treatment of unipolar and bipolar depression: a retrospective chart review. Ann Clin Psychiatry 2000; 12:137–140.
56. Lattanzi L, Dell'Osso L, Cassano P, Pini S, Rucci P, Houck PR, Gemignani A, Battistini G, Bassi A, Abelli M, Cassano GB. Pramipexole in treatment-resistant depression: a 16-week naturalistic study. Bipolar Disord 2002; 4(5): 307–314.
57. Perugi G, Toni C, Ruffolo G, Frare F, Akiskal H. Adjunctive dopamine agonists in treatment-resistant bipolar II depression: an open case series. Pharmacopsychiatry 2001; 34(4):137–141.
58. Menza MA, Kaufman KR, Castellanos AM. Modafinil augmentation of antidepressant treatment in depression. J Clin Psychiatry 2000; 61:378–381.
59. DeBattista C, Solvason HB, Flores BH, et al. Modafinil as an adjunctive agent in the treatment of fatigue and hypersomnia associated with depression. Presented at the 39th Annual Meeting of the American College of Neuropsychopharmacology, San Juan, Puerto Rico, 2000.
60. Ostroff RB, Nelson JC. Risperidone augmentation of selective serotonin reuptake inhibitors in major depression. J Clin Psychiatry 1999; 60:256–259.
61. Shelton RC, Tollefson GD, Tohen M, et al. A novel augmentation strategy for treating resistant major depression. Am J Psychiatry 2001; 158:131–134.
62. Nemets B, Mishory A, Levine J, et al. Inositol addition does not improve depression in SSRI treatment failures. J Neural Transm 1999; 106:795–798.
63. Papakostas GI, Petersen T, Nierenberg AA, Alpert JE, Murakami J, Rosenbaum JE, Fava M. Ziprasidone an augmentation for Major Depressive Disorder Resistant to SSRIs. Presented at the 156th Annual Meeting of the American Psychiatric Association, San Francisco, 2003.
64. Levine J, Mishori A, Susnosky M, et al. Combination of inositol and serotonin reuptake inhibitors in the treatment of depression. Biol Psychiatry 1999; 45: 270–273.
65. Stoll AL, Rueter S. Treatment augmentation with opiates in severe and refractory major depression [letter]. Am J Psychiatry 1999; 156:2017.

66. Bodkin JA, Zornberg GL, Lukas SE, et al. Buprenorphine treatment of refractory depression. J Clin Psychopharmacol 1995; 15:49–57.
67. Stahl SM. Basic psychopharmacology of antidepressants, pt 2: estrogen as an adjunct to antidepressant treatment. J Clin Psychiatry 1998; 59(suppl 4):15–24.
68. Stahl SM. Augmentation of antidepressants by estrogen. Psychopharmacol Bull 1998; 34:319–321.
69. Wolkowitz OM, Reus VI, Keebler A, et al. Double-blind treatment of major depression with dehydroepiandrosterone. Am J Psychiatry 1999; 156:646–649.
70. Pope HG Jr, Cohane GH, Kanayama G, Siegel AJ, Hudson JI. Testosterone gel supplementation for men with refractory depression: a randomized, placebo-controlled trial. Am J Psychiatry 2003; 160(1):105–111.
71. Alpert JE, Mischoulon D, Nierenberg AA, et al. Nutrition and depression: focus on folate. Nutrition 2000; 16:544–546.
72. Spillmann M, Fava M. S-adenosylmethionine (ademetionine) in psychiatric disorders: historical perspective and current status. CNS Drugs 1996; 6:416–425.
73. Alpert JE, Mischoulon D, Rubenstein GE, Bottonari K, Nierenberg AA, Fava M. Folinic acid (leucovorin) as an adjunctive treatment for SSRI-refractory depression. Ann Clin Psychiatry 2002; 14(1):33–38.
74. Carpenter LL, Jocic Z, Hall JM, Rasmussen SA, Price LH. Mirtazapine augmentation in the treatment of refractory depression. J Clin Psychiatry 1999; 60(1):45–49.
75. Carpenter LL, Yasmin S, Price LH. A double-blind, placebo-controlled study of antidepressant augmentation with mirtazapine. Biol Psychiatry 2002; 51(2):183–188.
76. Debonnel G, Gobbi G, Turcotte J, DeMontigny C, Blier P. The alpha-2 antagonist mirtazapine combined with the SSRI paroxetine induces a greater antidepressant response: a double-blind controlled study. Presented at the 39th Annual Meeting of the American College of Neuropsychopharmacology, San Juan, Puerto Rico, 2000.
77. Nelson JC, Mazure CM, Bowers MB, Jatlow P. A preliminary open study of the combination of fluoxetine and desipramine for rapid treatment of major depression. Arch Gen Psychiatry 1991; 48:303–307.
78. Nelson JC. Combined drug treatments: pros and cons. Presented at the 152nd Annual Meeting of the American Psychiatric Association, Washington DC, 1999.
79. Weilburg JB, Rosenbaum JF, Meltzer-Brody S, Shushtari J. Tricyclic augmentation of fluoxetine. Ann Clin Psychiatry 1991; 3:209–214.
80. Zajecka JM, Jeffries H, Fawcett J. The efficacy of fluoxetine combined with heterocyclic antidepressant in treatment-resistant depression: a retrospective analysis. J Clin Psychiatry 1995; 56(8):338–343.
81. Fava M. New approaches to the treatment of refractory depression. J Clin Psychiatry 2000; 61(suppl 1):26–32.
82. Hawley CJ, Sivakumaran T, Ochocki M, Bevan J. Co-administration of reboxetine and serotonin selective reuptake inhibitors in treatment-resistant patients with major depression. Presented at the 39th Annual Meeting of the American College of Neuropsychopharmacology, San Juan, Puerto Rico, 2000.

83. Dursun SM, Devarajan S. The efficacy and safety of reboxetine plus citalopram in treatment-resistant depression—an open, naturalistic case series. Presented at the 39th Annual Meeting of the American College of Neuropsychopharmacology, San Juan, Puerto Rico, 2000.

84. Lucca A, Serretti A, Smeraldi E. Effect of reboxetine augmentation in SSRI resistant patients. Hum Psychopharmacol 2000; 15(2):143–145.

85. Smith DL, Wenegrat BG. A case report of serotonin syndrome associated with combined nefazodone and fluoxetine. J Clin Psychiatry 2000; 61(2):146.

86. Bhatara VS, Magnus RD, Paul KL, Preskorn SH. Serotonin syndrome induced by venlafaxine and fluoxetine: a case study in polypharmacy and potential pharmacodynamic and pharmacokinetic mechanisms. Ann Pharmacother 1998; 32(4):432–436.

87. Benazzi F. Venlafaxine-fluoxetine interaction. J Clin Psychopharmacol 1999; 19(1):96–98.

88. McGrath PJ, Stewart JW, Harrison W, Quitkin FM. Treatment of tricyclic refractory depression with a monoamine oxidase inhibitor. Psychopharmacol Bull 1987; 23:169–172.

89. Thase ME, Mallinger AG, McKnight D, Himmelhoch JM. Treatment of imipramine resistant recurrent depression: IV. A double-blind crossover study of tranylcypromine in anergic bipolar depression. Am J Psychiatry 1992; 149: 195–198.

90. Thase ME, Blomgren SL, Birkett MA, Apter JT, Tepner RG. Fluoxetine treatment of patients with major depressive disorder who failed initial treatment with sertraline. J Clin Psychiatry 1997; 58(1):16–21.

91. Joffe RT, Levitt AJ, Sokolov ST, Young LT. Response to an open trial of a second SSRI in major depression. J Clin Psychiatry 1996; 57(3):114–115.

92. Thase ME, Feighner JP, Lydiard RB. Citalopram treatment of fluoxetine nonresponders. J Clin Psychiatry 2001; 62(9):683–687.

93. Fava M. Management of nonresponse and intolerance: switching strategies. J Clin Psychiatry 2000; 61(suppl 2):10–12.

94. Poirier MF, Boyer P. Venlafaxine and paroxetine in treatment-resistant depression. Double-blind, randomised comparison. Br J Psychiatry 1999; 175:12–16.

95. Nierenberg AA, Feighner JP, Rudolph R, Cole JO, Sullivan J. Venlafaxine for treatment-resistant unipolar depression. J Clin Psychopharmacol 1994; 14:419–423.

96. de Montigny C, Silverstone PH, Debonnel G, Blier P, Bakish D. Venlafaxine in treatment-resistant major depression: a Canadian multicenter, open-label trial. J Clin Psychopharmacol 1999; 19(5):401–406.

97. Nemeroff CB, Schatzberg AF, Goldstein DJ, Detke MJ, Mallinckrodt C, Lu Y, Tran PV. Duloxetine for the treatment of major depressive disorder. Psychopharm Bull 2002; 36(4):106–132.

98. Thase ME, Kremer C, Rodrigues H. Mirtazapine versus sertraline after SSRI nonresponse. Presented at the 154th Annual Meeting of the American Psychiatric Association. New Orleans, 2001.

99. Thase ME, Rush AJ, Howland RH, Kornstein SG, Kocsis JH, Gelenberg AJ, Schatzberg AF, Koran LM, Keller MB, Russell JM, Hirschfeld RM, LaVange LM, Klein DN, Fawcett J, Harrison W. Double-blind switch study of imipramine or sertraline treatment of antidepressant-resistant chronic depression. Arch Gen Psychiatry 2002; 59(3):233–239.

100. Nierenberg AA, Papakostas GI, Petersen T, Kelly KE, Iacoviello BM, Worthington JJ, Tedlow J, Alpert JE, Fava M. Nortriptyline for treatment-resistant depression. J Clin Psychiatry 2003; 64(1):35–39.

101. Fava M, Papakostas GI, Petersen T, Mahal Y, Quitkin F, Stewart J, McGrath P. Switching to bupropion in fluoxetine-resistant major depressive disorder. Ann Clin Psychiatry 2003; 15:17–22.

102. Fava M, McGrath PJ, Sheu WP, and the Reboxetine Study Group. Switching to reboxetine: an efficacy and safety study in patients with major depressive disorder unresponsive to fluoxetine. J Clin Psychopharm. In press.

103. McGrath PJ, Stewart JW, Nunes EV, Ocepek-Welikson K, Rabkin JG, Quitkin FM, Klein DF. A double-blind crossover trial of imipramine and phenelzine for outpatients with treatment-refractory depression. Am J Psychiatry 1993; 150(1):118–123.

104. Fava M, Rush AJ, Trivedi MH, Nierenberg AA, Thase ME, Sackeim HA, Quitkin FM, Wisniewski S, Lavori PW, Rosenbaum JF, Kupfer DJ, for the STAR*D Investigators Group. Background and rationale for the Sequenced Treatment Alternatives to Relieve Depression (STAR*D) study. Psychiatr Clinics of North Am 2003; 26:1–38.

12

Psychotherapy of Residual Symptoms

Giovanni A. Fava

University of Bologna
Bologna, Italy
and State University of New York at Buffalo
Buffalo, New York, U.S.A

Chiara Ruini

University of Bologna
Bologna, Italy

INTRODUCTION

The combination of psychotherapy and pharmacotherapy in the treatment of affective disorders has attracted considerable attention in the past two decades [1]. However, it has obtained limited support from controlled trials [2,3]. Indeed, also a detrimental effect (exposure and alprazolam in panic disorder) has been reported [4]. The underlying assumption of the integrated approach was that of an additive model of interaction between pharmacotherapy and psychotherapy, which could take place on the basis of specific changes to be induced by specific treatments. Further, the simultaneous administration of pharmacotherapy and psychotherapy is based on a cross-sectional, flat view of the disorders which ignores their longitudinal development [5]. An alternative way of integrating pharmacotherapy and psychotherapy involves their sequential administration according to the stages of the disorder.

Administration of treatments in sequential order is a common practice in clinical medicine when a treatment fails. If the physician prescribes antibiotic A to eradicate an infection and the ensuing response is judged to be unsatisfactory, the patient is switched to antibiotic B in the hope of a better outcome. The process is by approximation, applies only if treatment fails, and can be potentially avoided by appropriate pretreatment tests (e.g., in vitro determination of the susceptibility of bacteria to antimicrobial drugs). In clinical psychiatry, administration of treatment in sequential order has been mainly limited to instances of treatment resistance and involves different types of drugs, such as in drug-refractory depression [6]. However, cognitive behavioral strategies have been successful in the management of drug-resistant major depressive disorders [7] to the same extent that imipramine was found to be effective after unsuccessful cognitive therapy of depression [8]. Similar results have been obtained in other disorders, such as panic [9].

Within psychotherapeutic approaches, Emmelkamp et al. [10] deserve credit for suggesting the feasibility of applying different therapies consecutively instead of in combination and the need to compare the two approaches in controlled studies. A first attempt to demonstrate the effectiveness of the sequential approach (involving exposure in vivo followed by cognitive therapy) compared to a strategy where the two approaches were integrated from the start, did not yield significant differences in social phobia [11]. Similar disappointing results were obtained with application of cognitive therapy to panic disorder patients who failed to respond to exposure in vivo [12].

This type of sequential approach, however, was not targeted to the stages of illness [5] and particularly to residual symptoms [13]. The arbitrary nature of the clinical and research decisions along a response continuum that may range from treatment-resistant disorder to full remission via partial remission is not frequently acknowledged. In particular, treatment of depression by pharmacological means is likely to leave a substantial amount of residual symptomatology in most of patients [14].

The presence of residual symptoms after completion of drug or psychotherapeutic treatment has been correlated with poor long-term outcome [14].

Further, some residual symptoms of major depression may progress to become prodromal symptoms of relapse [15]. This has led to the development of a sequential strategy based on the use of pharmacotherapy in the acute phase of depression and cognitive therapy in its residual phase [16]. The preliminary results of this strategy, both in primary major depressive disorder [17,18] and recurrent depression [19], appear to be promising in terms of differential relapse rate. Its preventive effect appears to be related directly to the abatement of residual symptoms. In a study on recurrent depression [19], when patients after cognitive behavioral treatment or clinical management were classified as still presenting with residual symptoms or being fully asymptomatic, striking differences emerged during a 2-year follow-up in terms of relapse rate [20].

We will outline the most clinically significant findings concerned with residual symptoms of unipolar depression. We will then briefly describe the studies which developed the sequential approach in unipolar depression. Finally, we describe how this approach can be implemented in clinical practice.

RESIDUAL SYMPTOMS OF UNIPOLAR DEPRESSION

In 1973, Paykel and Weissman found social and interpersonal maladjustments in fully recovered depressed patients compared to controls despite considerable improvement in social adjustment upon treatment. Submissive dependency and family attachment improved almost completely, whereas two other personal dysfunctions, interpersonal friction and inhibited communication, showed little change and greatest residual impairment [21]. Residual social maladjustment was subsequently reported by other investigators [22–24] and was found to correlate with long-term outcome [24]. Similarly, dysfunctional attitudes and attributions were found to persist after recovery despite clinical and cognitive improvement [25–27]. These cognitive patterns were positively correlated with vulnerability to persistent depression or relapse [26,28,29]. Social maladjustments and dysfunctional attitudes may overlap with characterological traits assessed after clinical recovery [30–33] or premorbid personality features [34]. In any case, there appears to be a residual attributional interpersonal component which is refractory to otherwise successful treatment of depression. Such a component may entail considerable predictive value.

The notion that the majority of depressed patients experience mild but chronic residual symptoms or recurrence of symptoms after complete remission, which was well delineated in the 1970s [35], did not receive the attention it deserved in subsequent years. In fact, such a phenomenon was emphasized mainly in its etiological role in dysthymia. Akiskal [36] subdivided chronic depression into primary depression (usually of late onset and occurring as a sequela to one or more syndromal episodes of primary major depression), chronic secondary dysphoria (having a variable onset age and occurring in the setting of preexisting and incapacitating nonaffective disorder), and characterologic depression (with insidious and early developmental onset and fluctuating course). Hirschfeld et al. [37] suggested that chronicity in depression either results from an illness of minor nature with insidious onset in early adult life or is a function of an unresolved major depressive disorder. The presence of residual symptoms after completion of drug treatment [16,39–42] or cognitive behavioral therapy [43,44] of depression has been correlated with poor long-term outcome. However, methodological problems in the assessment of residual symptoms emerge. There are few psychometric studies addressing the phenomenology of depressed patients after benefiting from treatment, Recovered depressed patients displayed significantly more depression and anxiety than control subjects in one study [45] but not in another [46]. Differences in the sensitivity of the rating scales which were employed [47,48] may account for such discrepant results. Using an observer-rated scale, Paykel's Clinical Interview for Depression [49], which was found to be suitable and sensitive instrument for detecting subclinical symptomatology [48], only 6 (12%) of 49 patients with major depression successfully treated with antidepressant drugs and judged to be fully remitted had no residual symptoms [16]. The majority of residual symptoms were present also in the prodromal phase of illness. The most frequently reported symptoms involved anxiety and irritability. This was consistent with previous studies on prodromal symptoms of depression [50,51] and overlapped with findings concerned with interpersonal friction [21] and trait anxiety [32].

COGNITIVE BEHAVIORAL TREATMENT OF RESIDUAL SYMPTOMS

In a controlled therapeutic trial [16], 40 patients with major depressive disorder who had been successfully treated with antidepressants were randomly assigned to either cognitive behavioral treatment or clinical management of residual symptoms. In both cases, treatment consisted of 10 40-min sessions once every other week. In both groups, antidepressant drugs were tapered and discontinued. Cognitive therapy was conducted as described by Beck et al. [52,53]. The psychiatrist, an experienced therapist, used strategies and techniques designed to help depressed patients correct their distorted views and maladaptive beliefs. Whenever appropriate, as in the case of residual symptoms related to anxiety, exposure strategies based on Marks' guidelines [54] were planned with the patient. Clinical management consisted of monitoring medication tapering, reviewing the patient's clinical status, and providing the patient with support and advice if necessary. In clinical management, specific interventions such as exposure strategies, diary work, and cognitive restructuring were omitted. The group that received cognitive-behavioral treatment had a significantly lower level of residual symptoms after drug discontinuation in comparison with the clinical management group [16]. Cognitive-behavioral treatment also resulted in a lower rate of relapse [16] with achievement of statistical significance at a 4-year follow-up [17]. At a 6-year follow-up [18], when multiple relapses were taken into account, cognitive-behavioral treatment also resulted in a significantly lower number of depressive episodes. The rationale of this approach was to use cognitive-behavioral treatment resources when they are most likely to make a unique and separate contribution to patient well-being and to achieve a more pervasive recovery [55]. The target of psychotherapeutic work is thus no longer predetermined (e.g., cognitive triad) but varies according to the nature, characteristics, and intensity of residual symptomatology.

A combination of cognitive-behavioral therapy of residual symptoms and of a novel treatment strategy (well-being therapy) [56] was performed in a study on recurrent depression. Forty patients with recurrent depression according to the criteria used by Frank et al. [57] were randomly assigned to either a combination of cognitive-behavioral treatment of residual symptoms and well-being therapy or to clinical management. In both groups, antidepressant drug administration was tapered and discontinued. At a 2-year follow-up, psychotherapeutic treatment resulted in a significantly lower relapse rate (25%) than did clinical management (80%). The results of this preliminary investigation challenge the assumption that long-term drug treatment is the only tool available to prevent relapse in patients with recurrent depression [57].

Paykel et al. [58] provided an essential replication of the effectiveness of the sequential approach. One hundred fifty-eight patients with recent major depression, partially remitted with antidepressant drugs, were randomized to receive clinical management alone or clinical management supplemented by cognitive therapy of residual symptoms. They received continuation and maintenance antidepressant at the same dosage. Whereas the clinical management group had a relapse rate of 47% at 68 weeks, the group treated with cognitive therapy had a relapse rate of 29%.

STANDARD FORMAT OF SEQUENTIAL TREATMENT SESSIONS

Suitability and Motivation for Treatment

Before undergoing sequential treatment, patients should have displayed a satisfactory response to antidepressant drug treatment. They should thus have been treated with at least 3 months of drug treatment and no longer be presenting with depressed mood. During pharmacological treatment and clinical management it is, however, essential to introduce the subsequent part of treatment. A helpful example which was made [19] is the following. "When we first saw you, you were very depressed. You went off the road. We gave you antidepressant drugs and these put you back on the road. Things are much better now. However, if you keep on driving the way you did, you will go off the road again, sooner or later."

The example outlines the need for lifestyle modification and introduces a sense of control in the patients as to their depressive illness. This psychological preparation paves the way for subsequent psychotherapeutic approaches.

Standard Format

Psychotherapeutic intervention extends over 10 sessions of 30–45 min each every other week. The first session is mainly concerned with assessment and introduction of the psychotherapeutic treatment by the therapist, rehearsing the example provided before formal initiation of treatment. Sessions 2–6 are concerned with cognitive behavioral treatment of residual symptoms and lifestyle modification. The last 4 sessions involve well-being therapy.

Assessment

It is of the most importance to reassess the remitted patient as if he or she were a new patient. This means to go through symptoms in the most recent weeks in a careful way. Exploration should not concern only symptoms which characterize the diagnosis of major depressive disorder but also those which characterize anxiety disturbances (including phobic and obsessive-compulsive symptoms) and irritability. In the original studies [16,19], a modified version of Paykel's Clinical Interview for Depression [49] was employed, but other semistructured interviews may be used as long as these are sufficiently comprehensive as to anxiety and irritability. This is the first step in recognizing residual symptomatology.

The second deals with self-observation of the patient. The patient is instructed to report in a diary (Table 1) all episodes of distress which may ensue in the following 2 weeks. It is important to emphasize that distress (which is left unspecified) does not need to be prolonged, but may also be short lived. Patients are also instructed to build a list of situations which elicit

TABLE 1 Example of the Assessment Diary

Situation	Distress (0–100)	Thoughts
I am watching TV when the telephone rings	40	Something has certainly happened to....

distress and/or tend to induce avoidance. Each situation should be rated on a 0–100 point scale (0 = no problem; 100 = panic). Patients are instructed to bring the diary at the following visit.

Cognitive-Behavioral Treatment of Residual Symptoms

After the patient's assessment and reading the diary brought by the patient, a cognitive-behavioral package is formulated. This may encompass both exposure and cognitive restructuring. Exposure consists of homework exposure only. An exposure strategy is planned with the patient based on the list of situations outlined in the diary. The therapist writes an assignment per day, in the diary following a graded exposure [54]. The patient assigns a score from 0 to 100 for each homework assignment. At the following visit, the therapist reassesses the homework done and discusses the next steps and/or problems in compliance which may have ensued.

Cognitive restructuring follows the classic format of Beck et al. [52,53] and is based on introduction of the concept of automatic thoughts (second session) and of observer's interpretation (third session and on).

The problems which may be the object of cognitive restructuring strictly depend on the material offered by the patient. They may encompass insomnia (sleep hygiene instructions are added), hypersomnia, diminished energy and concentration, residual hopelessness, reentry problems (diminished functioning at work, avoidance, and procrastination), lack of assertiveness and self-care, perfectionism, and unrealistic self-expectations.

Well-Being Therapy

At the seventh session, well-being therapy is introduced [59]. Well-being therapy is a short-term psychotherapeutic strategy with sessions which may take place every week or every other week. The duration of each session may range from 30 to 50 min. It is a technique which emphasizes self-observation [60], with the use of a structured diary, and interaction between patients and therapists. Well-being therapy is based on Ryff's cognitive model of psychological well-being [61]. This model was selected on the basis of its easy applicability to clinical populations [62,63]. Well-being therapy is structured, directive, problem oriented, and based on an educational model. The development of sessions is as follows.

Seventh Session

The seventh session is simply concerned with identifying episodes of well-being and setting them into a situational context no matter how short lived they were. Patients are asked to report in a structured diary the circumstances surrounding their episodes of well-being, rated on a 0–100 scale, with 0 being absence of well-being and 100 the most intense well-being that could be experienced (Table 2). When patients are assigned this homework, they often object that they will bring a blank diary, because they never feel well. It is helpful to reply that these moments do exist but tend to pass unnoticed. Patients should therefore monitor them anyway.

Meehl [64, p 305] described "how people with low hedonic capacity should pay greater attention to the 'hedonic book keeping' of their activities than would be necessary for people located midway or high on the hedonic capacity continuum. That is, it matters more to someone cursed with an inborn hedonic defect whether he is efficient and sagacious in selecting friends, jobs, cities, tasks, hobbies, and activities in general."

Eighth Session

Once the instances of well-being are properly recognized, the patient is encouraged to identify thoughts and beliefs leading to premature interruption of well-being. For instance, in the example reported in Table 2, the patients added, "it is just because I brought two presents." The similarities with the search for irrational, tension-evoking thoughts in Ellis and Becker's rational-emotive therapy [65] and automatic thoughts in cognitive therapy [52] are obvious. The trigger for self-observation is, however, different, being based on well-being instead of distress.

This phase is crucial, since it allows the therapist to identify which areas of psychological well-being are unaffected by irrational or automatic thoughts and which are saturated with them. The therapist may challenge these thoughts with appropriate questions, such as, "what is the evidence for or against this idea?" or "are you thinking in all-or none terms?" [52]. The therapist may also reinforce and encourage activities that are likely to elicit well-being (for instance, assigning the task of undertaking particular pleasurable activities for a certain time each day). Such reinforcement may also result in graded task assignments [52]. However, the focus of this phase of well-being therapy is always on self-monitoring of moments and feelings of

TABLE 2   Self-Observation of Episodes of Well-Being

Situation	Feeling of well-being	Intensity (0–100)
I went to visit my nephews and they greeted me with great enthusiasm and joy.	They like me and care for me.	40

well-being. The therapist refrains from suggesting conceptual and technical alternatives unless a satisfactory degree of self-observation (including irrational or automatic thoughts) has been achieved.

Ninth Session

The monitoring of the course of episodes of well-being allows the therapist to realize specific impairments in well-being dimensions according to Ryff's conceptual framework. Ryff's six dimensions of psychological well-being are progressively introduced to the patients, as long as the material which is recorded lends itself to it. Errors in thinking and alternative interpretations are then discussed.

Cognitive restructuring in well-being therapy follows Ryff's conceptual framework [66]. The goal of the therapist is to lead the patient from an impaired level to an optimal level in the six dimensions of psychological well-being.

Environmental Mastery (Table 3). This is the most frequent impairment that emerges. It was expressed by a patient as follows, "I have got a filter that nullifies any positive achievement (I was just lucky) and amplifies any negative outcome, no matter how much expected (this once more confirms I am a failure)." This lack of sense of control leads the patient to miss surrounding opportunities with the possibility of subsequent regret over them.

Personal Growth (Table 3). Patients often tend to emphasize their distance from expected goals much more than the progress that has been made toward goal achievement. A basic impairment that emerges is the inability to identify the similarities between events and situations that were handled successfully in the past and those that are about to come (transfer of experiences). Impairments in perception of personal growth and environmental mastery thus tend to interact in a dysfunctional way. A university student who is unable to realize the common contents and methodological similarities between the exams they successfully passed and the ones that are to be given shows impairments in both environmental mastery and personal growth.

Purpose in Life (Table 3). An underlying assumption of psychological therapies (whether pharmacological or psychotherapeutic) is to restore premorbid functioning. In the case of treatments which emphasize self-help such as cognitive-behavioral therapy itself offers a sense of direction and hence a short-term goal. However, this does not persist when acute symptoms abate and/or premorbid functioning is suboptimal. Patients may perceive a lack of sense of direction and may devalue their function in life. This

TABLE 3 Modification of the Six Dimensions of Psychological Well-Being According to Ryff's Model

Dimensions	Impaired level	Optimal level
Environmental mastery	The subject has or feels difficulties in managing everyday affairs; feels unable to change or improve surrounding context; is unaware of surrounding opportunities; lacks sense of control over external world.	The subject has a sense of mastery and competence in managing the environment; controls external activities; makes effective use of surrounding opportunities; able to create or choose contexts suitable to personal needs and values.
Personal growth	The subject has a sense of personal stagnation; lacks sense of improvement or expansion over time; feels bored and uninterested with life; feels unable to develop new attitudes or behaviors.	The subject has a feeling of continued development; sees self as growing and expanding; is open to new experiences; has sense of realizing own potential; sees improvement in self and behavior over time.
Purpose in life	The subject lacks a sense of meaning in life; has few goals or aims, lacks sense of direction, does not see purpose in past life; has no outlooks or beliefs that give life meaning.	The subject has goals in life and a sense of directedness; feels there is meaning to present and past life; holds beliefs that give life purpose; has aims and objectives for living.
Autonomy	The subject is overconcerned with the expectations and evaluation of others; relies on judgment of others to make important decisions; conforms to social pressures to think or act in certain ways.	The subject is self-determining and independent; able to resist social pressures; regulates behavior from within; evaluates self by personal standards.
Self-acceptance	The subject feels dissatisfied with self; is disappointed with what has occurred in past life; is troubled about certain personal qualities; wishes to be different than what he or she is.	The subject has a positive attitude toward the self; accepts his or her good and bad qualities; feels positive about past life.
Positive relations with others	The subject has few close, trusting relationships with others; finds it difficult to be open and is isolated and frustrated in interpersonal relationships; not willing to make compromises to sustain important ties with others.	The subject has warm and trusting relationships with others; is concerned about the welfare of others; capable of strong empathy affection, and intimacy; understands give and take of human relationships.

Source: Ref. 61.

particularly occurs when environmental mastery and sense of personal growth are impaired.

Autonomy (Table 3).   It is a frequent clinical observation that patients may exhibit a pattern whereby a perceived lack of self-worth leads to unassertive behavior. For instance, patients may hide their opinions or preferences, go along with a situation that is not in their best interests, or consistently put their needs behind the needs of others. This pattern undermines environmental mastery and purpose in life and these, in turn, may affect autonomy, since these dimensions are highly correlated in clinical populations Such attitudes may not be obvious to the patients, who hide their considerable need for social approval. A patient who tries to please everyone is likely to fail to achieve this goal, and the unavoidable conflicts that may ensue result in chronic dissatisfaction and frustration.

Self-Acceptance (Table 3).   Patients may maintain unrealistically high standards and expectations driven by perfectionistic attitudes (that reflect lack of self-acceptance) and/or endorsement of external instead of personal standards (that reflect lack of autonomy). As a result, any instance of well-being is neutralized by a chronic dissatisfaction with oneself. A person may set unrealistic standards for their performance. For instance, it is a frequent clinical observation that patients with social phobia tend to aspire to outstanding social performances (e.g., being sharp or humorous) and are not satisfied with average performances (despite the fact that these latter would not put them under the spotlight, which could be seen as their apparent goal).

Positive Relations with Others (Table 3).   Interpersonal relationships may be influenced by strongly held attitudes of which the patient may be unaware and which may be dysfunctional. For instance, a young woman who recently got married may have set unrealistic standards for her marital relationship and find herself frequently disappointed. At the same time, she may avoid pursuing social plans which involve other people and may lack sources of comparison. Impairments in self-acceptance (with the resulting belief of being rejectable and unlovable) may also undermine positive relations with others.

Lifestyle Modification

One of the aims of therapy is also that of making the patient aware of allostatic loads (i.e., chronic and often subtle life stresses that exert harmful consequences on the individual over a certain amount of time). Examples may be excessive work loads, unawareness of the longer time that an increasing age requires for recovering from demanding days, inability to protect oneself from requests which exceed the potential of the individual, and inappropriate sleeping habits.

Such awareness (and the resulting lifestyle implementation) are pursued in all phases of psychotherapy, but particularly with well-being therapy. Patients are given instructions in the diary as to this implementation.

DRUG TAPERING AND DISCONTINUATION

Sequential treatment offers a unique opportunity for antidepressant drug tapering and discontinuation. It offers in fact the opportunity to monitor the patient in one of the most delicate aspects of treatment. In the original studies [16,19], antidepressant drugs were mainly tricyclics and were decreased at the rate of 25 mg of amitriptyline or its equivalents every other week. When selective serotonin receptake inhibitors (SSRIs) are involved, the more gradual tapering is, the better.

It is important to warn patients that they should not perceive "steps" (as one patient defined them) in this tapering (e.g., patients should not perceive substantial differences in their sleep, energy, mood, appetite from reducing 200 mg of amitriptyline per day to 175 mg). If they do, the appropriateness of tapering the antidepressant drug should be questioned. Indeed, in the original studies, drug discontinuation could not take place in a few patients.

The sequential format offers an ideal opportunity to support psychologically the patient when withdrawal syndromes (despite slow tapering, particularly with SSRIs) do occur.

At times, patients are fearful of drug discontinuation. It is then helpful to emphasize that a drug-free status is a step forward in therapy and may be associated with an increased quality of life. It is thus a sign of progress. Antidepressant drugs may be prescribed again if they are needed, in the setting of prodromal symptoms of mood deterioration, and patients should be reassured about this possibility which is always available.

CONCLUSION

This sequential model that was developed for preventing relapse in depression [16] may potentially apply to any type of psychiatric disorder [13] or when psychotherapy is associated with medical illness. Marks [67] suggested that current prevailing therapeutic mechanisms for explaining therapeutic effectiveness in psychotherapy are about to change. Foa and Kozak [68] wondered whether the slowing advance of cognitive behavior may be the result of an alienation from psychopathology. The sequential model introduces a conceptual shift in psychotherapy research and practice. The target of psychotherapeutic efforts is not predetermined and therapy driven (e.g., cognitive triad), but depends on the type and intensity of residual symptomatology [16,19] or the specific impairments in psychological well-being [19,69]. The cognitive-behavioral approach that is entailed by the sequential model is thus pragmatic, realistic instead of idealistic, with a strictly evidence-based appraisal of its components [70]. There is limited awareness that current techniques of treating affective disorders are geared to acute situations more than residual phases of illness [14] and neglect psychological well-being [66]. The model may be frustrating to the purist in its blurring of clear-cut interpretative instruments. However, it is more in keeping with the complexity of the balance of positive and negative affects [71] in health and disease and the clinical needs of patients with affective disorders.

ACKNOWLEDGMENTS

The work described in this paper was supported in part by grants from the Mental Health Evaluation Project (Istituto Superiore di Sanità, Rome) and the Ministero dell'Università e della Ricerca Scientifica e Tecnologica (Rome) to G.A.F.

REFERENCES

1. GA Fava. Conceptual obstacles to research progress in affective disorders. Psychother Psychosom 66:283–285, 1997.
2. BE Wexler, JC Nelson. The treatment of depressive disorders. Int J Mental Health 22:7–41, 1993.
3. MG Gelder. Treatment of the neuroses. Int J Mental Health 21:3–42, 1993.
4. M Basoglu. Pharmacological and behavioral treatment of panic disorder. Psychother Psychosom 58:57–59, 1992.
5. GA Fava, R Kellner. Staging. A neglected dimension in psychiatric classification. Acta Psychiatr Scand 87:225–230, 1993.
6. J Ananth. Treatment-resistant depression. Psychother Psychosom 67:61–70, 1998.
7. GA Fava, G Savron, S Grandi, C Rafanelli. Cognitive-behavioral management of drug-resistant major depression disorder. J Clin Psychiatry 58:278–282, 1997.
8. JW Stewart, MA Mercier, V Agosti, M Guardino, FM Quitkin. Imipramine is effective after unsuccessful cognitive therapy. J Clin Psychopharmacol 13:114–119, 1993.
9. MH Pollack, MW Otto, JF Rosenbaum, eds. Challenges in Clinical Practice. New York: Guilford Press, 1996.
10. PMG Emmelkamp, TK Bouman, A Scholing. Anxiety Disorders. Chichester, UK: Wiley, 1993.

11. A Scholing, PMG Emmelkamp. Cognitive and behavioral treatments of fear of blushing, sweating or trembling. Behav Res Ther 31:155–170, 1993.

12. GA Fava, G Savron, M Zielezny, S Grandi, C Rafanelli, S Conti. Overcoming resistance to exposure in panic disorder with agoraphobia. Acta Psychiatr Scand 95:306–312, 1997.

13. GA Fava. The concept of recovery in affective disorders. Psychother Psychosom 65:2–13, 1996.

14. GA Fava. Subclinical symptoms in mood disorders. Pathophysiological and therapeutic implications. Psychol Med 29:47–61, 1999.

15. GA Fava, R Kellner. Prodromal symptoms in affective disorders. Am J Psychiatry 148:823–830, 1991.

16. GA Fava, S Grandi, M Zielezny, R Canestrari, MA Morphy. Cognitive behavioral treatment of residual symptoms in primary major depressive disorder. Am J Psychiatry 151:1295–1299, 1994.

17. GA Fava, S Grandi, M Zielezny, C Rafanelli, R Canestrari. Four year outcome for cognitive behavioral treatment of residual symptoms in major depression. Am J Psychiatry 153:945–947, 1996.

18. GA Fava, C Rafanelli, S Grandi, R Canestrari, MA Morphy. Six year outcome for cognitive behavioral treatment of residual symptoms in major depression. Am J Psychiatry 155:1443–1445, 1998.

19. GA Fava, C Rafanelli, S Grandi, S Conti, P Belluardo. Prevention of recurrent depression with cognitive behavioral therapy. Arch Gen Psychiatry 55:816–820, 1998.

20. GA Fava, C Rafanelli, S Grandi, S Conti, P Belluardo. Letter to the editor. Arch Gen Psychiatry 56:765, 1999.

21. ES Paykel, MM Weissman. Social adjustment and depression. Arch Gen Psychiatry 28:659–664, 1973.

22. W Coryell, W Scheftner, MB Keller, J Endicott, J Maser, GL Klerman. The enduring psychosocial consequences of mania and depression. Am J Psychiatry 150:720–727, 1993.

23. F Bauwens, A Tray, D Pardoen, M Vander Elst, J Mendlewicz. Social adjustment of remitted bipolar and unipolar out-patients. Br J Psychiatry 159:239–244, 1991.

24. PN Goering, WJ Lancee, SJJ Freeman. Marital support and recovery from depression. Br J Psychiatry 160:76–82, 1992.

25. G Eaves, AJ Rush. Cognitive patterns in symptomatic and remitted unipolar major depression. J Abnorm Psychol 93:31–40, 1984.

26. JMG Williams, D Healy, JD Teasdale, W White, ES Paykel. Dysfunctional attitudes and vulnerability to persistent depression. Psychol Med 20:375–381, 1990.

27. GW Brown, A Bifulco, B Andrews. Self-esteem and depression. Soc Psychiatry Psychiatr Epidemiol 25:244–249, 1990.

28. MJ Power, CF Duggan, AS Lee, RM Murray. Dysfunctional attitudes in depressed and recovered depressed patients and their first degree-relatives. Psychol Med 25:97–93, 1995.

29. J Scott, D Eccleston, R Boys. Can we predict the persistence of depression? Br J Psychiatry 161:633–637, 1992.
30. ED Peselow, MP Sanfilipo, RR Fieve, G Gubelkian. Personality traits during depression and after clinical recovery. Br J Psychiatry 164:349–354, 1994.
31. M Fava, E Bouffides, JA Pava, MK McCarthy, RJ Steingard, JF Rosenbaum. Personality disorder comorbidity with major depression and response to fluoxetine treatment. Psychother Psychosom 62:160–167, 1994.
32. LO Murray, IM Blackburn. Personality differences in patients with depressive illness and anxiety neurosis. Acta Psychiatr Scandinav 50:183–191, 1974.
33. C Perris, M Eisemann, L von Knorring, H Perris. Personality traits in former depression patients and in healthy subjects without past history of depression. Psychopathology 17:178–186, 1984.
34. PJ Clayton, C Ernst, J Angst. Premorbid personality traits of men who develop unipolar or bipolar disorder. Eur Arch Psychiatry Clin Neurosci 243:340–346, 1994.
35. MM Weissman, SV Kasl, GL Klerman. Follow-up of depressed women after maintenance treatment. Am J Psychiatry 133:757–760, 1976.
36. HS Akiskal. Dysthymic disorder. Am J Psychiatry 140:11–20, 1983.
37. RMA Hirschfeld, GL Klerman, NC Andreasen, PJ Clayton, MB Keller. Psychosocial predictors of chronicity in depressed patients. Br J Psychiatry 148:648–654, 1986.
38. RH Mindham, C Howland, M Shepherd. An evaluation of continuation therapy with tricyclic antidepressants in depressive illness. Psychol Med 3:5–17, 1973.
39. C Faravelli, A Ambonetti, S Pallanti, A Pazzagli. Depressive relapses and incomplete recovery from index episode. Am J Psychiatry 143:888–891, 1986.
40. RF Prien, DJ Kupfer. Continuation drug therapy for major depressive episodes. Am J Psychiatry 143:18–23, 1986.
41. A Georgotas, RE McCue. Relapse of depressed patients after effective continuation therapy. J Affect Disord 17, 159–164, 1989.
42. M Maj, F Veltro, R Pirozzi, S Lobrace, L Magliano. Pattern of recurrence of illness after recovery from an episode of major depression. Am J Psychiatry 149:795–800, 1992.
43. AD Simons, GE Murphy, JL Levine, RD Wetzel. Cognitive therapy and pharmacotherapy of depression. Arch Gen Psychiatry 43:43–50, 1986.
44. ME Thase, AD Simons, J McGeary, JF Cabalane, C Hughes, T Harden, E Friedman. Relapse after cognitive behavior therapy of depression. Am J Psychiatry 149:1046–1052, 1992.
45. GA Fava, R Kellner, J Lisansky, S Park, GI Perini, M Zielezny. Rating depression in normals and depressives. J Affect Disord 11:29–33, 1986.
46. V Agosti, JW Stewart, FM Quitkin, K Ocepek-Welikson. How symptomatic do depressed patients remain after benefiting from medication treatment? Compr Psychiatry 34:182–186, 1993.
47. R Kellner. The development of sensitive scales for research in therapeutics. In: M Fava, JF Rosenbaum, eds. Research Design and Methods in Psychiatry. Amsterdam: Elsevier, 1992, pp 213–222.

48. GA Fava: Measurement of prodromal and subclinical symptoms. In: M Fava, and JF Rosenbaum, eds. Research Design and Methods in Psychiatry. Amsterdam: Elsevier, 1992, pp 223–230.

49. ES Paykel. The Clinical Interview for Depression. J Affect Disord 9: 85–96, 1985.

50. GA Fava, S Grandi, R Canestrari, G Molnar. Prodromal symptoms in primary major depressive disorder. J Affect Disord 19:149–152, 1990.

51. HM van Praag. About the centrality of mood disorders. Eur Neuropsychopharmacol 2:393–404, 1992.

52. AT Beck, AJ Rush, BF Shaw, G Emery. Cognitive Therapy of Depression. New York: Guilford Press, 1979.

53. AT Beck, G Emery. Anxiety Disorders and Phobias. New York: Basic Books, 1985.

54. IM Marks. Fears, Phobias, and Rituals: Panic, Anxiety and Their Disorders. New York: Oxford University Press, 1987.

55. JA Pava, M Fava, JA Levenson. Integrating cognitive therapy and pharmacotherapy in the treatment and prophylaxis of depression. Psychother Psychosom 61:211–219, 1994.

56. GA Fava, C Rafanelli, M Cazzaro, S Conti, S Grandi. Well-being therapy. Psychol Med 28:475–480, 1998.

57. E Frank, DJ Kupfer, JM Perel, C Cornes, DB Jarrett, AG Mallinger, ME Thase, AB McEacran, VJ Grochocinski. Three year outcomes for maintenance therapies in recurrent depression. Arch Gen Psychiatry 47:1093–1099, 1990.

58. ES Paykel, J Scott, JD Teasdale, AL Johnson, A Garlan, R Moore, A Jenaway, PL Cornwall, H Hayhurst, R Abbot, M Pope. Prevention of relapse in residual depression by cognitive therapy. Arch Gen Psychiatry 56:829–835, 1999.

59. GA Fava, C Ruini. The sequential approach to relapse prevention in unipolar depression. World Psychiatry 1:10–15, 2002.

60. PMG Emmelkamp. Self-observation versus flooding in the treatment of agoraphobia. Behav Res Ther 12:229–237, 1974.

61. CD Ryff. Happiness is everything, or is it? Explorations on the meaning of psychological well-being. J Pers Soc Psychol 57:1069–1081, 1989.

62. C Rafanelli, SK Park, C Ruini, F Ottolini, M Cazzaro, GA Fava. Rating well-being and distress. Stress Med 16:55–61, 2000.

63. GA Fava, C Rafanelli, F Ottolini, C Ruini, M Cazzaro, S Grandi. Psychological well-being and residual symptoms in remitted patients with panic disorder and agoraphobia. J Affect Disord 65:185–190, 2001.

64. PE Meehl. Hedonic capacity: some conjectures. Bull Menninger Clin 39:295–307, 1975.

65. A Ellis, I Becker. A Guide to Personal Happiness. Hollywood, CA: Melvin Powers, 1982.

66. CD Ryff, B Singer. Psychological well-being: Meaning, measurement, and implications for psychotherapy research. Psychother Psychosom 65:14–23, 1996.

67. I Marks. Is a paradigm shift occurring in brief psychological treatments? Psychother Psychosom 68:169, 1999.
68. EB Foa, MJ Kozak. Beyond the efficacy ceiling? Cognitive behavior therapy in search of theory. Behav Ther 28:601–611, 1997.
69. GA Fava. Well-being therapy. Psychother Psychosom 68:170–178, 1999.
70. GA Fava. Cognitive behavioral therapy. In: M Fink, ed. Encyclopedia of Stress. San Diego: C Academic Press, 2000, pp 484–487.
71. CD Ryff, B Singer. The contours of positive human health. Psychol Inquiry 9:1–28, 1998.

13

Diagnosis and Treatment of Depression During Pregnancy

Ruta Nonacs
Massachusetts General Hospital
Boston, Massachusetts, U.S.A.

Lee S. Cohen
Massachusetts General Hospital
and Harvard Medical School
Boston, Massachusetts, U.S.A.

INTRODUCTION

Mood disorders are common in women and typically emerge during the childbearing years (1). With the advent of effective and well-tolerated pharmacological treatments for psychiatric disorders, a growing number of women are treated with psychotropic medications during their reproductive years. Although pregnancy has traditionally been considered to be a time of emotional well-being, recent data indicate that about 10% of women experience clinically significant depressive symptoms during pregnancy (antenatal depression) (2–5). Furthermore, women with histories of major depression appear to be at high risk for recurrent depression during pregnancy, particularly in the setting of antidepressant discontinuation (6).

Frequently women with histories of major depression seek consultations regarding the use of antidepressant medications during pregnancy either prior to conception or early in the course of pregnancy. In other cases, women present with a recurrent or new onset of depressive symptoms during pregnancy. In both of these settings, the clinician faces certain challenges when making recommendations regarding the treatment of depression during pregnancy. All antidepressant medications diffuse readily across the placenta, and no psychotropic drug has yet been approved by the Food and Drug Administration (FDA) for use during pregnancy. Although data accumulated over the last 30 years suggest that some medications may be used safely during pregnancy (7–9), knowledge regarding the risks of prenatal exposure to psychotropic medications is incomplete. Thus, it is common for patients to avoid pharmacological treatment during pregnancy.

The clinical challenge for physicians who care for women with psychiatric disorders during pregnancy is to minimize risk to the fetus while limiting morbidity from untreated psychiatric illness in the mother. Because no decision is absolutely free of risk, it is imperative that these clinical decisions be made collaboratively with patients and their partners on a case by case basis. It is the physician's responsibility to provide accurate and up-to-date information on the reproductive safety of pharmacological treatment and to help the patient to select the most appropriate treatment strategy. Even when given comparable information, patients may make different decisions regarding the use of pharmacological therapy during pregnancy. In this chapter, we review the available information on antidepressant medication use during pregnancy and provide guidelines for the treatment of depression in pregnant women.

DEPRESSION DURING PREGNANCY (ANTENATAL DEPRESSION)

Although pregnancy has previously been described as a time during which women are at lower risk for psychiatric illness, recent studies indicate that about 10% of women suffer from clinically significant depressive symptoms during pregnancy (2–4). A personal history of affective illness significantly increases this risk (3,5); however, for about one-third of the women who become depressed during pregnancy, this represents the first episode of major depression (3). Other risk factor factors for antenatal depression include marital discord or dissatisfaction, inadequate psychosocial supports, recent adverse life events, lower socioeconomic status, and unwanted pregnancy (2,3,5).

Women with recurrent major depression who have been maintained on an antidepressant medication prior to conception appear to be at especially high risk for relapse during pregnancy (10). Although there are accumulating data to support the relative safety of using certain antidepressants during pregnancy, women commonly choose or are counseled to discontinue anti-depressant treatment during pregnancy. A large body of literature in non-gravid populations indicates that the discontinuation of maintenance pharmacological treatment is associated with high rates of relapse (11,12). Preliminary data suggest pregnancy does not protect against relapse in the setting of medication discontinuation. Among women with recurrent major depression who discontinue antidepressant medication proximate to conception, approximately 75% relapse during pregnancy, typically during the first trimester (8).

Although more severe forms of affective illness may be readily detected, depression that emerges during pregnancy is frequently overlooked. Many of the neurovegetative signs and symptoms characteristic of major depression (e.g., sleep and appetite disturbance, diminished libido, low energy) are also observed in nondepressed women during pregnancy. In addition, certain medical disorders commonly seen during pregnancy such as anemia, gestational diabetes, and thyroid dysfunction may be associated with depressive symptoms and may complicate the diagnosis of depression during pregnancy (13). Clinical features that may support the diagnosis of major depression include anhedonia, feelings of guilt and hopelessness, and suicidal thoughts. Suicidal ideation is often reported; however, risk of self-injurious or suicidal behaviors appears to be relatively low in the population of women who develop depression during pregnancy (14,15).

RISKS OF UNTREATED DEPRESSION IN THE MOTHER

Although clinicians have appropriate concern regarding the known and unknown risks associated with fetal exposure to psychiatric medications, the potential impact of untreated psychiatric illness on fetal well-being has frequently been overlooked. Depression increases the risk of self-injurious or suicidal behaviors in the mother but also may contribute to inadequate self-care and poor compliance with prenatal care. Women with depression often present with decreased appetite and consequently lower than expected weight gain in pregnancy, which are factors that have been associated with negative pregnancy outcomes (16). In addition, pregnant women with depression are also more likely to smoke and to use either alcohol or illicit drugs (16); which are behaviors that further increase risk to the fetus.

In addition, current research suggests that maternal depression itself may adversely affect the developing fetus. Although it has been difficult to assess the impact of antenatal depression on fetal development and neonatal well-being in humans, several studies have found an association between maternal depression and factors which predict poor neonatal outcome, including preterm birth, lower birth weight, smaller head circumference, and lower Apgar scores (17–21). The physiological mechanisms by which symptoms of depression might affect neonatal outcome are not clear. However, increased serum cortisol and catecholamine levels, which are typically observed in patients with depression, may affect placental function by altering uterine blood flow and inducing uterine irritability (22,23). Dysregulation of the hypothalamic-pituitary-adrenal (HPA) axis that is associated with depression may also have a direct effect on fetal development. Animal studies suggest that stress during pregnancy is also associated with neuronal death and abnormal development of neural structures in the fetal brain, as well as sustained dysfunction on the HPA axis in the offspring (23,24).

Maternal depression may also have a significant impact on the family unit. Depression is typically associated with interpersonal difficulties, and disruptions in mother-child interactions and attachment may have a profound impact on infant development. Recent research indicates that children of depressed mothers are more likely to have behavioral problems and to exhibit disruptions in cognitive and emotional development (25–27). Furthermore, depression during pregnancy significantly increases a woman' risk of postpartum depression (5,28). Thus, antenatal depression may have significant negative effects that extend well beyond the pregnancy.

NONPHARMACOLOGICAL TREATMENT OF ANTENATAL DEPRESSION

Until recently, there have been no clinical trials of nonpharmacological treatments for antenatal depression. Interpersonal therapy (IPT) is a short-term, manual-driven psychotherapy that deals primarily with four major problem areas: grief, interpersonal disputes, role transitions, and interpersonal deficits (29). Given the importance of interpersonal relationships in couples expecting a child and the significant role transitions that take place during pregnancy and subsequent to delivery, IPT is ideally suited for the treatment of depressed pregnant women. Spinelli (1997) has adapted IPT for the treatment of women with antenatal depression, focusing on the role transitions and interpersonal disputes characteristic of pregnancy and motherhood. In a pilot study of 13 women (30). IPT significantly reduced the severity of depressive symptoms and induced remission in all patients. Furthermore, none of the women followed after delivery (n = 10) developed postpartum depression. Although this study is limited by its small size and lack of a control group, its results are encouraging. Not only does this modality of treatment treat the acute symptoms of depression during pregnancy, it appears to decrease the risk for depression after delivery. Larger prospective studies of IPT during pregnancy are currently underway.

PHARMACOLOGICAL TREATMENT OF ANTENATAL DEPRESSION

When considering the use of a psychiatric medication during pregnancy, the clinician must address four primary types of risk with respect to the developing fetus: (1) risk of pregnancy loss or miscarriage, (2) risk of organ malformation or teratogenesis, (3) risk of neonatal toxicity or withdrawal syndromes during the acute neonatal period, and (4) risk of long-term neurobehavioral sequelae (8).

To provide guidance to physicians seeking information on the reproductive safety of various prescription medications, the FDA has established a system that classifies medications into five risk categories (A, B, C, D, and X) based of data derived from human and animal studies. Category A medications are designated as safe for use during pregnancy, whereas category X drugs are contraindicated and are known to have risks to the fetus that outweigh any benefit to the patient. Most psychotropic medications are classified as category C, agents for which human studies are lacking and for which "risk cannot be ruled out." No psychotropic drugs are classified as safe for use during pregnancy (category A).

Unfortunately, this system of classification is frequently ambiguous and may sometimes be misleading. For example, certain tricyclic antidepressants have been labeled as category D, indicating "positive evidence of risk," although the pooled available data do not support this assertion and, in fact, suggest that these drugs are safe for use during pregnancy (7). Therefore, the physician must rely on other sources of information when providing well-informed recommendations on the use of psychotropic medications during pregnancy. For obvious ethical reasons, it is not possible to conduct randomized, placebo-controlled studies on medication safety in pregnant populations. Therefore, much of the data on reproductive safety has been derived from retrospective studies and case reports, although more recent studies have utilized a prospective design (31,33–36).

Risk of Pregnancy Loss

Recent attention has focused on whether certain antidepressants may increase the risk of early pregnancy loss. Although most reports do not indicate that antidepressants increase the risk of miscarriage, several reports have suggested small increases in the rates of spontaneous abortion among women treated with selective serotonin reuptake inhibitor (SSRI) antidepressants and venlafaxine during the first trimester of pregnancy (31,35,36). In these reports, the observed differences have not reached statistical significance; rates of miscarriage in exposed women were in the range of what would be normally expected in women with no known exposure. An alternative explanation for this finding of slightly increased risk of miscarriage in antidepressant-exposed women is that depression itself is a factor that may contribute to an increasing risk of spontaneous abortion. Some researchers also suggest that the number of spontaneous abortions may have been overestimated, because when questioned during the follow-up interviews, some women taking medications at conception may have chosen to report a miscarriage when in fact they had decided to terminate their pregnancy (36). Further studies are needed to better define this risk.

Risk of Congenital Malformation

The baseline incidence of major congenital malformations in newborns born in the United States is estimated to be between 3 and 4% (37). During the earliest stages of pregnancy, formation of major organ systems takes place and is complete within the first 12 weeks after conception. A teratogen is defined as an agent that interferes with this process and produces some type of organ malformation or dysfunction. Exposure to a toxic agent before 2 weeks of gestation is not associated with congenital malformations and is more likely to result in a nonviable blighted ovum (38). For each organ or organ system there exists a critical period during which development takes place and may be susceptible to the effects of a teratogen (39). For example, formation of the heart and great vessels takes place from 4–9 weeks after conception. Formation of the lip and palate is typically complete by week 10. Neural tube folding and closure, which form the brain and spinal cord, occurs within the first 4 weeks of gestation.

Although early case reports suggested a possible association between first-trimester exposure to tricyclic antidepressants (TCAs) and limb malformation, 3 prospective and more than 10 retrospective studies have examined the risk of organ dysgenesis in over 400 cases of first-trimester exposure to TCAs (8,31,32,40–43). When evaluated on an individual basis and when pooled, these studies fail to indicate a significant association between fetal exposure to TCAs and risk for any major congenital anomaly. Among the TCAs, desipramine and nortriptyline are preferred, since they are less anticholinergic and are the least likely to exacerbate orthostatic hypotension that occurs during pregnancy.

Except for fluoxetine, information on the reproductive safety of SSRIs is limited. Four prospective studies have evaluated rates of congenital malformation in approximately 1100 fluoxetine-exposed infants (31,33,44,45). The postmarketing surveillance registry established by the manufacturer of fluoxetine and two other retrospective studies (41,46) complement these findings. These data collected from over 2500 cases indicate no increase in risk of major congenital malformation in fluoxetine-exposed infants.

Although no study observed an increase in the risk for *major* congenital anomaly, Chambers and colleagues noted an increase in the risk for multiple *minor* malformations in fluoxetine-exposed infants (33). In this study, minor anomalies were defined as structural defects that had no cosmetic or functional importance. In addition, this report suggested that late exposure to fluoxetine was associated with premature labor and poor neonatal adaptation. Interpretation of the findings in this study is limited by several methodological difficulties (47,48). For example, the fluoxetine-exposed women and control groups differed significantly in terms of important variables such as age, presence of psychiatric illness, and exposure to other medications. In addition, nonblinded raters were utilized, and only half of the fluoxetine-exposed infants were evaluated, which raises the question of selection bias. Although further data are needed to ensure clinical confidence, the data collected thus far on fluoxetine suggests that it is unlikely to be a significant human teratogen.

Information regarding the reproductive safety of sertraline, paroxetine, fluvoxamine, and citalopram use during pregnancy is gradually accumulating but is limited in terms of sample size (35,41,46,49,50). Two meta-analyses combining studies with exposures to tricyclic antidepressants and SSRIs did not demonstrate an increase in the risk of congenital malformation (51,52). One prospective study of 531 infants with first-trimester exposure to SSRIs (mostly citalopram, n = 375) did not demonstrate an increased risk of organ malformation (49). In a retrospective study of 63 infants with first-trimester exposure to paroxetine, no increase in teratogenic risk was observed (50). In a prospective, controlled cohort study, Kulin and colleagues (1998) reported on outcomes in neonates exposed in utero to fluvoxamine (n = 26), paroxetine (n = 97), and sertraline (n = 147) (35). Pregnancy outcomes did not differ between the exposed and nonexposed groups in terms of risk for congenital malformations. Birth weights and gestational age were similar in both groups. Although this information on these SSRIs is reassuring, one of the major limitations of this study is that the analysis grouped the three antidepressants together versus analyzing each antidepressant separately for teratogenic risk.

Prospective data on 150 women exposed to venlafaxine during the first trimester of pregnancy suggest no increase in the risk of major malformations as compared to nonexposed controls (36). GlaxoSmithKline, the manufacturer of bupropion (Wellbutrin), has set up a pregnancy registry, and preliminary analysis of the data includes 166 pregnancy outcomes involving first-trimester exposure to bupropion. Three infants were born with major malformations. This represents a 2.1% risk of congenital malformations, which is consistent with what is observed in the general population of women with no known exposure. Although these initial reports are reassuring, larger samples are required to establish the reproductive safety of these newer antidepressants. It is estimated that at least 500–600 exposures must be collected to demonstrate a twofold increase in risk for a particular malformation over what is observed in the general population (53).

To date, prospective data on the use of mirtazapine, nefazodone, and trazodone are not available. Scant information is available regarding the reproductive safety of monoamine oxidase inhibitors (MAOIs). One study in humans described an increase in congenital malformations after prenatal exposure to tranylcypromine and phenelzine, although the sample size was extremely small (54). Moreover, during labor and delivery, MAOIs may produce a hypertensive crisis should tocolytic medications, such as terbutaline, be used to forestall delivery. Given this lack of data, and the cumbersome restrictions associated with their use, MAOIs are typically avoided during pregnancy.

Risk of Neonatal Toxicity

Neonatal toxicity or *perinatal syndromes* refer to a spectrum of physical and behavioral symptoms observed in the acute neonatal period that are attributed to drug exposure at or near the time of delivery. Over the last two decades, a wide range of transient neonatal distress syndromes associated with exposure to (or withdrawal from) antidepressants in utero have been described; however, studies of larger samples suggest that the incidence of these adverse events is low. Anecdotal reports that attribute these syndromes to drug exposure must be cautiously interpreted, and larger samples must be studied in order to establish a causal link between exposure to a particular medication and a perinatal syndrome.

Various case reports have described perinatal syndromes in infants exposed to TCAs in utero. A TCA withdrawal syndrome with characteristic symptoms of jitteriness, irritability, and, less commonly, seizures (55–59) has been observed. Withdrawal seizures have been reported only with clomipramine (55,59). In addition, neonatal toxicity attributed to the anticholinergic effect of TCAs, including symptoms of functional bowel obstruction and urinary retention, has also been reported (60,61). In all cases, these symptoms have been transient.

The extent to which prenatal exposure to fluoxetine or other SSRIs is associated with neonatal toxicity is still unclear. Case reports and one prospective study have described perinatal complications in fluoxetine-exposed infants, including poor neonatal adaptation, respiratory distress, feeding problems, and jitteriness (33,62). Other prospective studies have not observed perinatal distress in infants exposed to fluoxetine or other SSRIs (35,63–65).

More recently, there has been a growing concern regarding the potential for withdrawal syndromes in neonates exposed to paroxetine. Case reports of neonatal withdrawal in neonates exposed to paroxetine have been published and describe transient symptoms of irritability, excessive crying, increased muscle tone, feeding problems, sleep disruption, and respiratory distress (66–69). In a prospectively ascertained sample of 55 neonates exposed to paroxetine proximate to delivery (dose range 10–60 mg, median 20 mg), 22% (n = 12) had complications necessitating intensive treatment (67). The most common symptoms included respiratory distress (n = 9), hypoglycemia (n = 2), and jaundice (n = 1), all of which resolved over 1–2 weeks without specific intervention. The extent to which other SSRIs (with longer half-lives) have similar neonatal toxicity profiles remains to be explored; however, most prospective studies have not demonstrated significant adverse events in exposed infants (35,44,49,64,65). Furthermore, it is crucial to investigate other factors that modulate vulnerability to neonatal toxicity (e.g., prematurity, low birth weight).

Risk of Neurobehavioral Sequelae

Because neuronal migration and differentiation occur throughout pregnancy and into the early years of life, the central nervous system (CNS) remains particularly vulnerable to toxic agents throughout pregnancy. However, insults that occur after neural tube closure produce changes in behavior and function as opposed to gross structural abnormalities. Behavioral teratogenesis refers to the potential of a psychotropic drug administered prenatally to cause long-term neurobehavioral sequelae. For example, are children who have been exposed to an antidepressant in utero at risk for cognitive or behavioral problems at a later point during development? Animal studies demonstrate changes in behavior and neurotransmitter function after prenatal exposure to a variety of psychotropic agents (70–72). The extent to which these findings are of consequence to humans has yet to be demonstrated.

With regard to long-term neurobehavioral sequelae in children exposed to either fluoxetine or TCAs, the data are limited but reassuring. In a landmark study, Nulman and colleagues (34) followed a cohort of children up to preschool age who had been exposed to either TCAs (n = 80) or fluoxetine (n = 55) during pregnancy (most commonly during the first trimester) and compared these subjects to a cohort of nonexposed controls (n = 84). Results indicated no significant differences in IQ, temperament, behavior, reactivity, mood, distractibility, or activity level between exposed and nonexposed children. A more recent report from the same group followed a cohort of children exposed to fluoxetine (n = 40) or tricyclic antidepressants (n = 47) for the *entire duration of the pregnancy* and yielded similar results (65). The investigators concluded that their findings support the hypothesis that fluoxetine and tricyclic antidepressants are not behavioral teratogens. However, these data are preliminary, and clearly further investigation into the long-term neurobehavioral effects of prenatal exposure to antidepressants, as well as other psychotropic medications, is warranted.

GUIDELINES FOR THE TREATMENT OF DEPRESSION DURING PREGNANCY

Only recently has attention focused on the treatment of depression during pregnancy (6,7,9); however, the management of antenatal depression is largely guided by practical experience, with few definitive data and no controlled treatment studies to inform treatment. The most appropriate treatment algorithm depends on the severity of the disorder and ultimately on the wishes of the patient. Clinicians must work collaboratively with the patient to arrive at the safest decision based on available information. A patient's past psychiatric history and current symptoms as well as her attitude toward the use of psychiatric medications during pregnancy must be carefully assessed.

Women with histories of major depression frequently present for consultation regarding the use of psychotropic medications during pregnancy, or they may seek treatment after recurrence of illness following conception. Not infrequently, women present with the first onset of psychiatric illness during pregnancy. All decisions regarding the continuation or initiation of treatment during pregnancy must reflect an assessment of the following risks: (1) risk of fetal exposure to medication, (2) risk of untreated psychiatric illness in the mother, and (3) risk of relapse associated with discontinuation of maintenance treatment. A discussion of each of these risks should be documented in the medical record, as well as the patient's competence to understand these issues regarding treatment.

With the advent of newer and better-tolerated antidepressants, a growing number of women are prescribed antidepressant medications during the childbearing years. For those women with recurrent major depression who are on maintenance treatment and plan to conceive, the clinician and patient must decide whether to maintain or discontinue antidepressant treatment during pregnancy. Ideally, decisions regarding the use of psychotropic medications during pregnancy should be made prior to conception. In this setting, the clinician must provide information regarding the patient's risk for relapse in the setting of medication discontinuation. One must also take into account the risk of chronic, recurrent depression and treatment resistance in patients who experience depressive relapse after medication discontinuation (73–75).

In patients with less severe depression, it is appropriate to consider discontinuation of pharmacological therapy during pregnancy. Interpersonal or cognitive behavioral therapy may be used prior to conception to facilitate the gradual tapering and discontinuation of an antidepressant medication in women planning to become pregnant. These modalities of treatment may reduce the risk of recurrent depressive symptoms during pregnancy, although this has not been studied systematically. Close monitoring during pregnancy is essential even if all medications are discontinued and there is no need for medication management. Psychiatrically ill women are at high risk for relapse during pregnancy, and early detection and treatment of recurrent illness may significantly reduce morbidity associated with antenatal affective disorder.

Many women who discontinue antidepressant treatment during pregnancy do experience recurrent depressive symptoms (6). Thus, for those women with more recurrent or refractory depressive illness, the patient and clinician may decide that the safest option is to continue pharmacological treatment during pregnancy. In this setting, the clinician should attempt to select medications for use during pregnancy that have a well-characterized reproductive safety profile. Often this may necessitate switching from one psychotropic agent to another with a better reproductive safety profile. An example of this would be switching from ncfazodone, a medication for which there are no data on reproductive safety, to an agent such as fluoxetine. In other situations, one may decide to use a medication for which information regarding reproductive safety is sparse. A scenario that highlights this is the woman with refractory depressive illness who has responded only to one antidepressant for which data on reproductive safety is limited (i.e., venlafaxine). She may choose to continue this medication during pregnancy rather than risk relapse if she discontinued this agent or switched to another antidepressant.

Women may also experience new onset of depressive symptoms during pregnancy. For women who present with minor depressive symptoms, nonpharmacological treatment strategies should be explored first. Interpersonal psychotherapy or cognitive behavioral therapy may be beneficial for reducing the severity of depressive symptoms and may either limit or obviate the need for medications (29,30,76). In general, pharmacological treatment is pursued when nonpharmacological strategies have failed or when it is felt that the risks associated with psychiatric illness during pregnancy outweigh the risks of fetal exposure to a particular medication.

In situations where pharmacological treatment is indicated, the clinician should attempt to select the safest medication regimen, using, if possible, medications with the safest reproductive profile. Fluoxetine, with the most extensive literature supporting its reproductive safety, is a first-line choice. The tricyclic antidepressants have been relatively well characterized in this setting and should be considered as first-line agents. Among the TCAs, desipramine and nortriptyline are preferred, since they are less anticholinergic and are the least likely to exacerbate orthostatic hypotension during pregnancy. There is a growing literature on the reproductive safety of the newer SSRIs, including citalopram, and these agents may be useful in certain settings (35,49). In patients with depression who have not responded to either fluoxetine or a TCA, these newer agents may be considered, acknowledging that information on their reproductive safety is limited. When prescribing medications during pregnancy, every attempt should be made to simplify the medication regimen. For instance, one may select a more sedating tricyclic antidepressant for a women who presents with depression and sleep disturbance rather than using an SSRI in combination with trazodone or a benzodiazepine.

In addition, the clinician must use an adequate dosage of medication. Frequently, the dosage of a medication is reduced during pregnancy in an attempt to limit risk to the fetus; however, this type of modification in treatment may instead place the woman at greater risk for recurrent illness. During pregnancy, changes in plasma volume, as well as increases in hepatic metabolism and renal clearance, may significantly affect drug levels (77,78). Several groups have described a significant reduction (up to 65%) in serum levels of tricyclic antidepressants during pregnancy (32,52). Subtherapeutic levels were associated with depressive relapse (32), therefore, the daily TCA dosage was increased during pregnancy to induce remission. Similarly, many women taking SSRIs during pregnancy require an increase in SSRI dosage to sustain euthymia (79).

Based on a number of anecdotal reports of toxicity in infants born to mothers treated with antidepressants, some investigators have recommended discontinuation of antidepressant medication several days or weeks prior to delivery to minimize the risk of neonatal toxicity. Given the low incidence of neonatal toxicity with most antidepressants, this practice carries significant risk, since it withdraws treatment from patients precisely as they are about to enter the postpartum period, a time of heightened risk for affective illness.

Severely depressed patients with acute suicidality or psychosis require hospitalization, and electroconvulsive therapy (ECT) is frequently the treatment of choice. Two recent reviews of ECT use during pregnancy note the efficacy and safety of this procedure (80,81). In a review of the 300 case reports of ECT during pregnancy published over the past 50 years, there have been four reports of premature labor. There have been no reports of premature rupture of membranes caused by ECT. Given its relative safety, ECT may also be considered as an alternative to conventional pharmacotherapy for women who wish to avoid extended exposure to psychotropic medications during pregnancy or for those women who fail to respond to standard antidepressant therapy.

CONCLUSION

Depression occurs commonly during pregnancy, and women with recurrent depression are at particularly high risk for depressive illness in this setting.

Although the use of psychotropic medications during pregnancy raises concerns, there are data to support the use of certain antidepressants, including fluoxetine and the tricyclic antidepressants. Data on the newer SSRI antidepressants is gradually accumulating and is encouraging. None of the SSRIs or TCAs has been associated with an increased risk of congenital malformation. However, our information on the long-term neurobehavioral effects of these medications remains limited. As depression during pregnancy carries a risk for both the mother and child, it is crucial to recognize depression in this setting and to provide appropriate treatment strategies. Further data on nonpharmacological and pharmacological strategies is clearly needed to aid in the treatment of this challenging clinical population.

REFERENCES

1. Kessler RC, McGonagle KA, Swartz M, Blazer DG, Nelson CB. Sex and depression in the National Comorbidity Survey I: lifetime prevalence, chronicity and recurrence. J Affect Dis 1993; 29:85–96.
2. O'Hara MW. Social support, life events, and depression during pregnancy and the pueperium. Arch Gen Psychiatry 1986; 43:569–573.
3. O'Hara MW. Postpartum Depression: Causes and Consequences. New York: Springer-Verlag, 1995.
4. Evans J, Heron J, Francomb H, Oke S, Golding J. Cohort study of depressed mood during pregnancy and after childbirth. BMJ 2001; 323(7307):257–260.
5. Gotlib IH, Whiffen VE, Mount JH, Milne K, Cordy NI. Prevalence rates and demographic characteristics associated with depression in pregnancy and the postpartum period. J Consult Clin Psychol 1989; 57:269–274.
6. Altshuler L, Cohen L, Moline M, Kahn D, Carpenter D, Docherty J. Treatment of depression in women: the expert consensus guidelines. Postgrad Med Spec Rep 2001; 1–116.
7. Altshuler LL, Cohen LS, Szuba MP, Burt VK, Gitlin M, Mintz J. Pharmacologic management of psychiatric illness in pregnancy: dilemmas and guidelines. Am J Psychiatry 1996; 153:592–606.
8. Cohen L, Altshuler L. Pharmacologic management of psychiatric illness during pregnancy and the postpartum period. In: Dunner D, Rosenbaum J, eds. Psychiatric Clinics of North America Annual of Drug Therapy. Philadelphia: Saunders, 1997:21–60.
9. Wisner KL, Gelenberg AJ, Leonard H, Zarin D, Frank E. Pharmacologic treatment of depression during pregnancy. JAMA 1999; 282(13):1264–1269.
10. Cohen L, Goldstein J, Grush L, Impact of pregnancy on risk for relapse of major depressive disorder. Presented at the American Psychiatric Association Annual Meeting, New York, May 7, 1996.
11. Baldessarini R, Tondo L. Effects of lithium treatment in bipolar disorders and post-treatment-discontinuation reccurence risk. Clin Drug Invest 1998; 15:337–351.

12. Kupfer D, Frank E, Perel J, Cornes C, Mallinger A, Thase M, McEachran A, Grochocinski V. Five-year outcome for maintenance therapies in recurrent depression. Arch of Gen Psychiatry 1992; 49(10):769–773.

13. Klein M, Essex M. Pregnant or depressed? The effects of overlap between symptoms of depression and somatic complaints of pregnancy on rates of major depression in the second trimester. Depression 1995; 2:308–314.

14. Marzuk M, Tardiff K, Leon AC, Hirsch CS, Portera L, Hartwell N, Iqbal MI. Lower risk of suicide during pregnancy. Am J Psychiatry 1997; 154:122–123.

15. Appleby L. Suicide during pregnancy and in the first postnatal year. BMJ 1991; 302(6769):137–140.

16. Zuckerman BS, Amaro H, Bauchner H, et al. Depression during pregnancy: retionship to prior health behaviors. Am J Obstet Gynecol 1989; 160:1107–1111.

17. Orr S, Miller C. Maternal depressive symptoms and the risk of poor pregnancy outcome. Review of the literature and preliminary findings. Epidemiol Rev 1995; 17(1):165–171.

18. Orr ST, James SA, Blackmore Prince C. Maternal prenatal depressive symptoms and spontaneous preterm births among African-American women in Baltimore, Maryland. Am J Epidemiol 2002; 156(9):797–802.

19. Dayan J, Creveuil C, Herlicoviez M, et al. Role of anxiety and depression in the onset of spontaneous preterm labor. Am J Epidemiol 2002; 155:293–301.

20. Steer RA, Scholl TO, Hediger ML, Fischer RL. Self-reported depression and negative pregnancy outcomes. J Clin Epidemiol 1992; 45(10):1093–1099.

21. Zuckerman B, Bauchner H, Parker S, Cabral H. Maternal depressive symptoms during pregnancy, and newborn irritability. J Dev Behav Pediatr 1990; 11(4): 190–194.

22. Teixeira JM, Fisk NM, Glover V. Association between maternal anxiety in pregnancy and increased uterine artery resistance index: cohort based study. BMJ 1999; 318(7177):153–157.

23. Glover V. Maternal stress or anxiety in pregnancy and emotional development of the child. Br J Med 1997; 171:105–106.

24. Alves SE, Akbari HM, Anderson GM, Azmitia EC, McEwen BC, Strand FL. Neonatal ACTH administration elicits long-term changes in forebrain monoamine innervation. Subsequent disruptions in hypothalamic-pituitary-adrenal and gonadal function. Ann NY Acad Sci 1997; 814:226–251.

25. Murray L, Cooper P. Effects of postnatal depression on infant development. Arch Dis Child 1997; 77(2):99–101.

26. Murray L. The impact of postnatal depression on infant development. J Child Psychol Psychiatry 1992; 33:543–561.

27. Weinberg M, Tronick E. The impact of maternal psychiatric illness on infant development. J Clin Psychiatry 1998; 59(suppl 2):53–61.

28. O'Hara MW, Neunaber DJ, Zekoski EM. A prospective study of postpartum depression: prevalence, course, and predictive factors. J Abnorm Psychol 1984; 93:158.

29. Klerman GL, Weissman MM, Rounsaville BJ, et al. Interpersonal Psychotherapy of Depression. New York: Basic Books, 1984.

30. Spinelli M. Interpersonal psychotherapy for depressed antepartum women: A pilot study. Am J Psychiatry 1997; 154:1028–1030.

31. Pastuszak A, Schick-Boschetto B, Zuber C, Feldkamp M, Pinelli M, Sihn S, Donnenfeld A, McCormack M, Leen-Mitchell M, Woodland C, Gardner A, Horn M, Koren G. Pregnancy outcome following first-trimester exposure to fluoxetine (Prozac). JAMA 1993; 269(17):2246–2248.

32. Altshuler LL, Hendrick VC. Pregnancy and psychotropic medication: changes in blood levels. J Clin Psychopharmacol 1996; 16:78–80.

33. Chambers C, Johnson K, Dick L, Felix R, Jones KL. Birth outcomes in pregnant women taking fluoxetine. N Engl J Med 1996; 335(14):1010–1015.

34. Nulman I, Rovet J, Stewart D, Wolpin J, Gardner HA, Theis JG, Kulin N, Koren G. Neurodevelopment of children exposed in utero to antidepressant drugs. N Engl J Med 1997; 336:258–262.

35. Kulin N, Pastuszak A, Sage S, et al. Pregnancy outcome following maternal use of the new selective serotonin reuptake inhibitors: a prospective controlled multicenter study. JAMA 1998; 279:609–610.

36. Einarson A, Fatoye B, Sarkar M, Lavigne SV, Brochu J, Chambers C, Mastroiacovo P, Addis A, Matsui D, Schuler L, Einarson TR, Koren G. Pregnancy outcome following gestational exposure to venlafaxine: a multicenter prospective controlled study. Am J Psychiatry 2001; 158(10):1728–1730.

37. Fabro SE. Clinical Obstetrics. New York: Wiley, 1987.

38. Langman J. Human development-normal and abnormals. In: Langman J, ed. Medical Embryology. Baltimore: Williams & Wilkins, 1985:123.

39. Moore K, Persaud T. The Developing Human: Clinically Oriented Embryology. Philadelphia: Saunders, 1993.

40. Loebstein R, Koren G. Pregnancy outcome and neurodevelopment of children exposed in utero to psychoactive drugs: the Motherisk experience. J Psychiatry Neurosci 1997; 22(3):192–196.

41. McElhatton P, Garbis H, Elefant E, Vial T, Bellemin B, Mastroiacovo P, Arnon J, Rodriguez-Pinella E, Schaefer C, Pexieder T, Merlob P, Verme SD. The outcome of pregnancy in 689 women exposed to theraputic doses of antidepressants. A Collaborative Study of the European Network of Teratology Information Services (ENTIS). Reprod Toxicol 1996; 10(4):285–294.

42. Misri S, Sivertz K. Tricyclic drugs in pregnancy and lactation: A preliminary report. Int J Psychiatry Med 1991; 21(2):157–171.

43. Simon G, Korff MV, Heiligenstein J, Revicki D, Grothaus L, Katon W, Wagner E. Initial antidepressant choice in primary care. Effectivness and cost of fluoxetine vs. tricyclic antidepressants. JAMA 1996; 275(24):1897–1902.

44. Goldstein DJ. Effects of third trimester fluoxetine exposure on the newborn. J Clin Psychopharmacol 1995; 15(6):417–420.

45. Nulman I, Koren G. The safety of fluoxetine during pregnancy and lactation. Teratology 1996; 53:304–308.

46. Simon GE, Cunningham ML, Davis RL. Outcomes of prenatal antidepressant exposure. Am J Psychiatry 2002; 159(12):2055–2061.

47. Cohen LS, Rosenbaum JF. Fluoxetine in pregnancy (letter). N Engl J Med 1997; 336(12):872.

48. Robert E. Treatment depression in pregnancy. N Engl J Med 1996; 335(14): 1056–1058.

49. Ericson A, Kallen B, Wiholm B. Delivery outcome after the use of antidepressants in early pregnancy. Eur J Clin Pharmacol 1999; 55(7):503–508.

50. Inman W, Kobotu K, Pearce G, et al. Prescription event monitoring of paroxetine. PEM Rep 1993; PXL 1206:1-44.

51. Addis A, Impicciatore P, Miglio D, Colombo F, Bonati M. Drug use in pregnancy and lactation: the work of a regional drug information center. Ann Pharmacother 1995; 29:632–633.

52. Wisner K, Perel J, Wheeler S. Tricyclic dose requirements across pregnancy. Am J Psychiatry 1993; 150:1541–1542.

53. Shepard T. Catalog of Teratogenic Agents. Baltimore: Johns Hopkins University Press, 1989.

54. Heinonen O, Sloan D, Shapiro S. Birth Defects and Drugs in Pregnancy. Littleton, MA: Publishing Services Group, 1977.

55. Cowe L, Lloyd D, Dawling S. Neonatal convulsions caused by withdrawal from maternal clomipramine. BMJ 1982; 284:1837–1838.

56. Eggermont E. Withdrawal symptoms in neonates associated with maternal imipramine therapy. Lancet 1973; 2:680.

57. Schimmel M, Katz E, Shaag Y, Pastuszak A, Koren G. Toxic neonatal effects following maternal clomipramine therapy. Clin Toxicol 1991; 29:479–484.

58. Webster PAC. Withdrawal symptoms in neonates associated with maternal antidepressant therapy. Lancet 1973; 2:318–319.

59. Bromiker R, Kaplan M. Apparent intrauterine fetal withdrawal from clomipramine hydrochloride. JAMA 1994; 272(22):1722–1723.

60. Falterman LG, Richardson DJ. Small left colon syndrome associated with maternal ingestion of psychotropics. J Pediatr 1980; 97:300–310.

61. Shearer WT, Schreiner RL, Marshall RE. Urinary retention in a neonate secondary to maternal ingestion of nortriptyline. J Pediatr 1972; 81:570–572.

62. Spencer M. Fluoxetine hydrochloride (Prozac) toxicity in the neonate. Pediatrics 1993; 92:721–722.

63. Goldstein DJ. Effects of third trimester fluoxetine exposure on the newborn. Clin Psychopharmacol 1995; 15:417–420.

64. Cohen LS, Heller VL, Bailey JW, Grush L, Ablon JS, Bouffard SM. Birth outcomes following prenatal exposure to fluoxetine. Biol Psychiatry 2000; 48(10): 996–1000.

65. Nulman I, Rovet J, Stewart DE, Wolpin, J, Pace-Asciak P, Shuhaiber S, Koren G. Child development following exposure to tricyclic antidepressants or fluoxetine throughout fetal life: a prospective, controlled study. Am J Psychiatry 2002; 159(11):1889–1895.

66. Stiskal JA, Kulin N, Koren G, Ho T, Ito S. Neonatal paroxetine withdrawal syndrome. Arch Dis Child Fetal Neonatal Ed 2001; 84(2):F134–F135.

67. Costei AM, Kozer E, Ho T, Ito S, Koren G. Perinatal outcome following third trimester exposure to paroxetine. Arch Pediatr Adolesc Med 2002; 156(11): 1129–1132.

68. Dahl M, al e. Paroxetine withdrawl syndrome in a neonate (letter). Br J Psych 1997; 171:391–392.
69. Nordeng H, Lindemann R, Perminov KV, Reikvam A. Neonatal withdrawal syndrome after in utero exposure to selective serotonin reuptake inhibitors. Acta Paediatr 2001; 90(3):288–291.
70. Ali S, Buelkesam J, Newport L. Early neurobehavioral and neurochemical alterations in rats prenatally exposed to imipramine. Neurotoxicology 1986; 7:365–380.
71. Vorhees C, Brunner R, Butcher R. Psychotropic drugs as behavioral teratogens. Science 1979; 205:1220–1225.
72. Vernadakis A, Parker K. Drugs and the developing central nervous system. Pharmacol Ther 1980; 11:593–647.
73. Keller MB, Lavori PW, Lewis C, Klerman GL. Predictors of relapse in major depressive disorder. JAMA 1983; 250:3299–3309.
74. Mueller TI, Leon AC, Keller MB, Solomon DA, Endicott J, Coryell W, Warshaw M, Maser JD. Recurrence after recovery from major depressive disorder during 15 years of observational follow-up. Am J Psychiatry 1999; 156(7):1000–1006.
75. Post R. Transduction of psychosocial stress into the neurobiology of recurrent affective disorder. Am J Psychiatry 1992; 149:999–1010.
76. Beck AT, Rush AJ, Shaw BF, Emery G. Cognitive Therapy of Depression. New York: Guilford Press, 1979.
77. Jeffries WS, Bochner F. The effect of pregnancy on drug pharmacokinetics. Med J Aust 1988; 149:675–677.
78. Krauer B. Pharmacotherapy during pregnancy: emphasis on pharmacokinetics. In: Eskes TKAB, Finster M, eds. Drug Therapy During Pregnancy. London: Butterworths, 1985:9–31.
79. Hostetter A, Stowe ZN, Strader JR Jr, McLaughlin E, Llewellyn A. Dose of selective serotonin uptake inhibitors across pregnancy: clinical implications. Depress Anxiety 2000; 11(2):51–57.
80. Ferrill MJ, Kehoe WA, Jacisin JJ. ECT during pregnancy: physiologic and pharmacologic considerations. Convul Ther 1992; 8(3):186–200.
81. Miller LJ. Use of electroconvulsive therapy during pregnancy. Hosp Commun Psychiatry 1994; 45(5):444–450.

14

Approaches to the Treatment of Chronic Late-Life Depression

William J. Apfeldorf
University of New Mexico School of Medicine
Albuquerque, New Mexico, U.S.A.

George S. Alexopoulos
Cornell Institute of Geriatric Psychiatry
Joan and Sanford I. Weill Medical College of Cornell University
White Plains, New York, U.S.A.

INTRODUCTION

Geriatric depressive disorders are health problems with important medical, social, and financial consequences. Geriatric depression causes suffering to patients and their families, exacerbates medical illnesses, and contributes to disability that requires expensive support systems. Although the prevalence of depression does not appear to increase with age (Regier et al., 1988), the highest rates of suicide have been found in men aged 75 years and older (Conwell and Brent, 1995): Psychological autopsy studies of suicides in late life have found that most older suicide victims suffered from a psychiatric illness, usually late-onset depression and that most methods of suicide were violent.

Depression in late life often follows a relapsing and chronic course (Alexopoulos and Chester, 1992; Callahan et al., 1994; Cole and Bellavance,

1997). Hence, approaches to treatment must include efforts for minimization of relapse, recurrence, and residual symptoms. Treating clinicians need to take a long-term view of the illness and its management, and to educate their patients accordingly if effective preventive treatment strategies are to be implemented and accepted by patients and their families. Over the past decade, much has been learned about how to treat illness episodes and prevent relapse, recurrence, and chronicity in geriatric depression, especially in recurrent unipolar depression, but little is known about primary prevention of depression in later life. In this chapter, we present (1) characterization of chronic geriatric depression and subtypes, (2) a public health rationale for intervening in the depression in old age, (3) which patients may benefit from long-term or maintenance treatment, and (4) the evidence base for clinical decision-making and recommendations about the use of specific agents.

Diagnostic Difficulties in Late-Life Depression

Current diagnostic criteria for psychiatric disorders are codified in *Diagnostic and Statistical Manual for Mental Disorders*, 4th ed–TR (American Psychiatric Association, 2000), based on epidemiological and field trials across age groups. However, diagnosis of psychiatric disorders in the elderly is complicated by several factors. First, the experience and expression of psychiatric symptoms are a function of age. Second, the criteria for psychiatric diagnosis must be applied age appropriately. Third, the presence of multiple comorbid conditions is the rule rather than the exception in geriatric patients. The signs and symptoms of psychiatric disorders may overlap with signs or symptoms of many medical illnesses and may complicate diagnostic assessments. Medical and neurological disorders may result in persistent psychiatric syndromes that will remit only when the underlying medical disorders are addressed. Fourth, psychiatric disorders may have a late onset, so clinicians cannot be guided by previous history. Fifth, elderly patients underreport psychological symptoms or ascribe symptoms to other somatic concerns. Finally, there are currently no biological gold standard assessments or markers generally accepted for geriatric psychiatric disorders. To overcome these factors, clinicians may use the reports of family informants or caregivers to supplement information provided by the patient. In addition, the adoption of an inclusive approach allows consideration and treatment of psychiatric disorders while a search for medical or neurological disorders is conducted.

Subtypes of Chronic Late-Life Depression

No single mechanism uniformly explains the development of late-life depression. It is becoming apparent that there are many subtypes of chronic late-life depression, and the differentiation of which subtype afflicts an individual may have future bearing on illness course and treatment.

Late-Onset Depression

Geriatric depression with onset of the first episode in late life (late-onset) is a heterogeneous entity that includes a large subgroup of patients who develop depression as part of a medical or neurological disorder that may or may not be clinically evident when the depression first appears. Compared to patients who first experienced depression in early or midlife (early-onset), those with late-onset depression have a higher frequency of neuropsychological (Alexopoulos et al., 1993) and neuroradiological abnormalities (Krishnan, 1993), higher level of disability, and lower familial prevalence of affective disorders (Jacoby and Levy 1980; Coffey et al., 1988; Alexopoulos, 1990; Alexopolous et al., 1992, 1993, 1996).

Vascular Depression

Cerebrovascular disease is frequent in elderly depressives. Post noted a high incidence of cerebrovascular disease in elderly depressed patients and suggested that the resultant brain damage predisposes late-life depression (Post and Schulman, 1985). Depression is highly prevalent in patients with hypertension (Rabkin et al., 1983), coronary artery disease (Carney et al., 1987), and vascular dementia (Sulzer et al., 1993). Depression is a frequent complication of stroke (Folstein et al., 1971; Robinson et al., 1984; Robinson and Spiker, 1985; Starkstein et al., 1988; Ebrahim et al., 1987). "Silent" cerebral infarction was observed in 94% of patients with onset of first depressive episode after 65 years of age (Fujikawa et al., 1993). On imaging, late-onset depressives exhibit white matter hyperintensities more frequently than non-depressed matched subjects (Krishnan et al., 1988, Coffey et al., 1989, Krishnan, 1993). Patients with vascular depression appear to have greater difficulty with initiation and perseveration, less insight, and less agitation and guilt than comparison depressed patients without vascular risk factors (Alexopoulos et al., 1997). The concept of vascular depression provides new avenues for studies that can determine if drugs used in the prevention and treatment of cerebrovascular disease can reduce the risk for depression in patients with vascular risk factors or reduce chronicity, recurrence, cognitive impairment, and disability. Moreover, the long-term efficacy of specific antidepressants can be investigated in depressed patients at risk for new vascular lesions, since animal studies suggests that some antidepressants, but not others, promote recovery after ischemic brain lesions.

Depression with "Pseudodementia"

Geriatric depression with reversible dementia, the syndrome usually called pseudodementia, as a rule is a severe depression accompanied by a mild reversible dementia syndrome. Depressed elderly patients with pseudo-dementia often have a late onset and a severe depressive syndrome characterized by psychomotor retardation and delusions (Alexopoulos et al., 1993). Although the dementia syndrome initially subsides after effective antidepressant treatment, in the long run, a high percentage of these patients develop irreversible dementia. With the advent of new pharmacological treatments for dementia syndromes, it remains to be studied whether the identification of pseudodementia provides an early opportunity to intervene pharmacologically and improve the course of the underlying dementing illness.

Depression-Executive Dysfunction Syndrome

Clinical, structural, and functional neuroimaging, and neuropathological studies suggest that frontostriatal dysfunction contributes to the pathogenesis of at least some late-life depressive syndromes. Based on these findings, the "depression-executive dysfunction" syndrome has been described and conceptualized as an entity with pronounced frontostriatal dysfunction (Alexopoulos, 2001). On a clinical level, the syndrome is characterized by psychomotor retardation, reduced interest in activities, suspiciousness, impaired instrumental activities of daily living, and limited vegetative symptoms. The clinical significance of identifying the depression-executive dysfunction syndrome of late life is that emerging evidence suggests that the syndrome has a poor or slow and unstable response to classic antidepressants (Kalayam and Alexopoulos 1999; Alexopoulos et al., 2000).

Mood Disorder Secondary to Other Medical Conditions

In elderly persons, medical and neurological illnesses may predispose to or even cause depression. Drugs, medical illnesses, and dementing disorders may lead to depression. Steroids, reserpine, methyldopa, anti-Parkinsonian drugs, and β-blockers can cause depression. Viral infections, endocrinopathies such as thyroid or parathyroid abnormalities, and malignancies, such as lymphoma or pancreatic cancer, often are complicated by depression. Although it is essential to diagnose and treat the underlying disease, depression may not remit until an antidepressant agent is used. Depression is especially common in patients with neurological brain diseases. Approximately 30–60% of stroke patients experience depression within 24 months after the stroke (Astrom et al., 1993). In Alzheimer's patients, major depression occurs in approximately 15% of patients and less severe depressive syndromes in 40–50% of patients (Wragg and Jeste, 1989).

PUBLIC HEALTH RATIONALE FOR INTERVENING IN CHRONIC GERIATRIC DEPRESSION

Within the United States, the number of persons aged 65 years and older will reach 13.3% of the estimated 298 million total by the year 2010 and the number of persons age 85 and older will be 1.91% (Malmgren, 1994). The prevalence of depression in community-residing elderly is between 1 and 3%; prevalence rates are higher in healthcare settings, with approximately 10% of elderly patients in primary care settings and 15% in acute care or nursing care facilities being clinically depressed (for review, see Mulsant and Ganguli, 1999). In addition to being a prevalent illness, depression in old age also has serious health consequences. For example, in a nursing home population, major depressive disorder increased the likelihood of death by 59% over 1 year independent of physical health (Rovner et al., 1991). In cardiac patients, depression increased by fivefold the risk of mortality 6 months after myocardial infarction (Frasure-Smith et al., 1993). The Medical Outcomes Study found that depression was almost as debilitating as advanced coronary artery disease (Wells and Burnam, 1991); of particular importance to geriatric populations, the effects of medical illness and depression on functioning are additive (Wells et al., 1989). The World Health Organization in collaboration with the World Bank and the Harvard School of Public Health developed a measure for years lived with disability (YLD) (WHO, 1996): YLD is derived from a calculation taking into consideration the incidence of a disorder, the average age of onset, the average duration of disability, and the severity weight of the condition. Unipolar depression has been found to be the leading cause of YLD worldwide and alone is responsible for more than one in every 10 years of life lived with disability worldwide. The Disability Adjusted Life Year (DALY) is a single measure of disease burden and expresses years of life lost to premature death and years lived with disability of specified severity and duration: One DALY is 1 lost year of healthy life. By this measure, major depression alone ranked second only to ischemic heart disease in magnitude of disease burden in established market economies, such as the United States (Murray and Lopez, 1996). Depression was found to be the fourth among the leading causes of disease burden (DALY) worldwide.

Depression is a chronic illness with relapses and recurrences: the term relapse denotes the reappearance of full syndromal depression within 6 months of remission of the index episode; and the term recurrence denotes the reappearance of depression beyond 6 months from the end of the index episode. In a large observational study of depressed patients, a cumulative recurrence rate of 85% was noted, with the majority of patients suffering a recurrence within 5 years (Mueller et al., 1999). Although most studies of recurrence risk have been conducted in midlife patients, available data in the elderly suggest that elderly patients have similar rates of recurrence; however, the time between episodes is shorter, with most relapses and recurrences occurring within 2 years (Zis et al., 1980; Georgotas and McCue, 1989; Reynolds et al., 1999). These observations highlight the importance of keeping patients well following the acute treatment of a depressive episode via continuation and maintenance therapy. The primary goal of continuation therapy is to prevent relapse and of maintenance therapy to prevent recurrence and to prolong recovery. As will be discussed below, maintenance treatment extends to 3 years in one controlled clinical trial (Reynolds et al., 1999) and to four years in one open pharmacotherapy trial (Flint and Rifat, 2000).

These data have led to the conclusion that within the clinical context of old-age depression are vulnerabilities to relapse, recurrence, and chronicity. In particular, the coexistence of depression in later life with chronic medical illnesses may represent a vulnerability to relapse and chronicity. The disability of chronic medical illnesses sets the stage for demoralization and depression; conversely, depression itself can and does amplify the disability of coexisting medical illnesses (for review, see Lenze et al., 2001). Advanced age, female gender, medical burden, severity of depression, and cognitive dysfunction predict disability (Alexopoulos et al., 1996). Further, the co-occurrence of depression in older adults with multiple personal losses and bereavement (Reynolds et al., 1999) to chronic insomnia (Ford and Kamerow, 1989), with risk factors of cerebrovascular disease and to neuro-degenerative disorders like Alzheimer's disease and Parkinson's disease (Alexopoulos et al., 1997), with progressive depletion of psychosocial resources (Dew et al., 1997), and with limited access to adequate treatment (Harman and Reynolds, 2000) may contribute to a relapsing, chronic illness course.

As noted above, studies by the World Health Organization have shown that unipolar major depression and suicide are currently the fourth most important contributors to the global burden of illness-related disability (WHO, 1996). Because illness burden contributors attributable to depression increase with age, depression is projected to become an even more important source of illness-related disability over the next decade, especially in the developed economies, where an increasing proportion of the population is elderly. Thus, employing treatments that prevent relapse and recurrence, and that reduce residual symptoms of depression and anxiety, are extremely important to diminishing depression's contribution to the global burden of disease.

TREATMENT CONSIDERATIONS

Goals of Treatment

The main goals of treatment for geriatric depression include (1) full remission of depression and (2) reduction in the risk of relapse and recurrence. Older patients can benefit from the same psychopharmacological agents as younger patients. However, the clinician must be aware that aging and medical conditions associated with aging can have an impact on pharmacokinetics and can increase the sensitivity to side effects even at low plasma concentrations of antidepressants. Aging-induced changes in hepatic metabolism prolong the clearance of many psychopharmacological agents in older people, thus increasing the likelihood that drugs and their active metabolites will accumulate and cause toxicity (Catterson et al., 1997).

There is currently a paucity of research studies guiding the selection of one type of antidepressant over another, and the choice is often made based on the drug's side effect profile and the potential for drug-drug interactions. The sensitivity of geriatric patients to interventions may lead to treatment complications or undertreatment. Compliance with a prescribed regimen is often problematic in geriatric patients struggling with comorbid conditions which both impair their ability to maintain adherence and require attention: It is estimated that 70% of elderly patients fail to take 25–50% of their medications as prescribed (Perel, 1994). Minimizing polypharmacy aids in preventing drug-drug interactions, iatrogenic illness, and compliance difficulties.

An orderly approach to the design of successive treatment trials is essential. When failure to respond to a specific treatment occurs, information is gained to guide the selection of the next intervention. Patients and their families benefit from education and participation in the treatment decision process. Sharing responsibility with patients and families for important treatment decisions may reduce the risk of undertreatment, improve compliance, provide relief to a family system stressed by the presence of a psychiatric disorder, and assist the patient and caregivers in monitoring the effects of treatments. Since geriatric psychiatric disorders often lead to permanent disability, undertreatment may have severe consequences.

Initial Treatment Strategies and Medication Selection

The 2001 report *Expert Consensus Guideline Series: Pharmacotherapy of Depressive Disorders in Older Patients* (Alexopoulos et al., 2001) provides practice guidelines developed to answer clinical questions that are not adequately or definitively answered by currently available research literature.

For severe unipolar nonpsychotic major depressive disorder, the guidelines recommend combining antidepressant medication and psychotherapy as the treatment of choice, with medication alone as an alternate first-line strategy. Electroconvulsive therapy (ECT) is an alternative treatment for severe depression for patients who have failed to respond to multiple adequate trials of antidepressants, who are at acute suicidal risk, or whose medical status precludes adequate medication trials. For unipolar psychotic major depressive disorder, the guidelines recommend either a combination of antidepressant and antipsychotic medications or ECT. For persistent dysthymic disorder or minor depressive disorder, the guidelines recommend beginning with antidepressant medications in combination with psychotherapy, but also consider medication alone or psychotherapy alone as acceptable alternatives.

The current recommended first-line therapy for depression in later life is a selective serotonin reuptake inhibitor (SSRIs), because, in comparison to tricyclic antidepressants (TCAs) like nortriptyline, SSRIs are safer in regard to overdose, better tolerated, and do not require blood level monitoring or electrocardiographic (EKG) analysis prior to initiation of therapy (for review, see Dunner, 1994; Menting et al., 1996; Montgomery, 1998; Montgomery and Kasper, 1998). Although multiple clinical trials have found similar efficacy between SSRIs and TCAs in the acute treatment of geriatric depression, with SSRIs being better tolerated (for review, see Schneider, 1999), their comparability during continuation and maintenance treatment in preventing relapse and recurrence of depression in the elderly has to date received relatively little attention. An open-trial study has recently reported similar rates of relapse for paroxetine and nortriptyline: 16 vs 10%, respectively, during an open 18-month follow-up study in the elderly (Bump et al, 2001). However, the investigators also observed a lower burden of residual depressive symptoms during continuation and maintenance treatment with nortriptyline. These data suggest that paroxetine and nortriptyline have similar efficacy in relapse and recurrence prevention in elderly depressed patients over an 18-month period but also raise the possibility that nortriptyline may do a better job in reducing residual symptoms. These findings are also relevant to current discussions of the cost of antidepressants. On the one hand, cost differential would favor the use of less expensive agents like nortriptyline over paroxetine if relapse and drop out rates are equivalent; on the other, the greater safety of SSRI agents like paroxetine, especially in very old patients, represents a compelling argument for their use in this population.

The Consensus Guidelines consider the SSRIs as the medications of choice for treating depression in older patients (Alexopoulos et al., 2001), and venlafaxine XR is another first-line option. High second-line alternatives are buproprion and mirtazapine. Tricyclic antidepressants (nortriptyline and desipramine) are also effective agents. The SSRIs have a better side effect

TABLE 1 Adequate Dose of Antidepressants for Late Life Chronic Depression

Antidepressant	Average daily target dose after 6 weeks of treatment (mg)
Citalopram	20–30
Paroxetine	20–30
Fluoxetine	20–30
Sertraline	100
Venlafaxine	150
Bupropion	200–300
Mirtazapine	30
Nefazodone	200–300

and safety profile. The guidelines also recommend avoiding the following antidepressants in older patients: amitriptyline, amoxapine, doxepin, imipramine, isocarboxazid, maprotiline, tranylcypromine, and trazodone. The guidelines recommend the use of atypical antipsychotics for the treatment of psychotic depression, which are preferred to the use of clozapine or conventional antipsychotics. In evaluating psychosocial interventions for the older depressed patient, the guidelines consider cognitive-behavior therapy, interpersonal therapy, problem-solving therapy, and supportive psychotherapy first line in efficacy and acceptability.

The current recommendations include beginning with lower doses of the various antidepressants than currently used in younger patients, and tend to avoid extremely high doses (Table 1).The guidelines also suggest that if an older patient is having an inadequate response to initial treatment, a change in the treatment regimen is indicated after 2–4 weeks if there is little or no response and 3–5 weeks if there is a partial response (Table 2). These

TABLE 2 Duration of Adequate Antidepressant Trial Before Changing Treatment Regimen for an Older Patient Who Is Having Inadequate Response to Initial Treatment

No Response:
 Minimum: 2.0–3.5 weeks
 Maximum: 4–6 weeks

Partial Response:
 Minimum: 3–4 weeks
 Maximum: 5–7.5 weeks

are shorter trials than recommended by the Agency for Healthcare Policy and Research (AHPR) guidelines for the treatment of depression in mixed-age adults.

Continuation and Maintenance Treatment

Depression is a relapsing and remitting illness; 50–80% of patients who have had one depressive episode can expect a recurrence. The recurrence rate increases with each successive episode. In mixed-age unipolar depressives, 34% of patients have a depressive episode during the year after recovery (Keller et al., 1983, 1984), with the relapse (within 6 months from recovery) rate being higher during the months immediately after recovery. The figures for relapse/recurrence in major depression (15–19%) in geriatric patients (Alexopoulos et al., 1989) are comparable to those of mixed-age populations (21%; Keller et al., 1983, 1984). In mixed-age populations, a history of three or more previous depressive episodes and late age of depression onset are the strongest predictors of relapse/recurrence (Keller et al., 1983, 1984). In geriatric populations, most studies suggest that the likelihood of relapse is increased in patients with a history of frequent episodes, intercurrent medical illnesses, and possibly high severity of depression (Georgatas et al., 1988, 1989; Alexopoulos et al., 1989). Once recovery is achieved, continuation treatment should be administered for at least 6 months with the same dosages of the antidepressant that were used during the acute treatment. Failure to provide continuation treatment results in relapse in 30–35% of cases.

Current practice also recommends long-term treatment of elderly patients with a history of frequent and/or multiple episodes of major depression, those who have a major depressive episode plus preexisting dysthymia, those with onset of major depression after the age of 60 years, those with long duration of individual episodes, with severe index episodes, with poor symptom control during continuation therapy, and those with comorbid anxiety disorders or substance abuse. The rationale for this recommendation is based primarily upon knowledge about the natural illness course of depression in later life, especially when complicated by psychiatric comorbidity. Patients with multiple prior episodes are at very high risk for recurrence, and the interepisode wellness interval and risk for nonresponse or chronicity increases with each succeeding episode. A proportion of patients with recurrence may fail to respond to reinitiation of treatment with the agent that induced remission: 10% of patients with a recurrence of major depression failed to respond to nortriptyline even though their index episodes had remitted with this agent (Reynolds et al., 1994). With each succeeding episode, there appears to be an increased risk for nonresponse and chronicity. Even patients whose first episodes of major depression occur at age 60 years or later appear to be at substantial risk for relapse and recurrence (Georgatas et al., 1988). Similarly, patients with prolonged index episodes, those who take longer to respond, and those who have residual symptoms of anxiety are all at high risk for recurrence (Flint and Rifat, 2000; Dew et al., 2001) and thus would benefit from maintenance treatment.

It is estimated that 70% of patients fail to take 20–25% of the dosages of their medications. Older patients and their families may not understand the importance of taking medications as prescribed. Concurrent medical illnesses can interfere with antidepressant response or attainment of adequate dosages. Alcoholism and other substance abuse may undercut pharmacotherapy. Difficulties accessing healthcare may hinder the ability of elderly, especially functionally impaired elderly, to obtain adequate treatment.

Choosing Continuation and Maintenance Treatment

The National Institutes of Health (NIH) consensus panel of the diagnosis and treatment of depression in later life recommended that depressed geriatric patients be continued on antidepressant medication for at least 6 months for first episodes of depression and maintained at least 1 year for recurrent depressive episodes (Lebowitz et al., 1997). Given concerns about high rates of relapse and recurrence, many investigators have advocated up to 2 years of maintenance antidepressant medication in the elderly (OADIG, 1993). The Consensus Guidelines (Alexopolous et al., 2001) recommend a variable duration of continuation and maintenance treatment, which is determined by the number of lifetime depressive episodes (Table 3).

Naturalistic studies of treatment intensity in later life have indicated that psychiatrists decrease the dose of pharmacotherapy even before patients

TABLE 3 Duration of Continuation/Maintenance Treatment for an Older Patient with a History of Severe Unipolar Depression

Number of depressive episodes (lifetime)	Duration of continuation/maintenance
One episode	1 year
Two episodes	2 years
Three episodes	> 3 years

The duration of continuation/maintenance treatment for demented patients should be similar to that of nondemented elderly patients.
[a]Consensus was only reached on treatment following for three prior episodes.

have completely responded (Alexopoulos et al., 1996). However, doses of antidepressant medication used during acute therapy are appropriate for use during long-term or maintenance treatment; that is, the dose that gets patients well is also the most likely to keep them well. In a randomized, doubled-blind study of full-dose versus half-dose maintenance nortriptyline, Reynolds and colleagues (1999) observed that half-dose nortriptyline (associated with plasma steady-state levels of 40–60 ng/mL) was associated with higher residual levels of depressive symptoms and more frequent minor depressive episodes than the use of full-dose nortriptyline (associated with plasma steady-state levels of 80–120 ng/mL). Therefore, for continuation and maintenance treatment, the Consensus Guidelines (Alexopolos et al., 2001) recommend using the dosages found effective during acute treatment.

Not all elderly depressed patients require antidepressant medication to remain well. Patients whose depressions are initially less severe (as indicated by Hamilton-17 depression ratings of less than 20) and who show a rapid resolution of depressive symptoms (i.e., within 6 weeks) may be able to remain well and depression free for at least 3 years with the use of monthly maintenance interpersonal psychotherapy (Reynolds et al., 1997; Dew et al., 2001). Interpersonal psychotherapy focuses on grief, role disputes, role transitions, and interpersonal deficits (Klerman et al., 1984); this form of treatment may be especially meaningful for elderly people facing multiple losses, role changes, social isolation, and helplessness associated with late-life depression.

Other psychosocial interventions that may be useful in treating geriatric depression or residual symptoms include problem-solving therapy or cognitive-behavior therapy (Klausner and Alexopoulos, 1999). Problem-solving therapy postulates that deficiencies in social problem-solving skills enhance the risk for depression. Through improving problem-solving skills, the elderly are given the tools to enable them to cope with stressors and thereby experience fewer symptoms of psychopathology (Hawton and Kirk, 1989). Problem-solving therapy was better able to reduce symptoms of depression in older patients when compared to reminiscence therapy or placement on a waiting list (Arean et al., 1993). Cognitive-behavior therapy is designed to modify automatic thought and action patterns, improve skills, and alter the emotional states that contribute to the onset and perpetuation of depression (Gallagher-Thompson et al., 1990). Group psychotherapies have demonstrated efficacy in the treatment of elderly depressives with partial response to prior treatment (Klausner et al., 1998).

Evaluating Efficacy of Treatment

In evaluating whether an intervention is successful, it is necessary to determine whether depressive symptoms have remitted, minimize the burden of any residual depressive symptoms, and minimize the likelihood of relapse. Continuing full-dose nortriptyline (i.e., doses used during acute treatment to produce steady-state levels of 80–120 ng/mL) for 16 weeks after remission of the index episode of major depression is associated with continuing improvement, or resolution, of residual depressive symptoms and improvement in scores of overall functioning (Opdyke et al., 1997). However, minor depressive episodes or brief mild elevations in depression ratings are common during this period, underscoring the need for continuing therapy to stabilize remission and to prevent relapse. In addition, residual symptoms of anxiety or sleep disturbance during this period may signify incomplete remission and increased hazard for relapse or recurrence (Reynolds et al., 1997; Flint and Rifat, 2000).

Special Treatment Issues

Combination Regimens

Combinations of antidepressant drugs have been used to improve the response of partially remitted geriatric depression. Lithium may augment tricyclic antidepressant response in elderly patients (Salzman, 1994). The dose of lithium required by depressed elderly patients receiving tricyclics may be one-third to one-half that of younger adults. In younger depressives, combinations of tricyclics with SSRIs have led to an antidepressant response sooner than tricyclics alone. Other augmentation techniques include combinations of antidepressants with thyroid hormones, psychostimulants, antidepressants with different mechanisms of action, pindolol, and other agents (Sussman and Joffe, 1998). Clinical experience suggests that augmentation techniques can be effective in some depressed geriatric patients with incomplete response to a single antidepressant agent. However, systematic studies of such combinations are lacking in the elderly.

Treatment of Psychotic Depression

Psychotic depression is rather frequent in the elderly population. It occurs in 3.6% of elderly depressives living in the community (Kivel and Pahkala, 1989) and in 20–45% of hospitalized elderly depressives (Meyers, 1992). Psychotic depression is a severe illness with profound depressive symptomatology accompanied by delusions and less frequently by hallucinations. Delusions occur in successive episodes of geriatric depression if the severity of episodes is high (Baldwin, 1988; Sands and Harrow, 1994). However, in geriatric patients, psychotic depression is not merely a consequence of high severity of depression, since high percentages of severely depressed elderly patients do not develop delusions (Baldwin, 1988; Sands and Harrow, 1994). Psychotic depression is associated with a risk for suicide (Roose et al., 1983), usually with violent means (Isometsa et al., 1994). For this reason, it is crucial to diagnose and treat psychotic depression.

The need for special treatment makes it crucial to diagnose psychotic depression. It often is difficult to distinguish depressive delusions from overvalued ideas of worthlessness and hopelessness. Nondelusional depressed patients, as a rule, are able to recognize the exaggerated nature of their overvalued ideas, although they are unable to stop being preoccupied with them. Depressive delusions can be distinguished from delusions of demented patients in that the latter are less systematized and less congruent to the affective disturbance (Greenwald et al., 1989). In contrast, depressive delusions usually are organized ideas of hypochondriasis, nihilism, guilt, persecution, or jealousy.

Threats to Adequate Treatment

The most frequent errors in clinical practice include underdosing, discontinuing treatment too soon, and not aiming for full remission and recovery; that is, settling for partial response. Additional threats to adequate treatment include the need for more than drug therapy (e.g., psychotherapy), as well as the need for more than one drug, to achieve and maintain wellness. Approximately one in five elderly depressed patients do not respond satisfactorily to a combination of antidepressant medication and psychotherapy (Little et al., 1998). About half of the treated patients also require the use of an adjunctive antidepressant or mood-stabilizing medication to achieve remission. If the adjunctive medication is discontinued and the patient is allowed to remain only on the primary antidepressant agent as continuation therapy, a substantial proportion of such patients will relapse relatively quickly (Reynolds et al., 1997). Thus, if adjunctive medication is needed to bring about remission, its continued use may be necessary to preserve remission and to ensure prolonged recovery in the elderly. Longer time to response and higher anxiety scores at the time of response have been shown to place patients at higher risk for recurrence (Flint and Rifat, 2000; Dew et al., 2001). Hence, such patients need careful surveillance.

The treatment of depression in old age takes place primarily in the general medical sector and not in the specialty mental health sector. Both the recognition and treatment of depression in elderly patients attending primary care clinics remains inadequate in the United States (Reynolds and Kupfer, 1999; Harman and Reynolds, 2000). A recent report from a multisite trial of paroxetine and problem-solving therapy for dysthymia and minor depression in 312 older patients (mean age 71 years) in primary care provides provocative data on the utility of treatment approaches but also the barriers to incorporating mental health care within primary care settings. (Williams et al., 2000). Currently, there are three ongoing multisite studies to provide services to older persons with psychiatric problems with mental health problems in primary care settings: (1) Improving Treatment of Late-Life Depression in Primary Care funded by the John A. Hartford and the California HealthCare Foundation; (2) Primary Care Research in Substance Abuse and Mental Health for Elders Study (PRISMe) funded by the Substance Abuse and Mental Health Services Administration; and (3) Prevention of Suicide in Primary Care Elderly Collaborative Trial (PROSPECT) funded by the National Institute of Mental Health. These models of care, which use different schema to incorporate effective treatments of depression as integral components of primary care services, show suggestive preliminary evidence that they are effective. However, incentives need to change in order to introduce these models of care into the primary care physician's office.

CONCLUSION

The treatment of geriatric patients with chronic depression presents the clinician with challenges and opportunities. Untreated geriatric psychiatric syndromes carry significant morbidity and mortality, and can also adversely impact on families and caregivers. Difficulties in recognizing psychiatric symptoms, medical and psychiatric comorbidity, altered pharmacokinetics, and sensitivity to side effects may complicate the treatment of the elderly. With advances in our knowledge of geriatric depression subtypes and the availability of studies investigation specific antidepressants in the elderly, antidepressant selection may be guided by the patient's specific clinical symptoms and comorbidity. Future directions for research and investigation include the development of interventions to prevent or abort the development of geriatric chronic depression.

REFERENCES

Alexopoulos GS (1990). Clinical and biological findings in late-onset depression. In: Tasman A, Goldfinger SM, Kaufman CA, eds. Review of Psychiatry. Vol 9. Washington, DC: American Psychiatric Press, pp 249–262.

Alexopoulos GS, Chester JG (1992). Outcomes of geriatric depression. Clin Geriatr Med 8:363–376.

Alexopoulos GS, Young RC, Abrams RC, et al. (1989). Chronicity and relapse in geriatric depression. Biol Psychiatry 26:551–564.

Alexopoulos GS, Young RC, Meyers BS (1991). Outcome of geriatric delusional depression (abst). American Psychiatric Association, Annual Meeting, New Orleans.

Alexopoulos GS, Young RC, Shindledecker R (1992). Brain computed tomography in geriatric depression and primary degenerative dementia. Biol Psychiatry 31:591–599.

Alexopoulos GS, Young RC, Meyers BS (1993). Geriatric depression: age of onset and dementia. Biol Psychiatry 34:141–145.

Alexopoulos GS, Meyers BS, Young RC, et al. (1996a). Recovery in geriatric depression. Arch Gen Psychiatry 53:305–312.

Alexopoulos GS, Vrontou C, Kakuma T, et al. (1996b). Disability in geriatric depression. Am J Psychiatry 153:877–885.

Alexopoulos GS, Meyers BS, Young RC, et al. (1997). Clinically defined vascular depression. Am J Psychiatry 154:562–565.

Alexopoulos GS, Meyers BS, Young RC, et al. (2000). Executive dysfunction and long-term outcomes of geriatric depression. Arch Gen Psychiatry 57: 285–290.

Alexopoulos GS, Katz IR, Reynolds CF, et al. (2001). The Expert Consensus Guideline Series: Pharmacotherapy of Depressive Disorders in Older Adults. Postgrad Med Spec Rep, 1–86.

American Psychiatric Association (2000). Diagnostic and Statistical Manual of Mental Disorders. (4th ed–TR). Washington, DC.

Antsey J, Brodaty H (1995). Antidepressants and the elderly: double-blind trials 1987–1992. Int J Geriat Psychiatry 10:265–279.

Arean PA, Perri MG, Nezu AM, et al. (1993). Comparative effectiveness of social problem-solving therapy and reminiscence therapy as treatments for depression in older adults. J Consult Clin Psychol 61:1003–1010.

Astrom M, Adofspm R, Asplund K (1993). Major depression in stroke patients. A three year longitudinal study. Stroke 24:976–982.

Baldwin RC (1988). Delusional and non-delusional depression in late life. Evidence for distinct subtypes. Br J Psychiatry 152:39–44.

Bump GM, Mulsant SH, Pollock SG, et al. (2001). Paroxetine versus nortriptyline in the continuation and maintenance treatment of depression in the elderly. Depression Anxiety 13:38–44.

Callahan CM, Hui SL, Nienaber NA, et al. (1994). Longitudinal study of depression and health services use among elderly primary care patients. J Am Geriatr Soc 42: 833–838.

Carney RM, Rich WM, Tevelde A, et al. (1987). Major depressive disorder in coronary artery disease. Am J Cardiol 60:1273–1275.

Catterson ML, Perskom SH, and Martin RL (1997). Pharmacodynamic and pharmacokinetic considerations in geriatric psychopharmacology. Psychiatr Clin North Am 20(1):205–218.

Coffey CE, Figiel GS, Djang WT, et al. (1988). Leukoencephalopathy in elderly depressed patients referred for ECT. Biol Psychiatry 24:143–161.

Coffey CE, Figiel GS, Djang WT, et al. (1989). White matter hyperintensity on MRI clinical and neuroanatomic correlates in the depressed elderly. J Neuropsychiatry Clin Neurosci 1:135–144.

Cole MG, Bellavance F (1997). The prognosis of depression in old age. Am J Geriatr Psychiatry 5:4–14.

Conwell Y, Brent D (1995). Suicide in aging, I: patterns of psychiatric diagnosis. Int Psychogeriatr 7:149–164.

Dew MA, Reynolds CF, Houck PR, et al. (1997). Temporal profiles of the course of depression during treatment: Predictors of pathways toward recovery in the elderly. Arch Gen Psychiatry 54:1016–1024.

Dew MA, Reynolds CF, Mulsant BH, et al. (2001). Initial recovery patterns may predict which maintenance therapies for depression will keep older adults well. J Affect Disord 65:155–166.

Dunner DL (1994). An overview of paroxetine in the elderly. Gerontology 40 (suppl 1):21–27.

Ebrahim S, Barer K, Nouri F (1987). Affective illness after stroke. Br J Psychiatry 154:170–182.

Finkel SI, Richter EM, Clary CM (1999). Comparative efficacy and safety of sertraline versus nortriptyline in major depression in patients 70 and older. Int Psychogeriatr 11:85–99.

Flint AJ (1998). Choosing appropriate antidepressant therapy in the elderly: a risk:benefit assessment of available agents. Drugs Aging 13:269–280.

Flint AJ, Rifat SL (1997). Two-year outcome of elderly patients with anxious depression. Psychiatry Res 66:23–31.

Flint AJ, Rifat SL (2000). Maintenance treatment for recurrent depression in late-life. Am J Geriatr Psychiatry 8:112–116.

Folstein MF, Maiberger R, McHugh PR (1971). Mood disorders as a specific complication of stroke. J Neurol Neurosurg Psychiatry 40:1018–1020.

Ford DE, Kamerow DB (1989). Epidemiologic study of sleep disturbances and psychiatric disorders. JAMA 262:1479–84.

Frasure-Smith N, Lesperance F, Talajic M (1993). Depression following myocardial infarction, impact on 6-month survival. JAMA 270:1819–1825.

Fujikawa T, Yarnawaki S, Touhouda Y (1993). Incidence of silent cerebral infarction in patients with major depression. Stroke 24:1631–1634.

Gallagher-Thompson D, Hanley-Peterson P, Thompson LW (1990). Maintenance of gains versus relapse following brief psychotherapy for depression. J Consult Clin Psychol 58:371–374.

Georgotas A, McCue RE (1989). Relapse of depressed patients after effective continuation therapy. J Affect Disord 17:159–164.

Georgotas A, McCue RE, Cooper TB, et al. (1988). How effective and safe is continuation therapy in elderly depressed patients? Arch Gen Psychiatry 45:929–932.

Georgotas A, McCue RE, Cooper TB (1989). A placebo-controlled comparison of nortriptyline and phenelzine in maintenance therapy of elderly depressed patients. Arch Gen Psychiatry 46:783–785.

Greenwald BS, Kramer-Ginsber E, Marin DB, et al. (1989). Dementia with co-existent major depression. Am J Psychiatry 146:1472–1478.

Harman JS, Reynolds CF (2000). Removing the barriers to effective depression treatment in old age. 48:1012–1013.

Hawton K, Kirk J (1989). Problem solving. In: Hawton K, Salkovskis PM, Kirk J, Clark DM, eds. Cognitive Behaviour Therapy for Psychiatric Patients: A Practical Guide. Oxford, UK: Oxford University Press.

Isometsa E, Henriksson M, Aro H, et al. (1994). Suicide in psychotic major depression. J Affect Disord 31:187–191.

Jacoby RJ, Levy R (1980). Computed tomography in the elderly. Affective disorder. Br J Psychiatry 136:270–275.

Kalayam B, Alexopoulos GS (1999). Prefrontal dysfunction and reatment response in geriatric depression. Arch Gen Psychiatry 56:713–718.

Keller M, Lavori PW, Lewis CE, et al. (1983). Predictors of. relapse in major depressive disorder. JAMA 250:3299–3304.

Keller MB, Klerman GL, Lavori PW, et al. (1984). Long-term outcome of episodes of major depression. JAMA 252:788–792.

Kivel SL, Pahkala K (1989). Delusional depression in the elderly: A community study. Gerontology 22:236–241.

Klausner EJ, Alexopoulos GS (1999). The future of psychosocial treatments for elderly patients. Psychiatr Serv 50:1198–1204.

Klausner EJ, Clarkin JF, Spielman L, et al. (1998). Late-life depression and functional disability: the role of goal-focused group psychotherapy. Int J Geriat Psychiatry 13:707–716.

Klerman GL, Weissman MM, Rounsaville BJ, Sherron ES (1984). Interpersonal Psychotherapy of Depression. New York: Basic Books.

Krishnan KRR (1993). Neuroanatonmic substrates of depression in the elderly. J Geriatr Psychiatr Neurol 6:39–58.

Krishnan KRR, Goli V, Ellinwood EH, et al. (1988). Leukoencephalopathy in patient diagnosed as major depressive. Biol Psychiatry 23:519–522.

Lebowitz BD, Pearson JL, Schneider LS, et al. (1997). Diagnosis and treatment of depression in late-life: Consensus statement update. JAMA 278: 1186–1190.

Lenze EJ, Rogers JC, Martire LM, et al. (2001). The association of late-life depression and anxiety with physical disability: A review of the literature and prospectus for future research. Am J Geriatr Psychiatry 9:113–135.

Little JT, Reynolds CF, Dew MA, et al. (1998). How common is resistance to treatment in recurrent, nonpsychotic geriatric depression? Am J Psychiatry 155: 1035–1038.

Malmgren R (1994). Epidemiology of aging. In: Coffey CE, Cummings JL, eds. The American Psychiatric Press Textbook of Geriatric Psychiatry. 2nd ed. Washington, DC: American Psychiatric Press, pp 433–459.

Menting JE, Honig A, Verhev FR, et al. (1996). Selective serotonin reuptake inhibitors (SSRIs) in the treatment of elderly depressed patients: a qualitative analysis of the literature on their efficacy and side-effects. Int Clin Psychopharmacol 11:165–175.

Meyers BS (1992). Geriatric delusional depression. Clin Geriatr Med 8:299–308.

Meyers BS, Gabrielle M, Kakuma T, et al. (1996). Anxiety and depression as predictors of recurrence in geriatric depression. Am J Geriatr Psychiatry 4:252–257.

Montgomery SA (1998). Efficacy and safety of the selective serotonin reuptake inhibitors in treating depression in elderly patients. Int Clin Psychopharmacol 13(suppl 5):S49–S54.

Montgomery SA, Kasper S (1998). Depression: a long-term illness and its treatment. Int Clin Psychopharmacol 13(suppl 6):S23–S26.

Mueller TI, Leon AC, Keller MB, et al. (1999). Recurrence after recovery from major depressive disorder during 15 years of observational follow-up. Am J Psychiatry 156:1000–1006.

Mulsant SH, Ganguli M (1999). Epidemiology and diagnosis of depression in late-life. J Clin Psychiatry 60(suppl):9–15.

National Institutes of Health Consensus Development Panel on Depression in Late Life (1992). Diagnosis and treatment of depression in late life. JAMA 268:1018–1024.

Old Age Depression Interest Group (OADIG) (1993). How long should the elderly take antidepressants? A double-blind, placebo-controlled study of continuation/prophylaxis therapy with dothiepin. Br J Psychiatry 162:175–182.

Opdyke KS, Reynolds CF, Begley AE, et al. (1997). The effects of continuation treatment on residual symptoms of late-life depression: How well is "well?" Depression Anxiety 4:312–319.

Perel JM (1994). Geropharmacokineties of therapeutics, toxic effects, and compliance. In: Schneider S, Reynolds CF, Lebowitz BD, eds. Diagnosis and Treatment of Depression in Late Life. Washington, DC: American Psychiatric Press, pp 245–255.

Plotkin DA, Gerson SG, Jarvik LF (1987). Antidepressant drug treatment in the elderly. In: Meltzer HY, ed. Psychopharmacology: The Third Generation of Progress. New York: Raven Press, pp 1149–1158.

Post F, Schulman K (1985). New views on old age affective disorder. In: Recent Advances in Psychogeriatrics. Aire T, ed. New York: Churchill Livingstone, pp 119–140.

Rabkin JG, Charles E, Kass F (1983). Hypertension and DSM III depression in psychiatric outpatients. Am J Psychiatry 140:1072–1074.

Regier DA, Boyd JH, Burke JD, et al. (1988). one-month prevalence of mental disorders in the United States based on five Epidemiologic Catchment Area sites. Arch Gen Psychiatry 45:977–986.

Reynolds CF, Kupfer DJ (1999). Depression and aging: a look to the future. Psychiatr Serv 50:1167–1172.

Reynolds CF, Perel JM, Frank E, et al. (1989). Open trial maintenance pharmacotherapy in late life depression: survival analysis. Psychiatry Res 27:225–231.

Reynolds CE, Frank E, Perel JM, et al. (1992). Combined pharmacotherapy and psychotherapy in the acute and continuation treatment of elderly patients with recurrent major depression: a preliminary report. Am J Psychiatry 149: 1687–1692.

Reynolds CF, Frank E, Perel JM, et al. (1994). Treatment of consecutive episodes of major depression in the elderly. Am J Psychiatry 151:1740–1743.

Reynolds CF, Frank E, Perel JM, et al. (1996). High relapse rates after discontinuation of adjunctive medication in elderly patients with recurrent major depression. Am J Psychiatry 153:1418–1422.

Reynolds CF, Frank E, Houck PR, et al. (1997). Which elderly patients with remitted depression remain well with continued interpersonal psychotherapy after discontinuation of antidepressant medication? Am J Psychiatry 154:958–962.

Reynolds CF, Frank E, Dew MA, et al. (1999a). Treatment in 70 + year olds with major depression: Excellent short-term but brittle long-term response. Am J Geriat Psychiatry 7:64–69.

Reynolds CF, Perel JM, Frank E, et al. (1999b). Three year outcomes of maintenance nortriptyline treatment in late-life depression: a study of two fixed plasma levels. Am J Psychiatry 156:1177–1181.

Reynolds CF, Frank, E, Perel JP, et al. (1999c). Nortriptyline and interpersonal psychotherapy as maintenance therapies for recurrent major depression: a randomized controlled trial in patients older than 59 years. JAMA 281:39–45.

Reynolds CF, Miller MD, Pasternak RE, et al. (1999d). Treatment of bereavement-related major depressive episodes in later life: a controlled study of acute and continuation treatment with nortriptyline and interpersonal psychotherapy. Am J Psychiatry 156:202–208.

Robinson DG, Spiker DG (1985). Delusional depressions: one year followup. JAffect Disord 9:79–83.

Robinson RG, Kubos KL, Starr LB, et al. (1984). Mood disorders in stroke patients: importance of location of lesion. Brain 107:81–93.

Roose SP, Glassman AH, Walsh T, et al. (1983). Depression, delusions, and suicide. Am J Psychiatry 140:1150–1162.

Rovner BW, German PS, Brant LJ, et al. (1991). Depression and mortality in nursing homes [published erratum appears in JAMA 1991 May 22–29; 265(20):2672] [see comments]. JAMA 265:993–996.

Salzman C (1994). Pharmacological treatment of depression in elderly patients. In: Schneider LS, Reynolds CF, Lebowitz BD, eds. Diagnosis and Treatment of Depression in Late Life. Washington, DC: American Psychiatric Press.

Sands JR, Harrow M (1994). Psychotic unipolar depression at followup: factors related to psychosis in the affective disorders. Am J Psychiatry 151:995–1000.

Satel SL, Nelson IC (1989). Stimulants in the treatment of depression: a critical overview. J Clin Psychiatry 50:241–249.

Schneider LS (1999). Treatment of depression in late life. Dial Clin Neurosci 1: 113–124.

Spiker DG, Weiss JC, Dealy RS, et al. (1985). The pharmacological treatment of delusional depression. Am J Psychiatry 142:430–436.

Starkstein SE, Robinson RG, Berthier ML, et al. (1988). Depressive disorders following posterior circulation as compared with middle cerebral artery infarcts. Brain 111:387.

Sulzer DL, Levin HS, Mahler ME, et al. (1993). A comparison of psychiatric symptoms in vascular dementia and Alzheimer's disease. Am J Psychiatry 150: 1806–1812.

Sussman N, Joffe RT (1998). Augmentation of antidepressant medications: conclusions and recommendations. J Clin Psychiatry 59(suppl 5):70–73.

U.S. Department of Health and Human Services. Mental Health: A Report of the Surgeon General—Older Adults and Mental Health. (1999). Rockville, MD: U.S. Department of Health and Human Services, Substance Abuse and Mental Health Services Administration, Center for Mental Health Services, National Institutes of Health, National Institute of Mental Health, 1999.

Wells KB, Burnam MA (1991). Caring for depression in America: Lessons learned from early findings of the Medical Outcomes Study. Psychiatr Med 9:503–519.

Wells KB, Stewart A, Hays RD, et al. (1989). The functioning and well-being of depressed patients.

Results from the Medical Outcomes Study [see comments]. JAMA 262:914–919.

World Health Organization (WHO) (1996). Global Health Statistics: A Compendium of Incidence, Prevalence and Mortality Estimates for Over 200 Conditions: The Global Burden of Disease. Cambridge, MA: Harvard University Press.

Williams JW, Barrett J, Oxman T, et al. (2000). Treatment of dysthymia and minor depression in primary care: a randomized controlled trial in older adults. JAMA 284:1519–1526.

Wragg RE, Jeste DV (1989). Overview of depression and psychosis in Alzheimer's disease. Am J Psychiatry 146:577–589.

Zis AP, Grof P, Webster M (1980). Predictors of relapse in recurrent affective disorders. Psychopharmacol Bull 16:47–49.

15

Approaches to Chronic Depression in Children and Adolescents

Daniel J. Pilowsky and Myrna M. Weissman
New York State Psychiatric Institute
and Columbia University
New York, New York, U.S.A.

Boris Birmaher
Western Psychiatric Institute and Clinic
University of Pittsburgh Medical Center
Pittsburgh, Pennsylvania, U.S.A.

INTRODUCTION

During the past 20 years there has been increasing recognition of depression in children and adolescents. Research in this area has focused on phenomenology (e.g., Carlson and Kashani, 1988; Mitchell et al., 1988), continuity with adult depression (e.g, Garber et al., 1988; Lewinsohn et al., 1999; Weissman et al., 1999a, 1999b), familial aggregation (e.g., Williamson et al., 1995; Klein et al., 2001), and identifying children at high risk (e.g., Orvaschel et al., 1988; Hammen et al., 1990; Weissman et al., 1997). The accumulated evidence has shown that the core symptoms of depression in childhood and adulthood are similar, with developmentally determined variations in their clinical presentation; that children of depressed parents are at increased risk for depression and a variety of nonmood disorders; and depression in adolescence often recurs or continues into adulthood.

Prior to 1970, pediatric depression was seldom mentioned, and some believed that children could not experience a clinical depression. Since then several developments have led to an increased interest in depression in childhood and adolescence. This increased interest can be attributed to the development of rating scales and structured interviews which led to an increasing recognition of depressive symptoms and disorders in this age group; and epidemiological studies which revealed that depression often begun in adolescence or early adulthood. More recently, in the 1990s, the Food and Drug Administration (FDA) mandated the inclusion of children in medication trials, thus leading to clinical trials of antidepressants in this age group.

This chapter will highlight diagnostic, epidemiological, risk factors, and treatment issues. In keeping with the focus of this volume, we will address issues relevant to chronic depression. Since the field of pediatric depression is relatively new, there is limited information specifically about chronic depression. Nevertheless, there are data on recurrent major depression, dysthymia, and double depression, which are all manifestations of chronicity and can be extrapolated to chronic depression.

For clarity, *pediatric depression* is used here to refer to depression in either childhood or adolescence. *Childhood* or *adolescent depression* refer specifically to depressive disorders with an onset in childhood or adolescence, respectively. This chapter considers only unipolar depression.

DIAGNOSTIC ISSUES

DSM-IV criteria for depressive disorders in children parallels adult criteria, with a few exceptions (APA, 1994). An irritable mood can substitute for a depressed mood, and a failure to make expected weight gains can substitute for a significant weight loss. The duration criteria for the diagnosis of dysthymia is at least one year for children and adolescents, instead of two. According to DSM IV, somatic complaints, irritability, and social withdrawal are common in children, whereas psychomotor retardation, hypersomnia, and delusions are less common in prepuberty than adolescence or adulthood.

The *Diagnostic and Statistical Manual of Mental Disorders*, 4th ed (DSM-IV) defines a major depressive episode as being chronic if full criteria have been met continuously for at least 2 years, and does not provide definitions of subtypes. The DSM-III Revised (DSM-III-R) definition of chronic depression includes three subtypes: (1) a major depressive episode lasting at least 2 years (chronic major depression); (2) partial remission of a major depressive episode with less severe symptoms persisting for at least 2 years (major depression in partial remission); and

(3) dysthymia. With the exception of dysthymia, relatively few chronic cases (i.e., chronic major depression and major depression in partial remission) can be identified until late adolescence or early adulthood. Thus, the DSM-III-R definition of chronic depression is not fully applicable to pediatric depression. Instead, we will focus on correlates and predictors of recurrence, as well as pediatric dysthymia.

The study of depression in children and adolescents is complicated by high comorbidity, making it difficult to study the effects of or risk for "pure" depression and by lack of specificity of putative risk factors. In young people, comorbidity is the rule rather than the exception: major depressive disorder (MDD) often co-occurs with other affective disorders (e.g., dysthymia) and with anxiety and disruptive behavior disorders (Angold et al., 1999a). The study of risk factors for depression has often led to the discovery of factors whose association with depression in youngsters is well documented but nonspecific. For example, parental depression, a well-established risk factor for depression in childhood and adolescence, also increases the risk for other psychopathology, including anxiety and disruptive behavior disorders (Weissman et al., 1997).

EPIDEMIOLOGY

The current prevalence of prepubertal depression is low, typically less than 1%. For example, Costello et al. (1988) found a 0.4% 1-year prevalence in a community sample (n = 789) of children aged 7–11 years, and others have reported similar as well as higher prevalences (for a review, see Angold and Costello, 2001). As puberty approaches, and even more markedly after the onset of puberty, the prevalence of MDD and other depressive disorders increases in both genders but more dramatically in girls (Wickramaratne and Weissman, 1998), leading to the higher female prevalence of unipolar depression typical of adult populations across different cultures (Weissman et al., 1996). Whereas depression prevalence (2.6%) was identical for 4- to 11-year-old boys and girls participating in the Ontario Child Health Study (Boyle et al., 1987; Fleming et al., 1989; Garrison et al., 1990), the rates for 12- to 16-year-old participants increased twofold to threefold (6.9 and 8.8% for boys and girls, respectively). By late adolescence MDD prevalence and gender distribution is comparable to that reported in adults, with point prevalence rates of 2–5% (Lewinsohn et al., 1993; Verhulst et al., 1997).

Both biological and psychosocial hypotheses have been proposed to explain the rapid shift from an absence of gender disparity in the prevalence rates of depression in prepubertal children to the female predominance observed in adolescence and adulthood. Briefly, recent evidence suggests that exposure to increased levels of testosterone and estrogen in puberty, especially in the presence of psychosocial stress, may independently increase risk for depression in vulnerable girls (Angold et al., 1999b; Silberg et al., 1999).

RISK FACTORS FOR CHILDHOOD AND ADOLESCENT-ONSET DEPRESSION

Even though the specific causes of mood disorders remain unknown, several promising hypotheses have emerged. Clearly, the genetic contribution to depression is likely to be significant and complex. Additionally, exposure to adverse and traumatic environmental circumstances may contribute to precipitating depressive episodes in vulnerable individuals. Among the risk factors for pediatric depression, parental depression has the most evidence to support its detrimental impact on children.

Parental Depression

There is abundant evidence that parental depression increases the risk for depression, anxiety disorders, and disruptive behavior disorders, as well as drug abuse in the offspring (e.g., see Weissman et al., 1997; Hammen et al., 1990, 1991; Goodman and Gotlib, 1999). Furthermore, there is some evidence that rates of depressive, conduct, and substance-use disorders are higher in children of unipolar mothers than among children of bipolar mothers (e.g., see Hammen et al., 1990). The association of offspring psychopathology and parental MDD is strongest for childhood-onset psychopathology and particularly for childhood-onset MDD (Orvaschel et al., 1988; Wickramaratne and Weissman, 1998). These findings, when considered in the context of familial aggregation research, suggest that childhood-onset MDD may have a higher familial loading than adolescent- and adult-onset MDD (for a discussion of this hypothesis, see Wickramaratne and Weissman, 1998).

The evidence that parental depression increases the risk for depression and other psychopathology among affected children is indisputable; however, our understanding of the mechanisms is limited. While there is evidence of heritability of unipolar depression, twin studies suggest that heritability is only moderate, with an heritability of liability to major depression approaching 40%, with the remaining liability (slightly over 60%) due to individual-specific environments (Kendler and Prescott, 1999; Sullivan et al., 2000). A host of modifiable psychosocial factors appear to mediate or moderate the effects of parental depression on children.

Psychosocial Risk Factors

There is evidence that impaired parenting is a risk factor for pediatric depression. Most of the research on parenting is based on observations of depressed mothers. They may be unavailable to their children or unresponsive, or they may be critical and rejecting (e.g., see a review by Downey and Coyne, 1990). In a study of children of depressed mothers, stressful life events had a greater detrimental impact (i.e., more depressive symptoms) among children of depressed mothers as compared to children of nondepressed mothers. The investigators concluded that depressed mothers were not able to "buffer" the impact of stressful life events on their children (Hammen et al., 1991). These findings are consistent with the hypothesis that support buffers the effects of stress as suggested by Cohen and Wills (1985). Others have reported that family risk factors impact offspring of nondepressed and depressed parents differently (Fendrich et al., 1990). The family risk factors they examined (parents' marital discord, parent-child discord, affectionless control, low family cohesion, and parental divorce) were associated with MDD only in children of nondepressed parents. Children of depressed parents developed MDD regardless of the presence of family risk factors. These investigators suggested that children of depressed parents may become depressed before family risk factors have a chance to exert their influence.

There is some evidence that stress, child maltreatment, and childhood adversity, broadly defined, are risk factors for pediatric depression. Stress may range from daily hassles and stressful life events to chronic adversity that is not associated with a specific event; for example, extreme poverty. Stress may include parental stress as well as stressful events that directly impact the child (Williamson et al., 1998). For example, maltreated children are at risk for major depression and dysthymia (Kaufman, 1991). Furthermore, an association of childhood physical and sexual abuse and adult depression and suicidality has been reported (McCauley et al., 1997). There is some evidence that responsive caretakers may buffer risk for depression and other forms of psychopathology (Nachmias et al., 1996), and that the quality of the caregiver-infant interaction is critical to normal development of affect regulation in the offspring (Kaufman et al., 2000).

In addition to stress and parenting, there is some evidence that the following may increase the risk for adolescent-onset MDD: negative cognitions, lack of social support from family, emotional reliance (a construct that reflects dependence on approval from others, and anxiety about being alone and about abandonment), poor physical health, and a past history of episodes of depression and anxiety disorders (Lewinsohn et al., 1995a).

A major problem with psychosocial risk factors research is that these factors are often studied independently of a family history of MDD. Since family history is a powerful predictor of pediatric MDD, the putative risk factors may be a reflection of this history. For example, impaired parenting may be a consequence of MDD in one or both parents rather than an independent risk factor. Warner et al. (1995) dealt with this problem by assessing the impact of a chaotic family environment on children's diagnoses while controlling for parental diagnosis. They found that a chaotic family environment independently predicted dysthymia in the offspring. Thus, future studies should estimate the impact of psychosocial stressons separately among children with and without a family history of depression.

A limitation of studies of psychosocial risk factors in high-risk samples (e.g., children of depressed parents or children with depressive symptoms) is that these children often already have a psychiatric disorder (e.g., anxiety disorders or depression) when they are assessed. Consequently, interpretation can not preclude the possibility that family risk variables are a consequence, rather than the cause, of the child's psychopathology. Additionally, many psychosocial risk factors are nonspecific; that is, they increase the risk for multiple disorders. Since each approach has limitations, longitudinal research with both community-based and high-risk samples is needed. Future research should also compare risk factors for depression to those for other highly prevalent childhood and adolescent-onset disorders (e.g., anxiety and disruptive behavior disorders) in order to assess the specificity of psychosocial risk factors.

Biological Risk Factors

Very few studies have evaluated the biological correlates associated with increased likelihood for recurrences or chronic child and adolescent depression. Rao and colleagues (1996) reported that youth with elevated plasma cortisol around sleep onset appear to be more likely to have a recurrence of depression. Goodyear and colleagues (1998, 2001) found that higher cortisol/dehydroepiandrosterone (DHEA) ratios together with one or more disappointing life events predicted persistent MDD at 9 months of follow-up. This study indicated the importance of simultaneously assessing clinical, environmental, and biological factors and examining their combined importance for developing MDD. Finally, Goetz and colleagues (2001) reported that sleep disruption around sleep onset and during the first 100 min of sleep in depressed adolescents were associated with recurrent depressions.

In adults, abnormalities in the sleep electroencephalogram and growth hormone and cortisol secretion have also been found to be associated with more chronic and recurrent depressions (e.g., see Franz et al., 1995; Thase et al., 1995; Harris et al., 2001), but the clinical use of these findings has not been well investigated.

Follow-up studies of children and adolescents, who at intake did not have any psychiatric disorders, have reported that rapid increase of nocturnal growth hormone secretion following sleep onset (Coplan et al., 2000); high density of rapid eye movements (REMs) (Rao et al., 1996); and the additive effects of high saliva cortisol and DHEA levels, subsyndromal depressive symptoms, and negative life events are associated with new onset of MDD (Goodyear et al., 2000). Whether these biological changes are also associated with recurrent or chronic depression is unclear.

CHRONIC DEPRESSION IN CHILDHOOD AND ADOLESCENCE

We shall now address antecedents and correlates of episodes of pediatric depression of longer than average duration and of recurrence. We will also deal with comorbidity, as well as pediatric dysthymia and its consequences.

Duration of MDD Episodes

Typically, clinically referred children and adolescents appear to recover faster from an MDD episode than their adult counterparts (Kovacs, 1996). In clinical samples, the average duration of an episode of pediatric MDD is about 9 months compared to 12 months in adults (Kovacs, 1996; Kovacs et al., 1997) and to about 6–7 months in community samples of adolescents. For example, in a community-based study of adolescent-onset MDD, mean duration of MDD episodes was 26.4 weeks (Lewinsohn et al., 1994). In the same study, longer episodes were observed in those whose depression occurred in early adolescence (at or before age 15 years), whose depression had been accompanied by suicidal ideation and for whom treatment was sought. These findings are consistent with those reported by other investigators (McCauley et al., 1993; Kovacs et al., 1997; and among adults, Coryell et al., 1994), and suggest that treatment is more likely to be sought when an MDD episode persists.

Age of onset has been found to affect duration of MDD episodes in some studies (Kovacs et al., 1984b; Warner et al., 1992; Lewinsohn et al., 1994) but not in others (McCauley et al., 1993; Kovacs et al., 1997). Overall, the evidence suggests that an earlier age of onset of MDD may be associated with longer duration of episodes, but further clarification of this issue is needed. Other factors, such as gender, social class, and episode severity, do not seem to correlate with episode duration (Kovacs et al., 1997).

MDD Recurrence

The term *recurrent depression* will be used here to refer to an episode of MDD or dysthymia that is followed by another episode of either condition, and between episodes the child or adolescent does not meet criteria for either disorder. During the interval between episodes, however, subsyndromal symptoms may be evident, and may be associated with psychosocial impairment (Lewinsohn et al., 2000a). In this section, we will consider MDD recurrence in childhood and adolescence, as well as recurrence in adulthood of pediatric-onset MDD. A methodological problem to keep in mind is that rates of recurrence are influenced by the length of follow-up. The longer patients are followed, the more likely the researchers are to find a higher rate of recurrence.

Does an episode of pediatric MDD predispose to recurrence in childhood or adolescence? There is evidence that pediatric MDD often recurs. Childhood depression, although rare, is often associated with 30–50% rates of recurrence in adolescence (Kovacs et al., 1984b; Garber et al., 1998; Pine et al., 1998). Brief multiple MDD episodes are common in adolescence (Angst et al., 1990).

Does an episode of pediatric depression predisposes to recurrence in adulthood? Longitudinal studies that followed up depressed adolescents to adulthood (Rao et al., 1995, 1999; Pine et al., 1998; Weissman et al., 1999; Lewinsohn et al., 2000b) have consistently demonstrated an increased risk for major depression in adulthood associated with an episode of major depression in adolescence. The accumulated evidence suggests that in clinical samples 60% or more of depressed adolescents followed into adulthood develop another depressive episode and about 50% in community samples. For example, Harrington et al. (1990) followed up 63 depressed children and adolescents on average 18 years after their initial clinical contact. They found that 60% of depressed adolescents and 27% of controls had one or more episodes of MDD in adulthood. In a community sample of 274 subjects with adolescent-onset MDD followed to early adulthood (19–23 years of age), 45.7% were found to have had one or more MDD episodes (Lewinsohn et al., 2000b). Additionally, adolescent-onset MDD is associated with adult suicidality. For example, Weissman et al.'s study of 91 adolescents who were diagnosed with MDD in adolescence and followed prospectively into adulthood and compared with children without any psychiatric disorder revealed a twofold increase of MDD, but not other psychiatric disorders, and a fivefold increase of the risk for first suicide attempts by adulthood (1999a).

Only two studies of depressed prepubertal children followed to adulthood are available (Harrington et al., 1990; Weissman et al., 1999b). Both found an increased risk of poor functioning. Nevertheless, compared to adolescent follow-up studies, weaker associations emerged between prepubertal depression and episodes of depression later in life. The retrospective nature of Harrington et al.'s study (adolescent depression data was obtained from medical records) limits the significance of the findings. Weissman et al.'s prospective study revealed that prepubertal-onset MDD was associated with a poor adult outcomes, but there was a lack of diagnostic specificity in adulthood. As adults, children with prepubertal-onset MDD went on to have high rates of substance abuse, conduct disorder, and bipolar I disorders. Adult recurrence of MDD was associated with family history of MDD.

In Lewinsohn et al.'s (2000b) study of 274 subjects with adolescent-onset MDD, about a third (31.8%) did not experience any psychiatric disorders in early adulthood (19–23 age period), 45.7% experienced an episode of major depression (with or without a comorbid nonmood disorder), and 22.6% experienced a nonmood disorder. The following factors predicted a recurrence of MDD in early adulthood: having had an MDD episode in adolescence, multiple MDD episodes in adolescence (as compared to one), female gender, family history of recurrent MDD, elevated borderline personality disorder symptoms, and conflicts with parents (females only). Among subjects with adolescent-onset MDD, as compared to controls, there was an increased risk of developing a nonaffective disorder in early adulthood. However, when compared to adolescents with nonaffective disorders, there was no evidence of increased risk. This finding is consistent with other studies which found a higher rate of nonaffective disorders in young adulthood among formerly depressed juveniles than in normal controls, but a similar rate compared with children and adolescents with nonaffective disorders (Harrington et al., 1990; Rao et al., 1995).

The accumulated evidence suggests that adolescent depression is likely to recur in adulthood, and prepubertal depression is associated with poor adult functioning but not specifically with adult depression.

Dysthymia and Double Depression

According to DSM-IV, dysthymia requires at least a 2-year duration in adults and 1 year in children. Thus, even though symptoms of dysthymia are less severe than those required to receive a diagnosis of MDD, dysthymia is by definition a form of chronic depression. It has a more protracted course than MDD: Available estimates suggest a median first episode length of 3.9 years in clinical samples (Kovacs et al., 1997) and between 2.5 and 3.4 years in community samples (Lewinsohn et al., 1991). Children who receive a dysthymia diagnosis are at increased risk of a subsequent MDD episode. In fact, the course of dysthymia is often punctuated by superimposed MDD episodes: Dysthmia and MDD coexist in about 30% of pediatric cases, a condition known as double depression. This proportion parallels the findings reported in the adult literature (Kovacs, 1996). The duration of both adult and pediatric MDD episodes superimposed on dysthymia may be shorter than the duration of MDD episodes in the absence of underlying dysthymia (Keller et al., 1982; Kovacs et al., 1997).

The Pittsburgh longitudinal study of childhood-onset depressive disorders generated the first reports of dysthymia in childhood. These reports (Kovacs et al., 1984a, 1984b, 1997) are based on a prospectively followed cohort of clinically ascertained children aged 8–13 years at study onset (n = 142). Of these, 55 had a dysthmia diagnosis at entry (23 with pure dysthymia and 32 with double depression), and form the basis for the findings summarized here. Dysthymic episodes had an earlier onset than first MDD episodes (8.7 vs 10.9 years), a finding also observed in a community sample (Lewinsohn et al., 1991). Most (69.1%) of the children had at least one superimposed MDD episode during the follow-up interval of 3–12 years. About half of the dysthymic children (53%), and 62% of the MDD group, had one or more preexisting conditions, including attention deficit–hyperactivity disorder (ADHD), enuresis/encopresis and anxiety disorders. In this cohort dysthymia, compared to MDD, was characterized by the rarity of anhedonia (5.6%) and of reduced appetite (5.6%) and by relatively low rates of neurovegetative symptoms (hyposomnia, 22%; fatigue 22%) (Kovacs, 1997).

The duration of dysthymic episodes may be influenced by comorbidity. In The Pittsburgh longitudinal study, first dysthymic episodes lasted 2.5 years longer in the presence of preexisting disorders (conduct disorder, oppositional defiant disorder, ADHD) than otherwise (Kovacs et al., 1997). Additionally, complications were frequent among dysthymia diagnosed children, with a cumulative probability of 81% of developing MDD 8.5 years after dysthymia onset, and a cumulative probability of 21% of developing a bipolar disorder, with dysthymia preceding MDD, and MDD eventually culminating in bipolar disorder (Kovacs, 1997). Even though other complicating conditions were observed, for example, anxiety and conduct disorders, affective disorders remained the most likely unfavorable outcome. Overall, the clinical course of childhood-onset dysthymia is characterized by "recovery followed by subsequent affective episodes and sporadic symptom-free intervals" (Kovacs, 1997, p 215). A few limitations of the Pittsburgh study are noteworthy: The sample included an overrepresentation of low socioeconomic status children, mostly from nonintact families (Kovacs, 1997), thus limiting generalizability to other populations.

Bipolar disorder seems to be the second (after MDD) most frequent complication of dysthymia. This worrisome finding parallels the association of dysthymia and bipolar disorder often described in the adult literature (e.g., see Klein et al., 1988; Wicki and Angst, 1991) Thus, dysthymic youngsters need to be targeted in efforts to prevent MDD and bipolar illness.

Pediatric-onset dysthymia, as well as double depression and recurrent MDD, are likely to impact negatively the development of children. Since depressed children and adolescents are often withdrawn and irritable, it may be difficult for them to establish and maintain social relationships. Additionally, poor concentration and psychomotor retardation may interfere with learning, and thus lead to academic failure and low self-esteem (Kovacs and Goldston, 1991; Harrington and Dubicka, 2001). There is some evidence of impairment in peer relationships after recovery from depression (Puig-Antich et al., 1985a, 1985b), and in multiple areas of functioning among adults who had been depressed as adolescents, including marital relationships (Garber et al., 1998), delinquent activities, and intimate relationships (Kandel and Davies, 1986). Since comorbidity is pervasive, it is hard to ascertain whether and to what extent associated impairments are related to depression per se or to comorbid conditions. Harrington et al. (1991) noted that most of the impact of juvenile depression on adult social functioning was associated with comorbid conduct disorder.

We have shown that MDD and bipolar disorder are common complications of childhood dysthymia. Therefore, these children remain at risk long after the episode that brought them to treatment is resolved. From a clinical, perspective, the most important feature of double depression is that it results in more severe and longer episodes, more suicidal attempts, and greater psychosocial impairment than MDD or dysthymia alone (Ferro et al., 1994; Kovacs et al., 1994).

COMORBIDITY

The most common comorbid psychiatric disorders in pediatric samples are affective, anxiety, and externalizing disorders. Comorbidity is the rule rather than the exception (Fleming et al., 1989; Hammen et al., 1990; Harrington et al., 1991). MDD and dysthymia often coexist as discussed above. About a third of depressed children and adolescents suffer from an anxiety disorder and about 15% from conduct disorder (Kovacs, 1996). A meta-analysis revealed that, controlling for other comorbidities among disorders, anxiety disorders were 8.2 times as common in depressed compared to nondepressed children and adolescents, conduct and oppositional disorders were 6.6 times as common, and ADHD was 5.5 times as common (Angold et al., 1999a). The onset of unipolar depression typically follows the onset of other disorders, with the exception of substance-abuse and panic disorders, which usually emerge in mid to late adolescence or early adulthood (Rohde et al., 1991; Kessler and Walters, 1998; Costello et al., 1999).

Comorbid anxiety disorders may increase the severity and duration of depressive disorders (McCauley et al., 1993; Emslie et al., 1998a), and may result in higher prevalence of suicidal behavior and psychosocial problems (Kovacs et al., 1989; Brent et al., 1990). Studies of adolescent depression suggest greater severity manifested by increased recurrence, in comorbid as compared to "pure" MDD cases (Sanford et al., 1995). However, findings are not uniform. For example, Harrington et al. (1991) reported that comorbid childhood conduct disorder is associated with lower rates of adult depression. Nevertheless, assessments of adult social functioning showed that childhood comorbid cases (depression and conduct disorder) had an increased risk of adult criminality. Others have reported that the presence of comorbid conduct disorder more than doubles the risk of suicide in depressed children (Kovacs et al., 1993). Brent et al. (1990) reported that among depressed patients who had attempted suicide, the degree of intent was associated with comorbid conduct disorder and comorbid substance abuse.

The significance of comorbidity differs across different disorders and outcome measures (Lewinsohn et al., 1995b). Additionally, comorbidity impacts children at different developmental periods. In spite of these sources of variability, some tentative generalizations can be made. The presence of comorbid disorders appears to be associated with a more severe course of depression manifested by longer duration of depressive episodes, increased likelihood of recurrence, or more severe impairment of social functioning. The combination of conduct disorder and depression, with its associated impairment of social functioning and increased suicidal risk, may comprise a distinct clinical and etiological subgroup (Birmaher et al., 1996).

Among children of depressed parents, Weissman et al. (1997) have described a sequence of disorders, starting with anxiety and conduct disorders in childhood, major depression in early to late adolescence, and substance abuse in young adulthood. Furthermore, in Weissman et al.'s cohort, grandchildren of depressed, compared to those of nondepressed grandparents, were at increased risk for anxiety disorders (fivefold). It is noteworthy that grandparent MDD had a stronger effect on the risk for anxiety in grandchildren than parent MDD (Warner et al., 1999). A number of investigators have reported that early anxiety increases the risk for later MDD (e.g., see Parker et al., 1997; Pine et al., 1998). Thus, the accumulating evidence suggests that early-onset anxiety may well indicate a vulnerability for the later development of depressive disorders and perhaps for chronicity. This vulnerability might also underlie the intergenerational transmission of a liability to develop depressive disorders.

APPROACHES TO TREATMENT

Evidence-based information on the efficacy of treatment for pediatric MDD is only beginning to emerge. Older medication trials with tricyclic antidepressants did not demonstrate efficacy in children or adolescents. More recent trials have demonstrated efficacy using selective serotonin reuptake inhibitors (SSRIs), but these trials are few and efficacy is limited. Even though psychoanalytically informed approaches to psychotherapeutic treatment of pediatric depression are used extensively in clinical practice (e.g., see Zaslow, 2000), no clinical trials are available. A few clinical trials of both psychotherapy and medication with adolescents are available. There have been no clinical trials of psychotherapy with prepubertal children with diagnosed depressive disorders, and few of these children have been included in recent medication trials. It should be noted that this chapter does not specifically address treatment of pediatric chronic depression, as little is known about such treatment. Nevertheless, a few trials have generated some information about relapse prevention, which should be the aim of treatment approaches to chronic depression.

Psychotherapy Trials

Only a few psychotherapies have been tested in controlled trials with children and adolescents. We will focus on cognitive-behavior therapy (CBT) and interpersonal therapy (IPT), as most of the available clinical trials have used these treatments. CBT has been the most frequently investigated treatment for depression in young people (Curry, 2001). CBT assumes that depression is caused or maintained by faulty cognitions or maladaptive coping behaviors. The specific techniques used in CBT vary, with some using primarily either behavioral or cognitive techniques. Children in the six available controlled studies of CBT targeting children below age 12 years (cited in Curry, 2001) were not clinically diagnosed as having depressive disorders. Instead, investigators relied on self-reported depression. These studies were all school based. All but one of the six studies that compared CBT to no treatment in this age group or to a waiting list condition demonstrated short-term efficacy in reducing depressive symptoms (Curry, 2001), and Weisz et al. (1997) demonstrated that the beneficial effects of CBT were maintained 9 months later.

In contrast to the children's studies, several CBT studies targeted clinically diagnosed adolescents. Additionally, most of these studies were done in clinical settings. We will review selected recent studies (for a comprehensive review, see Curry, 2001). Clarke et al. (1999) compared outcomes among 123 adolescents aged 14–18 years with diagnoses of major depression or dysthymia, treated using two variations of CBT, one with and one without a parental component, to those observed among adolescents in a waiting-list condition. After 8 weeks of treatment, about two-thirds of adolescents receiving either type of CBT no longer met criteria for a diagnosis of depression versus 48% of adolescents in the waiting-list condition. After the acute phase, those who had received active treatment were randomized to one of three follow-up conditions for the next 2 years: booster sessions and assessments every 4 months, assessments only every 4 months, or assessments every year. For those adolescents whose depression had remitted after 8 weeks of treatment, there was no significant difference in the rate of relapse as a function of booster sessions. In contrast, among adolescents still depressed at the end of acute treatment, after 1 year of follow-up, none receiving booster sessions met diagnostic criteria for a depressive disorder versus 50% for those receiving only assessments. By 2 years, these rates of remission were almost equalized at 100 and 90%. The investigators concluded that booster sessions facilitated remission among adolescents still depressed after treatment of the acute episode.

Brent and his colleagues (1997) in a clinical trial with 107 adolescents (aged 13 to 18 years) with major depression compared CBT to systemic behavioral family therapy (SBFT) and to nondirective supportive therapy (NST). Remission, which was defined as no longer meeting diagnostic criteria, was greatest with CBT (60%) compared to 38 and 39% for SBFT and NST, respectively. Recently, the same group of investigators completed a 2-year follow-up of these patients (Birmaher et al., 2000). There were no significant differences in the long-term outcomes among the three treatment conditions. Recurrence of depression during follow-up was associated with parent-child conflict or familial discord, suggesting the need for addressing these areas during maintenance treatment.

Two clinical trials of IPT for adolescents (IPT-A) are available in the literature. Interpersonal therapy is a well-established treatment for adult depression (Weissman et al., 2000). It is based on the theory that interpersonal disputes, life transitions, or losses cause or maintain depression (Weissman et al., 2000). Mufson et al, conducted a clinical trial of IPT-A (Mufson et al., 1999) that included 48 adolescents with major depression, aged 12–18 years. Among IPT-A adolescents at the end of treatment, 88% no longer met diagnostic criteria for major depression compared to 58% among adolescents assigned to clinical monitoring. A second study of IPT was conducted with 71 Puerto Rican adolescents with major depression, aged 13–18 years (Rossello and Bernal, 1999). They were assigned to CBT, IPT, or a waiting-list condition. Both IPT and CBT had a significant impact on depressive symptoms. Additionally, improvements in self-esteem and social adaptation were evident among IPT-treated adolescents.

Both CBT and IPT are efficacious in the short-term treatment of major depression in adolescents. There are no long-term follow-up data for IPT treatment. CBT follow-up data indicate that CBT is not superior to other psychotherapies with regard to rates of remission (Birmaher et al., 2000; Curry, 2001). However, rates of remission are high, suggesting a possible ceiling effect for all psychotherapies. Future directions for psychotherapy research may include the use of combined treatment (medication and psychotherapy) for severe or recurrent depression, the inclusion of a family component, as family conflict increases the rate of relapse (Birmaher et al., 2000), and the need to address all phases of the depression, not just acute episodes.

Medication Trials

The optimal pharmacological management of child and adolescent MDD may also involve some educative and psychosocial interventions. The rate of treatment response appears to be equivalent in SSRIs or either of the two psychotherapies discussed above (CBT and IPT), and the types of cases that do not respond to either medication or psychotherapy alone are similar (Brent et al., 1998; Emslie et al., 1998b; Mufson et al., 1999). Older medication studies targeting children and adolescents focused on tricyclic antidepressants (TCAs) and recent ones on SSRIs. Other antidepressants have not been well studied for the treatment of MDD in children and adolescents. Therefore, the focus here is on the use of TCAs and SSRIs for youth with MDD.

TCAs

Outpatient adult studies, involving thousands of subjects, have shown approximately a 50–70% response to TCAs, with drug-placebo differences ranging from 20 to 40% (APA, 2000). In contrast, only 13 double-blind psychopharmacological trials, which include approximately 330 depressed children and adolescents comparing TCAs (nortriptyline, imipramine, desipramine, amitriptyline) with placebo have been reported. These studies showed a similar response to both the TCAs and placebo (for a review, see Birmaher et al., 1996). Moreover, a recent study comparing imipramine, paroxetine, and placebo (Keller et al., 2001) in adolescents with MDD reported no significant differences between a TCA (imipramine) and placebo. Thus, efficacy as a treatment for MDD or dysthymia has not been demonstrated for the TCAs among children or adolescents.

SSRIs

The reports that SSRIs are efficacious for the treatment of adults with MDD (APA, 2000) together with the findings that SSRIs are efficacious and safe for other childhood psychiatric disorders (e.g., see Leonard et al., 1997), have a relatively safe side effect profile, very low lethality after an overdose, and easy administration have favored the SSRIs as the first-line medications for the treatment of MDD. A double-blind placebo-controlled study in a very small sample of adolescents with MDD did not find significant differences between placebo and fluoxetine (Simeon et al., 1990). However, a large 8-week double blind study for the treatment of children and adolescents with MDD showed that patients on 8-weeks of fluoxetine (20 mg/day) were more likely to show improvement than those on placebo (58 vs 32% on the clinical global improvement scale; CGI) (Emslie et al., 1997). A second study also using fluoxetine (20 mg/day) for 9 weeks replicated the above results (Emslie et al., 2002). In both studies, there were no age and sex effects and patients tolerated fluoxetine well. Despite the significant response to fluoxetine, many patients had only partial improvement and a substantial proportion did not remit.

Recently, a multicenter study comparing the effects of 12-week paroxetine, imipramine, and placebo for the treatment of a large sample of outpatient adolescents with MDD, aged 12 to 18 years (n = 275) was completed (Keller et al., 2001). Adolescents taking paroxetine showed significantly better response than those taking placebo. Among those receiving paroxetine, the CGI scores were "very much improved" or "improved" in 65.6% cases vs 52.1% for imipramine and 48.3% for placebo ($P = .02$). Hamilton scores (HAM-D) at or below 8, which are considered indicative of remission, were present in 63.3, 50.0, and 46.9% of adolescents who received paroxetine, imipramine, and placebo, respectively. Differences between youth taking imipramine and placebo were not significant for any of the outcomes assessed in this study.

Currently, the antidepressants of choice are the SSRIs, because they have been shown to be efficacious and safe for the treatment of adolescents with MDD, and safe for use with both children and adolescents. Further research for the other new antidepressants (e.g., bupropion, venlafaxine, nefazodone, mirtazepine) is needed. Patients should be treated with adequate doses for at least 6 weeks before declaring lack of response to treatment (treatment of nonresponders is described below). It is important to mention that specific psychotherapies (CBT or IPT) (Brent et al., 1997; Mufson et al., 1999) are also reasonable initial choices for the acute treatment of most youth with the first episode of major depression. Nevertheless, clinical experience suggests that more severe and chronic depressions, those with significant comorbid disorders, and those with parental conflict and psychopathology often fail respond to either medication or psychotherapy alone (Clarke et al., 1992; Brent et al., 1998; Emslie et al., 1998b). Therefore, severe and chronic depressions in adolescents should be treated with both antidepressants and psychotherapy, and other risk factors for poor outcome (e.g., parent depression, childhood ADHD) should be addressed with additional psychosocial and pharmacological interventions.

CONCLUSION

The epidemiological and clinical evidence suggests that adolescent depression is a distinct psychopathological entity, and that adolescent-onset MDD is continuous with adult depression. The recurrence rate of adolescent-onset MDD is substantial, and being female increases the risk of recurrence. Comorbidity is often associated with depression recurrence, greater functional impairment, or both. Comorbid conduct disorder and substance abuse may increase the risk of suicide.

Dysthymia has a protracted clinical course and is often complicated by MDD (double depression) and later bipolar disorder. Double depression often results in more severe and longer episodes, more suicide attempts, and psychosocial impairment than MDD or dysthymia alone.

Early-onset MDD is strongly associated with familial aggregation of depressive disorders. Individuals with early-onset MDD may constitute a relatively homogeneous group from a clinical and a genetic perspective. Clinically, early-onset MDD may be associated with a more chronic form of depression than late-onset MDD. Individuals with early-onset MDD may have an increased genetic vulnerability for developing depressive disorders. Psychosocial risk factors are likely to play an important role in the etiology of depression, but to advance the field they need to be studied among individuals with low and high familial aggregation for affective disorders.

Psychotherapeutic treatments of adolescent depression with demonstrated efficacy include CBT and IPT. Most other psychotherapies have not been studied using the rigorous methodology of clinical trials, and therefore we do not have empirical evidence for their effectiveness or lack thereof. Additionally, recent evidence suggests that the SSRIs are somewhat effective in the treatment of adolescent depression. Tricyclic antidepressants are not effective treatments for pediatric depression as demonstrated in several trials. Overall, with the exception of severe or complicated adolescent MDD (see Medication Trials above), a trial of psychotherapy seems an appropriate first approach to the treatment of adolescent depression. Cases of severe depression, those not responding to a trial of psychotherapy, and those with history of recurrence may be good candidates for medication or combined treatment.

Approaches to the treatment of prepubertal depression lack empirical validation, as no psychotherapeutic or psychopharmacological interventions have been proven to be effective in the treatment of MDD or dysthymia in this age group. The available SSRI trials (summarized above) included few prepubertal subjects. A few points can be made nevertheless. First, dysthymia of prepubertal onset is a serious condition that requires treatment beyond the remission of the episode that brought the child to treatment. Second, in this age group, a trial of psychotherapy is almost universally the first approach, because, in contrast to adolescent depression, conclusive evidence of medication efficacy is lacking. Such evidence may emerge as more children are included in SSRI trials.

ACKNOWLEDGMENTS

This work was partially supported by the following National Institute of Mental Health grants: MH63852 (Myrna M. Weissman and Daniel J. Pilowsky); and MH70008 (Boris Birmaher).

REFERENCES

American Psychiatric Association (APA) (1994). Diagnostic and Statistical Manual of Mental Disorders. 4th ed. Washington, D.C.

American Psychiatric Association (APA) (2000). Practice for the treatment of patients with major depressive disorder (revision). Am J Psychiatry 157 (Suppl.):1–45.

Angold A, Costello EJ, Erkani A (1999a). Comorbidity. J Child Psychol Psychiatry 40:57–87.

Angold A, Costello EJ, Worthman CM, (1999b). Pubertal changes in hormone levels and depression in girls. Psychol Med 29:1043–1053.

Angold A, Costello EJ (2001). The epidemiology of depression in children and adolescents. In: IM Goodyer, ed. The Depressed Child and Adolescent. 2nd ed. Cambridge, UK: Cambridge University Press, pp 143–178.

Angst J, Merikangas K, Scheidegger P, Wicki W (1990). Recurrent brief depression: a new subtype of affective disorder. J Affect Disord 19:87–98.

Birmaher B, Ryan ND, Williamson DE, et al. (1996). Childhood and adolescent depression: a review of the past 10 years. J Am Acad Child Adol Psychiatry 35:1427–1439.

Birmaher B, Brent DA, Kolko DJ, et al. (2000). Clinical outcome after short-term psychotherapy for adolescents with major depressive disorder. Arch Gen Psychiatry 57:29–36.

Boyle MH, Offord D, Hofman HG, et al. (1987). Ontario Child Health Study: I. Methodology. Arch Gen Psychiatry 44:826–831.

Brent DA, Kolko DJ, Allan MJ, et al. (1990). Suicidality in affectively disordered adolescent inpatients. J Am Acad Child Adol Psychiatry 29:586–593.

Brent DA, Holder D, Kolko DJ, et al. (1997). A clinical psychotherapy trial for adolescent depression comparing cognitive, family, and supportive therapy. Arch Gen Psychiatry 54:877–885.

Brent, D.A., Kolko, D., Birmaher, B., et al. (1998). Predictors of treatment efficacy in a clinical trial of three psychosocial treatments for adolescent depression. J Am Acad Child Adolesc Psychiatry 37:906–914.

Carlson GA, Kashani JH (1988). Phenomenology of major depression from childhood through adulthood: analyses of three studies. Am J Psychiatry 145:1222–1225.

Clarke GN, Hops, H., Lewinsohn, P.M., et al. (1992). Cognitive behavioral group treatment of adolescent depression: Prediction of outcome. Behav Ther 23:341–354.

Clarke GN, Rohde P, Lewinsohn PM, et al. (1999). Cognitive-behavioral treatment of adolescent depression: Efficacy of acute group treatment and booster sessions. J Am Acad Child Adol Psychiatry 38:272–279.

Cohen S, Wills T (1985). Stress, social support and the buffering hypothesis. Psychol Bull 98:310–357.

Coplan JD, Wolk SI, Goetz RR, et al. (2000). Nocturnal Growth hormone secretion studies in adolescents with and without major depression reexamined: integration of adult and clinical data. Biol Psychiatry 47:594–604.

Coryell W, Akiskal HS, Leon AC, et al. (1994). The time course of nonchronic major depressive disorder. Uniformity across episodes and samples. National Institute of Mental Health collaborative program on the psychobiology of depression-clinical studies. Arch Gen Psychiatry 51:405–410.

Costello EJ, Costelo AJ, Edelbrock C, et al. (1988). Psychiatric disorders in pediatric primary care. Arch Gen Psychiatry 45:1107–1116.

Costello EJ, Erkanil A, Federman E, Angold A (1999). Development of psychiatric comorbidity with substance abuse in adolescents: effects of timing and sex. J Clin Child Psychol 28:298–311.

Curry JF (2001). Specific psychotherapies for childhood and adolescents depression. Biol Psychiatry 49:1091–1100.

Downey G, Coyne JC (1990). Children of depressed parents: an integrative review. Psychol Bull 108:50–76.

Emslie G, Rush AJ, Weinberg AW, et al. (1997). A double-blind, randomized placebo-controlled trial of fluoxetine in depressed children and adolescents. Arch Gen Psychiatry 54:1031–1037.

Emslie GJ, Rush AJ, Weinberg WA, et al. (1998a). Fluoxetine in child and adolescent depression: acute and maintenance treatment. Depression Anxiety 7:32–39

Emslie GJ, Rush, AJ, Weinberg, WA, et al. (1998b). Fluoxetine in child and adolescent depression: acute and maintenance treatment. Depression Anxiety 7:32–39.

Emslie GJ, Heiligenstein JH, Wagner KD, et al. (2002). Fluoxetine for acute treatment of depression in children and adolescents: a placebo controlled, randomized clinical trial. J Am Acad Child Adol Psychiat 41:1205–1215.

Fendrich M, Warner V, Weissman MM, (1990). Family risk factors, parental depression, and psychopathology in offspring. Dev Psychopathol 26:40–50.

Ferro T, Carlson GA, Grayson P, et al. (1994). Depressive disorders: distinctions in children. J Am Acad Child Adol Psychiatry 33:664–670.

Fleming JE, Offord DR, Boyle MH (1989). Prevalence of child and adolescent depression in the community: Ontario Child Health Study. Br J Psychiatry 155:647–654.

Franz B, Kupfer DJ, Miewald JM, et al. (1995). Growth hormone secretion timing in depression: clinical outcome comparisons. Biol Psychiatry 38:720–729.

Garber J, Little S, Hilsman R, et al. (1998). Family Predictors of suicidal symptoms in young adolescents. J Adolesc 21:445–457.

Garber J, Kris MR, Koch M, Lindholm L (1988). Recurrent depression in adolescents: a follow-up study. J Am Acad Child Adol Psychiatry 27:49–54.

Garrison CZ, Jackson KL, Marsteller F, et al. (1990). A longitudinal study of depressive symptomatology in young adolescents. J Am Acad Child Adolesc Psychiatry 29:581–585.

Goetz RR, Wolk SI, Copla JD, et al. (2001). Premorbid polysomnographic signs in depressed adolescents: a reanalysis of EEG sleep after longitudinal follow-up in adulthood. Biol Psychiatry 49:930–942.

Goodman SH, Gotlib IH (1999). Risk of psychopathology in children of depressed mothers: a developmental model for understanding mechanisms of transmission. Psychol Rev 106:458–490.

Goodyear IM, Herbert J, Altham PME (1998). Adrenal steroid secretion and major depression in 8- to 16-years old, III. Influence of cortisol/DHEA ratio at presentation and subsequent rates of disappointing life vents and persistent major depression. Psychol Med 28: 265–273.

Goodyear IM, Herbert J, Tamplin A, Altham PME (2000). First episode major depression in adolescents: Affective, cognitive, and endocrine characteristics of risk status and predictors of onset. Br J Psychiatry 176:142–149.

Goodyear IM, Herbert J, Tamplin A, Altham PME (2001). Recent life events, cortisol, dehydroepiandrosterone, and the onset of major depression in high-risk adolescents. Br J Psychiatry 177:499–504.

Hammen C, Burge D, Bumey E, Adrian C (1990). Longitudinal study of diagnoses in children of women with unipolar and bipolar affective disorder. Arch Gen Psychiatry 47:1112–1117.

Hammen C, Burge D, Adrian C (1991). Timing of mother and child depression in a longitudinal study of children at risk. J Consul Clin Psychol 59:341–345.

Harrington RC, Fudge H, Rutter ML, Pickles A, Hill J (1990). Adult outcomes of childhood and adolescent depression. I: Psychiatric status. Arch Gen Psychiatry 47:465–473.

Harrington RC, Fudge H, Rutter ML, et al. (1991). Adult outcomes of childhood and adolescent depression. II: Risk for antisocial disorders. J Am Acad Child Adol Psychiatry 30:434–439.

Harrington RC, Dubicka B (2001). Natural History of mood disorders in children and adolescents. In: IM Goodyear, ed. The Depressed Child and Adolescent. 2nd ed. Cambridge, UK: Cambridge University Press, pp 353–371.

Harris TO, Borsanyi S, Messari S, et al. (2001). Morning cortisol as a risk factor fro subsequent major depressive disorder in adult women. Br J Psychiatry 177, 505–510.

Kandel DB, Davies M (1986). Adult sequelae of adolescent depressive symptoms. Arch Gen Psychiatry 43:255–262.

Kaufman J (1991). Depressive disorders in maltreated children. J Am Acad Child Adol Psychiatry 30:257–265.

Kaufman J, Plotsky PM, Nemeroff CB, et al. (2000). Effects of early adverse experiences on brain structure and function: clinical implications. Biol Psychiatry 48:778–790.

Keller MB, Shapiro RW, Lavori PW, Wolfe N (1982). Recovery in major depressive disorder. Arch Gen Psychiatry 39:905–910.

Keller MB, Ryan ND, Strober M, et al. (2001). Efficacy of paroxetine in the treatment of adolescent major depression: a randomized, controlled trial. J Am cad Child Adol Psychiatry 40:762–772.

Kendler KS, Prescott CA (1999). A population-based twin study of lifetime major depression in men and women. Arch Gen Psychiatry 56:39–44.

Kessler RC, Walters EE (1998). Epidemiology of DSM-III-R major depressions and minor depression among adolescents and young adults in the National Comorbidity Survey. Depression Anxiety 7:3–14.

Klein DN, Taylor EB, Harding K, et al. (1988). Double depression and episodic major depression: demographic, clinical familial, personality, and socio-environmental characteristics and short-term outcome. Am J Psychiatry 145:1226–1231.

Klein DN, Lewinsohn PM, Seeley JR, et al. (2001). A family study of major depressive disorder in a community sample of adolescents. Arch Gen Psychiatry 58:13–20.

Kovacs M, Feinberg TL, Crouse-Novack M, et al. (1984a). Depressive disorders in childhood: I. A longitudinal prospective study of characteristics and recovery. Arch Gen Psychiatry 41:229–237.

Kovacs M, Feinberg TL, Crouse-Novack M, et al. (1984b). Depressive disorders in childhood: II. A longitudinal study of the risk for a subsequent major depression. Arch Gen Psychiatry 40:643–649.

Kovacs M, Gatsonis C, Paulauskas SL, et al. (1989). Depressive disorders in childhood: IV. A longitudinal study of comorbidity with and risk for anxiety disorders. Arch Gen Psychiatry 46:776–782.

Kovacs M, Godlston D (1991). Cognitive and social cognitive development of depressed children and adolescents. J Am Acad Child Adolesc Psychiatry 30:388–392.

Kovacs M, Godlston D, Gatsonis C (1993). Suicidal behaviors and childhood-onset depressive disorders: a longitudinal investigation. J Am Acad Child Adol Psychiatry 32:8–20.

Kovacs M, Akiskal HS, Gatsonis C, et al. (1994). Childhood-onset dysthymic disorder. Arch Gen Psychiatry 51:365–374.

Kovacs M (1996). Presentation and course of major depressive disorder during childhood and later years of the life span. J Am Acad Child Adol Psychiatry 35:705–715.

Kovacs M (1997). Chronic depression in childhood. In: HS Akiskal, GB Cassino, eds. Dysthymia and the Spectrum of Chronic Depressions. New York: Guilford Press, pp 208–219.

Kovacs M, Obrosky S, Gatsonis C et al. (1997). First-episode major depressive and dysthymic disorder in childhood: clinical and sociodemographic factors in recovery. J Am Acad Child Adol Psychiatry 36:777–784.

Leonard HL, March J, Rickler KC, et al. (1997). Review of the pharmacology of the selective serotonin reuptake inhibitors in children and adolescents. J Am Acad Child Adolesc Psychiatry 36:725–736.

Lewinsohn PM, Rohde P, Seeley JR, Hops H (1991). Comorbidity of unipolar depression. I: major depression with dysthymia. J Abnorm Psychol 100: 205–213.

Lewinsohn PM, Hops H, Roberts RE, et al. (1993). Adolescent Psychopathology I. Prevalence and incidence of depression and other DSM-III-R disorders in high school students. J Abnorm Psychol 102:133–144.

Lewinsohn PM, Clarke GN, Seeley JR, Rohde P (1994). Major depression in community adolescents: age at onset, episode duration and time to recurrence. J Am Acad Child Adolesc Psychiatry 33:809–818.

Lewinsohn PM, Gotlib IH, Seeley JR (1995a). Adolescent psychopathology: IV. Specificity of psychosocial risk factors for depression and substance abuse in older adolescents. J Am Acad Child Adol Psychiatry 34:1221–1229.

Lewinsohn PM, Rohde P, Seeley JR (1995b). Adolescent psychopathology: the clinical consequences of comorbidity. J Am Acad Child Adol Psychiatry 34:510–519.

Lewinsohn PM, Rohde P, Klein DN, Seeley JR (1999). The natural course of adolescent major depressive disorder. I: Continuity into young adulthood. J Am Acad Child Adol Psychiatry 38:56–63.

Lewinsohn PM, Seeley JR, Solomon A, et al. (2000a). Clinical implications of "subthershold" depressive symptoms. J of Abnorm Psychol 109:345–351.

Lewinsohn PM, Rohde P, Seeley JR, et al. (2000b). Natural course of adolescent major depressive disorder in a community sample: predictors of recurrence in young adults. Am J Psychiatry 157:1584–1591.

McCauley E, Myers K, Mitchell J, et al. (1993). Depression in young people: initial presentation and clinical course. J Am Acad Child Adolesc Psychiatry 32:714–722.

McCauley J, Kern DE, Kolodner K, et al. (1997). Clinical characteristics of women with a history of childhood abuse: unhealed wounds. JAMA 277:1362–1368.

Mitchell J, McCauley E, Burke P (1988). Phenomenology of depression in children and adolescents. J Am Acad Child Adol Psychiatry 27:12–20.

Mufson L, Weissman MM, Moreau D, et al. (1999). Efficacy of interpersonal psychotherapy for depressed adolescents. Arch Gen Psychiatry 56:573–579.

Nachmias M, Gunnar M, Mangelsdorf S (1996). Behavioral inhibition and stress reactivity: the moderating role of attachments security. Child Dev 67:508–522.

Orvaschel H, Walsh Allis G, Ye W (1988). Psychopathology among children of parents with recurrent depression. J Abnorm Child Psychol 16:17–28.

Parker G, Wilhelm K, Asghari A (1997). Early onset depression: the relevance of anxiety. Soc Psychiatry Psychiatr Epidemiol 32:30–37.

Pine DS, Cohen P, Gurley D, et al. (1998). The risk for early adulthood anxiety and depressive disorders in adolescents with anxiety and depressive disorders. Arch Gen Psychiatry 55:56–64

Puig-Antich J, Lukens E, Davies M, et al. (1985a). Psychosocial functioning in prepubertal major depressive disorders. I. Interpersonal relationships during the depressive episode. Arch Gen Psychiatry 42:500–507.

Puig-Antich J, Lukens E, Davies M, et al. (1985b). Psychosocial Functioning in prepubertal major depressive disorders. II. Interpersonal relationships after sustained recovery from affective episode. Arch Gen Psychiatry 42:511–517.

Rao U, Ryan ND, Birmaher B, et al. (1995). Unipolar depression in adolescents: Clinical outcome in adulthood. J Am Acad Child Adol Psychiatry 34:566–577.

Rao U, Dahl RE, Ryan ND, et al. (1996). The relationship between longitudinal clinical course and sleep and cortisol changes in adolescent depression. Biol Psychiatry 40:474–484.

Rao U, Hammen C, Daley SE (1999). Continuity of depression during the transition to adulthood: a 5-year longitudinal study of young women. J Am Acad Child Adol Psychiatry 38:908–915.

Rohde P, Lewinsohn PM, Seeley JR (1991). Comorbidity of unipolar depression: II. Comorbidity with other mental disorders in adolescents and adults. J Abnorm Psychol 100:214–222.

Rossello J, Bernal G (1999). The efficacy of cognitive-behavioral and interpersonal treatments for depression in Puerto Rican adolescents. J Consult Clin Psychol 67:734–745.

Sanford M, Szatmari P, Spinner M, et al. (1995). Predicting the 1-year course of adolescent depression. J Am Acad Child Adol Psychiatry 34: 1618–1628

Silberg J, Pickles A, Rutter M, et al. (1999). The influence of genetic factors and life stress on depression among adolescent girls. Arch Gen Psychiatry 56:225–232.

Simeon J, Dinicola V, Ferguson H, et al. (1990). Adolescent depression: a placebo-controlled fluoxetine treatment study and follow-up. Prog Neuropsychopharmacol Biol Psychiatry 14:791–795.

Sullivan PF, Neale MC, Kendler KS (2000). Genetic epidemiology of major depression: review and meta-analysis. Am J Psychiatry 157:1552–1562.

Thase ME, Kupfer DJ, Buyssee DJ, et al. (1995). Electroencephalographic sleep profiles in single-episode and recurrent unipolar forms of major depression I: Comparison during acute depressive states. Biol Psychiatry 38:506–515.

Verhulst FC, van der Ende J, Ferdinand RF, et al. (1997). The prevalence of DSMIII-R diagnoses in a national sample of Dutch adolescents. Arch Gen Psychiatry 54:329–336.

Warner V, Weissman MM, Fendrich M, et al. (1992). The course of major depression in the offspring of depressed parents: incidence, recurrence, recovery. Arch Gen Psychiatry 49:795–801.

Warner V, Mufson L, Weissman MM (1995). Offspring at high and low risk for depression and anxiety: mechanisms of psychiatric disorder. J Am Acad Child Adolesc Psychiatry 34:786–797.

Warner V, Weissman MM, Mufson L, Wickramaratne PJ (1999). Grandparents, parents, and grandchildren at high risk for depression: a three-generation study. J Am Acad Child Adolesc Psychiatry 38:289–296.

Weissman MM, Bland RC, Canino GJ, et al. (1996). Cross-national epidemiology of major depression and bipolar disorder. JAMA, 276:293–299.

Weissman MM, Warner V, Wickramaratne P, et al. (1997). Offspring of depressed parents: 10 years later. Arch Gen Psychiatry 54:932–990.

Weissman MM, Wolk S, Goldstein RB, et al. (1999a). Depressed adolescents grown up. JAMA 281:1707–1713.

Weissman MM, Wolk S, Wickramaratne P, et al. (1999b). Children with pre-pubertal-onset major depressive disorder and anxiety grown up. Arch Gen Psychiatry 56:794–801.

Weissman MM, Markowitz JC, Klerman GL (2000). Comprehensive guide to interpersonal psychotherapy. New York: Basic Books.

Weisz JR, Thurber CA, Sweeney L, et al. (1997). Brief treatment of mild to moderate child depression using primary and secondary control enhancement training. J Consult Clin Psychol 65:703–707.

Wickramaratne PJ, Weissman MM (1998). Onset of psychopathology in offspring by developmental phase and parental depression. J Am Acad Child Adolesc Psychiatry 37(9):933–942.

Wicki W, Angst J (1991). The Zurich study: X. Hypomania in a 28 to 30 year old cohort. Eur Arch Psychiatry Clin Neurosci 240:339–348.

Williamson DE, Ryan ND, Birmaher B, et al. (1995). A case-control family history study of depression in adolescents. J Am Acad Child Adol Psychiatry 34:1596–1607.

Williamson DE, Birmaher B, Frank E, et al. (1998). Nature of life events and difficulties in depressed adolescents. J Am Acad Child Adol Psychiatry 37:1049–1057.

Zaslow S (2000). Depressed adolescents. In: JD O'Brien, DJ Pilowsky, OW Lewis, eds. Psychotherapies with children and adolescents. Adapting the psychodynamic process. Northvale, NJ: Jason Aronson, pp 209–230.

16

Chronic Depression in Patients with Medical Illness

Donald L. Rosenstein and Kambiz Soleymani
National Institute of Mental Health
National Institutes of Health
Bethesda, Maryland, U.S.A.

June Cai
Miriam Hospital and Brown University
Providence, Rhode Island, U.S.A.

INTRODUCTION

Psychiatric syndromes are both underappreciated and inadequately treated in medically ill patients. This is particularly true for individuals with medical problems who also suffer from chronic depression. The most prevalent medical illnesses in the United States (e.g., heart disease, cancer, cerebrovascular disease) are associated with higher rates of depressive disorders than are seen in the general population [1–4]. Increasingly, psychiatrists are being asked to evaluate and treat patients who are older, have serious medical problems, and take multiple medications, many of which cause central nervous system (CNS) adverse effects and precipitate drug-drug interactions. It is therefore not surprising that these patients present the consulting psychiatrist with multiple diagnostic and psychopharmacologic challenges. This chapter is intended to provide clinicians with general principles and specific recommendations regarding the optimum diagnostic and therapeutic approaches to chronic depression in selected medical illnesses.

GENERAL PRINCIPLES IN THE DIAGNOSIS AND MANAGEMENT OF COMORBID MEDICAL ILLNESS AND CHRONIC DEPRESSION

Begin with a Broad and Medically Oriented Differential Diagnosis

Patients with a medical illness can look depressed when they are not. One of the first questions that a psychiatrist should ask when evaluating a patient who is medically ill and on several medications is: "Is this depression or something else?" The patient with disseminated cancer undergoing chemotherapy is likely to suffer from fatigue, anorexia, weight loss, and insomnia whether a clinical depression is present or absent. A fundamental diagnostic task in the psychiatric evaluation of medically ill patients is teasing apart those symptoms attributable to a primary psychiatric disorder from those symptoms that are due to the underlying medical illness or its treatment.

A wide variety of medical conditions and multiple therapeutic interventions are associated with symptoms of depression. Endocrinopathies (e.g., Cushing's syndrome, hyperthyroidism or hypothyroidism), electrolyte abnormalities (e.g., hypercalcemia, hypomagnesemia), CNS lesions (e.g., stroke, lymphoma), and adverse medication effects (e.g., cytokine or glucocorticoid-induced neuropsychiatric toxicity) are just a few of the many conditions that can produce syndromes phenomenologically indistinguishable from those associated with primary depression. Whenever an underlying medical or metabolic abnormality is judged to be causing or exacerbating a depression, every effort should be made to correct that problem or discontinue/reduce the offending medication prior to (or in some cases, simultaneously with) psychopharmacological intervention. Often in these situations, the adage "less is more" should guide the psychopharmacological management of patients with depression suspected to be due to a general medical condition or medication. Too frequently, the addition of an antidepressant or anxiolytic to a patient's complicated pharmacological regimen results in worsening the clinical picture (e.g., precipitating a delirium or drug-drug interaction) rather than improving it.

Adverse CNS effects of medications are commonly mistaken for depression and anxiety. For example, several antiemetics used routinely by internists and surgeons have clinically significant dopamine-blocking effects (e.g., prochlorperazine, metoclopramide, trimethobenzamide, promethazine, droperidol) and can produce debilitating extrapyramidal system (EPS) effects. Patients treated with these agents can present with either an agitated depression (in the case of akathisia) or a more classic depression with psychomotor retardation (in the case of Parkinsonian symptoms) [5,6]. In one study in which cancer patients were asked about symptoms of akathisia [7], half of the study group treated with prochlorperazine (Compazine) or metoclopramide (Reglan) had experienced akathisia, and 75% of those patients noted that they would not have mentioned it to the hospital staff if they had not been specifically asked. The more recently released 5-HT3–blocking antiemetics (e.g., ondansetron [Zofran] and granisetron [Kytril]) are not associated with akathisia.

Delirium and pain also create diagnostic confusion regarding depressive symptoms observed in both hospitalized and ambulatory medically ill patients. Although the acutely agitated and floridly disorganized patient is usually correctly diagnosed with delirium, the patient with a more chronic, withdrawn, hypoactive delirium [8] is often mistakenly thought to be depressed and inappropriately treated with antidepressants. Similarly, patients who are irritable and short tempered because of inadequate pain control are often judged to be depressed and referred for psychiatric evaluation. That the pain associated with cancer and other chronic illnesses is frequently undertreated is one of the most well-established, enduring, and unfortunate practices in medicine [9]. Often it falls to the psychiatric consultant to elicit a careful pain history and communicate to the primary care provider the need for more aggressive analgesia.

Research approaches to the differential diagnosis of depression in the medically ill have been "inclusive" (counting all depressive symptoms toward a diagnosis of major depression [10] irrespective of their suspected etiopathogenesis), "exclusive" (counting only those symptoms judged not to be attributable to the medical condition), and "substitutive" (substituting other depressive symptoms for the neurovegetative symptoms of anorexia, sleep disturbance, anergia, and difficulty concentrating) [11]. In clinical practice, constantly changing medical and pharmacological circumstances can frustrate even the most rigorous diagnostic efforts to determine if a syndromal depression is present or not. In borderline cases, a personal or family history of major depression and the presence of symptoms such as excessive guilt, poor self-esteem, anhedonia, and ruminative thinking strengthen the argument for a diagnosis of comorbid depression. Our approach is to deemphasize the importance of arbitrary diagnostic thresholds and instead focus on interventions that alleviate specific target symptoms.

When Depression Is Present, It Should Be Considered a Serious and Compelling Complication of Medical Illness

Unfortunately, there is a pervasive tendency on the part of healthcare professionals, family members, and patients to view symptoms of depression, regardless of their severity and duration, as "understandable" and "appropriate" reactions to serious medical illness. Too often this perspective functions as a barrier to therapeutic interventions and patients suffer unnecessarily. While sadness, demoralization, worry, and difficulty concentrating are all predictable and normative responses to illness, major depression is a neurobiological complication of medical illness that should be treated aggressively with all of our psychotherapeutic and psychopharmacological tools. Unless there are specific contraindications (see below), we recommend an empiric trial of antidepressant pharmacotherapy, preferably in the setting of a supportive psychotherapy, for medically ill patients with a clinically significant depression. Furthermore, as the number of well-tolerated, safe, and effective antidepressants has grown, we have lowered our threshold for employing pharmacotherapy in the treatment of chronic and subsyndromal depression in the medical setting.

Anticipate Drug-Drug Interactions

Since polypharmacy is the rule rather than the exception in medically ill patients, the likelihood of medication intolerance or an adverse drug-drug interaction is a constant concern in this population. Although many drug-drug interactions are problematic, few are life threatening (e.g., the use of monamine oxidase inhibitors with meperidine [Demerol] or selective serotonin reuptake inhibitors). In some respects, the proliferation of preclinical data suggesting *potential* drug interactions has had a disorienting and paralyzing effect on clinicians. For medically ill patients on multiple medications, the risk of an adverse drug-drug interaction is real but not sufficient in most cases to withhold treatment.

Knowledge of drug metabolism and drug-drug interactions is growing at an astounding pace. A number of excellent reviews of the cytochrome P450 system and its importance in psychopharmacology have been published in the last few years [12–16]. There is also an extensive internet-based clinical pharmacology resource maintained by David Flockhart, M.D., Ph.D., from the Division of Clinical Pharmacology at the Indiana University School of Medicine. This website, which includes an up-to-date drug interaction chart and search mechanism, can be found at http://www.drug-interactions.com.

Since it is neither desirable nor possible to remember all the possible drug interactions our patients may be exposed to, the many available summary tables of cytochrome P450 isoenzyme drug interactions have become indispensable to psychiatrists. In Table 1 (provided by Terence Ketter, M.D.), the major hepatic cytochrome (CYP) P450 isoenzymes are listed across the top of the table. A substrate is a medication metabolized by a given isoenzyme. Two medications that are both substrates for the same isoenzyme are competitive inhibitors of that isoenzyme. In addition to being substrates for given isoenzymes, medications (as well as nicotine and even grapefruit juice) can function as specific inhibitors and inducers of isoenzymes. It should be stressed that Table 1 is neither complete nor necessarily indicative of harmful drug interactions. For example, an interaction may change the blood level of a medication within a range that is without clinical consequences. Often a simple preemptive dose reduction will allow for the safe combination of medications. Indeed, certain drug interactions can be exploited for clinical benefit. For instance, nefazodone can be used to relieve alprazolam interdose rebound anxiety [17].

Chronic Depression Results in Deleterious Medical Consequences

In addition to the direct psychosocial suffering associated with depression, recent clinical studies provide several examples of pathophysiological consequences of chronic depression. A recent supplement to the *American Heart Journal* [18] examined the extensive evidence establishing major depression as an independent risk factor for ischemic heart disease (IHD). Michelson et al. [19] demonstrated that women with a history of major depression had significantly lower mean bone mineral density compared with women without a history of depression. This same research group at the National Institute of Mental Health is currently pursuing preliminary indications that chronic depression is associated with alterations in intermediate glucose metabolism. These examples are compelling reminders that chronic depression can be both a consequence of and contributing factor in the development of medical illness. Whether specific therapeutic interventions will mitigate these pathological effects remains an important and unanswered question.

Chronic Depression Is Difficult to Treat in the Medically Ill: Patience and Persistence Are Necessary

Several factors make the treatment of chronic depression in patients with medical problems particularly problematic. As described in earlier chapters chronic depression, even in the absence of complicating medical problems, tends to be less responsive to psychotherapeutic and pharmacological

TABLE 1 Major CYP Isoenzymes and Their Respective Substrates, Inhibitors, and Inducers

CYP	CYP1A2	CYP2C9/10	CYP2C19ᵃ	CYP2D6ᵃ	CYP2E1	CYP3A3/4
% of all CYPᵇ	13	20 (for all 2C)		2	7	30 (for all 3A)
Substrates	Fluvoxamine 3° Amine TCAs (N-demethylation) Clozapine (major) Olanzapine Caffeine Methadone Tacrine Acetaminophen Phenacetin Propranolol Theophylline	THC NSAIDs Phenytoin (major) Tolbutamide S-warfarin	Citalopram (partly) Moclobemide 3° amine TCAs (N-demethylation) Diapezam (N-demethylation) Hexobarbital Mephobarbital Lansoprazole Omeprazole (5-hydroxylation) Rabeprazole (demethylation) Phenytoin (minor) S-mephenytoin Nelfinavir	Fluoxetine (partly) Mirtazapine (partly) Paroxetine Venlafaxine (O-de-methylation) 2° and 3° amine TCAs (2,8,10-hydroxylation) Trazodone Clozapine (minor) Haloperidol (reduction) Fluphenazine Perphenazine Risperidone Sertindole Thioridazine	Ethanol Acetaminophen Chlorzoxazone Halothane Isoflurane Methoxyflurane Savoflurane	Carbamazepine Alprazolam Diazepam (hydroxylation and N-demethylation) Midazolam Triazolam Zolpidem Buspirone Citalopram (partly) Mirtazepine(partly) Nefrazodone Reboxetine Sertraline 3° amine TCAs (N-demethylation) Sertindole Quetiapine Ziprasidone Amiodarone Disopyramide Lidocaine Propafenone Quinidine Erythromycin (macrolides) Androgens Dexamethasone Estrogens (steroids) Astemizole Loratadine Terfenadine Lovastatin Simvastatin Atorvastatin Cerivastatin (HMG-CoAR Inhib)

	Substrates	Inhibitors
		Fluvoxamine, Moclobemide, Cimetidine, Fluoroquinolines (ciprofloxacin, norfloxacin), Naringenin (grapefruit), Ticlopidine
		Fluvoxamine, Disulfiram, Amiodarone, Azapropazone, d-Propoxyphene, Fluconazole, Fluvastatin, Miconazole, Phenylbutazone, Stiripentol, Sulfaphenazole, Zafirlukast
		Fluoxetine, Fluvoxamine, Imipramine, Moclobemide, Tranylcypromine, Diazepam, Felbamate, Phenytoin, Topiramate, Cimetidine, Omeprazole
	Codeine (hydroxylation, C-demethylation), Dextromethorphan (O-demethylation), Hydrocodone, Oxycodone, Mexiletine, Propafenone (1C-antiarrhythmics), Beta blockers, Donepezil (partly), d- and l-fenfluramine	Bupropion, Fluoxetine, Fluvoxamine (weak), Hydroxybupropion, Paroxetine, Sertraline (weak), Moclobemide, Fluphenazine, Haloperidol, Perphenazine, Thioridazine, Amiodarone, Cimetidine, Methadone, Quinidine, Ritonavir
		Diethyldithiocarbamate (disulfiram metabolite)
	Diltiazem, Felodipine, Nimodipine, Nifedipine, Nisoldipine, Nitrendipine, Verapamil, Acetaminophen, Alfentanil, Codeine (demthylation), Fentanyl, Sufentanil, Ethosuximide, Tiagabine, Cyclophosphamide, Tamoxifen, Vincristine, Vinblastine, Ifosfamide, Cyclosporine, Tacrolimus, Cisapride, Donepezil (partly), Lovastatine, Omeprazole/rabeprazole (sulfonation), Protease inhibitors, Sildenafil	Fluoxetine, Fluvoxamine, Nefazodone, Sertraline (weak), Diltiazem, Verapamil, Dexamethasone, Gestodene, Clarithromycin, Erythromycin, Troleandomycin (macrolides), Fluconazole, Itraconazole, Ketoconazole (azole antifungals), Ritonavir, Indinavir (protease inhibitors), Amiodarone, Cimetidine, Mibefradil, Naringenin (grapefruit)

Inhibitors

TABLE 1 Continued

CYP	CYP1A2	CYP2C9/10	CYP2C19[a]	CYP2D6[a]	CYP2E1	CYP3A3/4
% of all CYP[b]	13	20 (for all 2C)		2	7	30 (for all 3A)
Inducers	Tobacco Omeprazole	Barbiturates Phenytoin Rifampin	Rifampin		Ethanol Isoniazid	Carbamazepine Barbiturates Phenobarbital Phenytoin St. John's wort
Substrates	Haloperidol Phenothiazines Thiothixene Verapamil	Diazepam Methadone 3°TCAS	Propranolol	Ecanide Flecanide Maprotiline Sertraline		Clonazepam Dapsone Lidocaine Methadone Guinidine Venlafaxine
Inhibitors	Isoniazid Enoxacin Ofloxacin Ritinovir St. John's wort	Cimetidine		Isoniazid		Nelfinavir Delavirdine
Inducers	Brussel sprouts Cabbage Charbroiled food	Carbamazepine	Barbiturates Carbamazepine Phenytoin			Nevirapine

[a] Clinically significant human polymorphism reported.
[b] CYP percentages from Ref. 13a.
Source: Adapted from Ref. 13.

intervention than an acute episode of major depression. It has also been the experience of many clinicians who work at the interface of medicine and psychiatry that depression, whether acute or chronic, is somewhat less likely to respond to treatment when comorbid medical problems are present [20]. A central problem in this regard is the fact that most medical problems are not stable over time and therefore make it more difficult to evaluate therapeutic interventions. An additional concern is that, whether appropriate or not, medical problems tend to be viewed as more pressing and important than depression. Consequently, significant depressive symptoms may be tolerated for long periods of time by physicians and patients simply because somatic symptoms are viewed as more worthy of attention. Even when a diagnosis of major depression is made correctly, understandable pharmacotherapeutic caution in debilitated patients often leads to medication trials that are inadequate in terms of antidepressant dose and duration. Although "start low and go slow" is a wise approach in this population, persistence in achieving the usual clinical outcomes is just as important for these patients as for patients who are medically healthy but psychiatrically ill. The net result of these factors is that by the time patients receive an appropriate evaluation for depression, they may well have endured unnecessarily long and severe suffering. One of the most important challenges for the consulting psychiatrist is to convince the patient and their primary care provider that the depression is not a necessary component of their medical condition. Finally, for all of the reasons discussed above, close communication with colleagues from medicine, surgery, nursing, and other disciplines is essential for the optimum management of the chronically depressed and medically ill.

SELECTED MEDICAL DISORDERS AND CHRONIC DEPRESSION

Cancer

Major depression and subsyndromal depressive disorders are very common in patients with cancer. Prevalence rates vary from as low as 5% to greater than 50% depending on how depression is defined, whether study samples are drawn from outpatient clinics or hospital wards, and the type of cancer involved [2,21,22]. Untreated depression has been linked to poor compliance with medical care, increased pain and disability [23], and a greater likelihood to consider euthanasia and physician-assisted suicide [24]. Whether the benefits of treating depression extend beyond quality of life issues [25] and can improve immunocompetence and survival is an intriguing possibility.

Although there are some preliminary data in support of this hypothesis, the existing evidence is far from conclusive [26].

The impetus for psychopharmacological interventions in cancer patients is often the presence of severe neurovegetative symptoms (e.g., anorexia, weight loss, sleep disturbance, fatigue, and weakness). In this context, choosing an antidepressant becomes a process of matching these target symptoms with anticipated adverse effects of medications. Mirtazepine (Remeron) has several properties (i.e., sedation, weight gain, antiemesis, low drug-drug interaction potential) that make it a first-line choice for patients with cancer or other wasting illnesses (e.g., AIDS). For the patient with a profound sleep disturbance and who is free of cardiovascular disease, a sedating tricyclic antidepressant (TCA) such as imipramine or amitriptyline can also be very effective. Alternatively, to minimize anticholinergic effects and orthostatic hypotension, nortriptyline (start at 10 or 25 mg per day and increase as tolerated) combined with a sedative-hypnotic (e.g., lorazepam, 0.5–2.0 mg q HS) is an established and well-tolerated treatment approach. In addition to their mood-enhancing effects, TCAs are associated with weight gain, have well-established analgesic properties, and allow for therapeutic blood level monitoring.

Selective serotonin reuptake inhibitors (SSRIs) are frequently useful for depressed cancer patients as long as gastrointestinal symptoms are not prominent. It is particularly important for patients with chemotherapy-related nausea to start with low doses of SSRIs and gradually advance the dose as tolerated. For oncology patients, SSRI-related drug interactions (in particular, interactions due to fluvoxamine and fluoxetine) are often clinically relevant. This is also true for nefazodone (Serzone), which is a potent inhibitor of CYP 3A3/4 (see Table 1).

Although there have only been a few prospective, double-blind, placebo-controlled studies of psychostimulants (i.e., methylphenidate and dextroamphetamine) in medically ill depressed patients [27–29], the literature is replete with large series of case reports and retrospective studies suggesting rapid (within days) and significant mood improvement in medically ill patients treated with psychostimulants [30]. The two main concerns many internists have regarding psychostimulant use in the oncology setting are appetite suppression and abuse potential. In practice, there is compelling evidence that appetite and weight changes due to depression are more likely to be improved than impaired with stimulants [30]. Medically ill patients are also unlikely to become tolerant of or to abuse stimulants [30]. Psychostimulant dosage ranges 5–20 mg twice a day (8:00 am and noon) for methylphenidate (Ritalin) and dextroamphetamine (Dexedrine).

Heart Disease

Numerous associations have been reported between depression and cardiovascular disease [4,31–33]. One of the most compelling series of studies to emerge in recent years links depression with mortality from cardiovascular disease [4,34,35]. For example, Frasure-Smith and colleagues, at the Montreal Heart Institute, demonstrated that depression at the time of a myocardial infarction (MI) is an independent risk factor for post-MI mortality at 6 and 18 months [36,37]. Furthermore, depressed patients who also had ≥ 10 PVCs per hour at the time of their MI had the highest subsequent mortality. One explanation for the increased cardiac mortality in depressed patients may be a higher prevalence of ventricular tachycardia (in depressed patients with coronary artery disease) compared with coronary artery disease patients who are not depressed [38]. Another potential explanation for this observation is abnormalities in platelet aggregation [35]. Whether the effective treatment of depression in this setting will increase survival time is an answerable question currently under investigation. In the meantime, the alleviation of depression improves both quality of life and functional outcome [39], and thus provides a compelling justification for a proactive treatment approach regardless of whether survival time is prolonged.

The safety and effectiveness of antidepressant pharmacotherapy in patients with IHD has received considerable attention in recent years [40–42]. TCAs have been studied most extensively in these patients and have been shown to be effective but less well tolerated and associated with significantly more serious adverse effects as compared with SSRIs. In addition to the common cardiovascular side effects of orthostatic hypotension and tachycardia, the principal concern with TCAs has been their potential life-threatening proarrhythmic effects. TCAs are class I antiarrhythmics (similar to quinidine). However, like other antiarrhythmics, they can induce arrhythmias under some circumstances. The first phase of the Cardiac Arrhythmia Suppression Trial (CAST I) was stopped in 1989 when it became clear that two class IC antiarrhythmic agents (flecainide and encainide) were associated with more deaths than placebo [43]. A few years later, CAST II was also stopped early when a class IA antiarrhythmic, moricizine, also increased mortality [44]. One explanation for this phenomenon is that these agents are antiarrhythmic in healthy myocardium but proarrhythmic in ischemic myocardium [45]. The practical consequences of these findings are that TCAs should be used with great caution, if at all, in patients with known or suspected heart disease.

Because SSRIs are essentially free of the cardiovascular adverse effects seen with TCAs and are generally well tolerated, they have emerged as the antidepressants of first choice for depressed patients with heart disease.

Despite one comparative study [46] of severely depressed elderly patients with cardiovascular disease that demonstrated a significantly greater response rate to nortriptyline than to fluoxetine, recent trials of SSRIs for comorbid depression and IHD are encouraging [41,42]. Potential SSRI drug interactions with beta blockers and antiarrhythmics (see Table 1) are indications for lower starting doses of SSRIs (fluoxetine [Prozac], 10 mg, sertraline [Zoloft], 25 mg, paroxetine [Paxil], 10 mg, citalopram [Celexa] 10 mg) and careful monitoring of cardiovascular status.

Experience with other recently released antidepressants in patients with heart disease is quite limited. Bupropion (Wellbutrin) can cause increases in blood pressure but has not been associated with cardiac conduction effects [47]. While nefazodone (Serzone) also appears to have a relatively benign cardiovascular side effect profile, isolated case reports have described asymptomatic bradycardia with its use. A more likely problem with nefazodone in cardiac patients on multiple medications is the potential for drug-drug interactions (see Table 1) that may lead to cardiac conduction disturbances. Venlafaxine (Effexor) raises blood pressure in a dose dependent fashion but appears to be relatively free of significant drug interactions [48]. Similarly, citalopram (Celexa) and mirtazapine (Remeron) appear to be associated with few clinically significant drug interactions, and although not studied extensively in patients with heart disease, to date they have not been associated with clinically significant cardiovascular adverse effects. Nonetheless, since so few data are available concerning the effectiveness of the newer antidepressants in patients with heart disease, treatment recommendations in this clinical setting must be considered preliminary.

Psychostimulants, such as methylphenidate and dextroamphetamine, have been used safely and successfully in patients with stable heart disease but should be avoided in patients with hypertension and arrhythmias [30]. Similarly, MAOIs are generally poor choices for patients with comorbid heart disease because of orthostatic hypotension and the potential for a hypertensive crisis and other drug interactions.

Cerebrovascular Disease

Several lines of investigation suggest that depression and cerebrovascular disease are related to each other in clinically relevant ways. First, it appears that some depressions that develop later in life are secondary to multiple small brain infarcts (vascular depression) [49]. Second, preliminary evidence suggests that depression may be a risk factor for stroke [50]. Third, post–stroke depression affects 30–50% of patients and can profoundly impede rehabilitation efforts. Even when patients do not develop depression in the aftermath of a stroke, apathy and pathological crying are two frequent symptoms that bring patients to the attention of a psychiatrist.

Although numerous studies have demonstrated the superiority of antidepressants to placebo for post–stroke depression [51], the psychopharmacological management of these patients is complicated by a number of factors. TCAs are effective but poorly tolerated because of anticholinergic effects, such as excessive sedation and orthostatic hypotension. Nortriptyline has been the TCA studied most often and with the greatest success in post–stroke depression. Nonetheless, many patients are still unable to complete a trial of nortriptyline owing to adverse effects. Two common concerns in the treatment of post–stroke patients are risk of seizures, making bupropion and to some extent TCAs problematic choices [52], and delirium, which should preclude treatment with any antidepressant. When the post–stroke clinical presentation is not complicated by delirium, SSRIs and psychostimulants (especially methylphenidate) are attractive antidepressant choices. Once again, drug-drug interactions are important to monitor in these patients who are likely to be on anticonvulsants for treatment or prophylaxis of seizures.

Parkinson's Disease

Parkinson's disease (PD) is a progressive and disabling neurological disorder with typical onset later in life. The prevalence of depression in PD has been estimated to be as high as 40% depending on how depressive symptoms are defined with respect to severity and duration [53]. Unfortunately, depression is often not adequately identified and managed in this group of patients. The accurate diagnosis of depression in patients with PD is complicated by considerable overlap of clinical signs and symptoms (e.g., early morning awakening, anxiety, motor slowing, fatigue, weight loss, and poor concentration). Early onset of Parkinsonian symptoms and a family history of PD are risk factors for depression [54]. Other risk factors include previous episodes of depression and greater functional disability due to PD. Patients with PD and comorbid depression show faster deterioration of their cognitive and physical skills than nondepressed PD patients [55].

Given the high prevalence of depression in PD patients and the observation that depression contributes to deterioration in their activities of daily living [56], psychiatric evaluation and active treatment of chronic depression should be considered standard of care in this population. Once again, since most PD patients are elderly and on multiple medications, drug-drug interactions are often clinically relevant. Because SSRIs have a better tolerability profile, they are the first-line choice for treatment of depression in PD. Nonetheless, some patients find that SSRIs can exacerbate symptoms such as tremors and rigidity. Although TCAs have been shown to be effective in the treatment of depression in PD, they should be used with caution in this setting because of their anticholinergic properties (especially in patients with concomitant heart disease, prostatic enlargement, and glaucoma). Consequently, low starting doses of any antidepressant should be employed in PD patients. Additionally, there have been a few reports of an interaction between selegiline and SSRIs causing the patients to exhibit signs of the serotonin syndrome. Finally, Wellbutrin is an appealing antidepressant for patients with PD because of its indirect dopaminergic properties. In one clinical trial, Wellbutrin improved not only symptoms of depression but also some of the Parkinsonian motor symptoms [57]. In pharmacologically unresponsive patients with depression and PD, electroconvulsive therapy can be effective for both depressive symptoms and the muscle rigidity associated with PD [54].

ELECTROCONVULSIVE THERAPY

Electroconvulsive therapy (ECT) is one of the safest and most effective treatments available for the treatment of depression. Unfortunately, ECT is frequently considered a treatment of last resort, if it is considered at all, for depressed patients in the medical setting. For the medically ill patient who has suffered from a severe and chronic depression, particularly for the elderly and delusional patient, ECT should be considered a first-line therapeutic option. Patients who have failed several adequate medication trials, develop intolerable medication adverse effects, or are actively suicidal are particularly good candidates for ECT. The following medical conditions have traditionally been considered contraindications for ECT: space-occupying intracerebral lesions; recent (with the past few months) myocardial infarction; cerebral aneurysm; recent cerebral hemorrhage; and patients for whom general anesthesia is considered high risk. In recent years, the thinking about ECT has shifted away from lists of absolute medical contraindications to a case-by-case approach to risk-benefit determinations [58].

CONCLUSION

There is ample room to improve both our conceptual and therapeutic armamentarium in the treatment of chronic depression associated with medical illness. As the physiological consequences of chronic depression become ever clearer, we are moving toward a more integrated approach to the prevention, diagnosis, and management of comorbid psychiatric and medical illness. Both compassionate care and compelling science argue for a more proactive and aggressive therapeutic approach to these patients. A systematic, safe, and effective approach to these challenging patients can be summarized as follows:

1. Focus the initial work-up on physiological and pharmacological sources of depressive symptoms.
2. Correct metabolic abnormalities and remove or decrease offending pharmacological agents.
3. Set the same treatment goals for the patient with comorbid depression and medical illness as you would for the patient with a primary depressive illness (albeit with greater caution regarding dose initiation and escalation).
4. Choose medications on the basis of therapeutic effects, adverse effects, and predicted CYP isoenzyme interactions with current medications.

For many patients with comorbid medical illness and chronic depression, especially for patients with cardiovascular illness, SSRIs have become first-line agents. However, the adverse effect profile of SSRIs makes them intolerable for many cancer patients and others with gastrointestinal symptoms and weight loss. Although mirtazepine (Remeron) has not been extensively studied in medically ill patients, it possesses several properties (i.e., it is sedating, causes increased appetite and weight gain, has antiemetic effects, and has a favorable drug-drug interaction profile) that make it an attractive antidepressant in this population. TCAs are still excellent choices in selected patients provided they are free of IHD. Psychostimulants continue to be underutilized because of largely unfounded concerns about appetite suppression, weight loss, tolerance, and abuse. Additionally, psychostimulants have one substantial advantage over other antidepressants in the medical setting: more rapid onset of effectiveness.

Rapidly evolving knowledge of drug metabolism by cytochrome P450 enzymes promises a more rational basis for medication selection. Much work remains in differentiating potential and unimportant drug interactions from clinically relevant interactions. As psychiatrists care for sicker and more complicated patients, the need for well-designed studies to guide the pharmacological management of depressed and medically ill patients will become increasingly important.

REFERENCES

1. Kessler RC, McGonagle KA, Zhao S, Nelson CB, Hughes M, Eshleman S, Wittchen H, Kendler KS. Lifetime and 12-month prevalence of DSM-III-R psychiatric disorders in the United States: results from the National Comorbidity Survey. Arch Gen Psychiatry 1994; 51:8–19.

2. Cassem EH. Depressive disorders in the medically ill: an overview. Psychosomatics 1995; 36:S2–S10.

3. Wells KB, Golding JM, Burnam MA. Psychiatric disorder in a sample of the general population with and without chronic medical conditions. Am J Psychiatry 1988; 145:976–981.

4. Musselman DL, Evans DL, Nemeroff CB. The relationship of depression to cardiovascular disease: epidemiology, biology, and treatment. Arch Gen Psychiatry 1998; 55:580–592.

5. Ferrando SJ, Eisendrath SJ. Adverse neuropsychiatric effects of dopamine antagonist medications: misdiagnosis in the medical setting. Psychosomatics 1991; 32:426–432.

6. Dukoff R, Horak ID, Hassan R, Rosenstein DL. Akathisia associated with prochlorperazine as an antiemetic: a case report. Ann Oncol 1996; 7:103–104.

7. Fleishman SB, Lavin MR, Sattler M, Szarka H. Antiemetic-induced akathisia in cancer patients receiving chemotherapy. Am J Psychiatry 1994; 151: 763–765.

8. Meagher DJ, Trzepacz PT. Motoric subtypes of delirium. Semin Clin Neuropsychiatry 2000; 5:75–85.

9. Jacox A, Carr DB, Payne R, Berde CB, Brietbart W, Cain JM, Chapman CR, Cleeland CS, Ferrell BR, Finley RS, Hester NO, Hill CS, Jr, Leak WD, Lipman AG, Logan CL, McGarvey CL, Miaskowski CA, Mulder DS, Paice JA, Shapiro BS, Silberstein EB, Smith RS, Stover J, Tsou CV, Vecchiarelli L, Weissman DE. Management of cancer pain. Clinical practice guideline no. 9 AHCPR publication no. 94-0592. Rockville, MD: US Department of Health and Human Services, Public Health Service, 1994.

10. Diagnostic and Statistical Manual of Mental Disorders. 4th ed. Washington, DC: American Psychiatric Association, 1994.

11. Endicott J. Measurement of depression in patients with cancer. Cancer 1984; 53:2243–2248.

12. Nemeroff CB, DeVane CL, Pollock BG. Newer antidepressants and the cytochrome P450 system. Am J Psychiatry 1996; 153:311–320.

13. Ketter TA, Flockhart DA, Post RM, Denicoff KD, Pazzaglia PJ, Marangell LA, George MS, Callahan AM. The emerging role of cytochrome P450 3A in psychopharmacology. J Clin Psychopharmacol 1995; 15:387–398.

13a. Shimada T, Yamazaki H, Mimura M, Inui Y, Guengerich FP. Interindividual variations in human liver cytochrome P-450 enzymes involved in the oxidation of drugs, carcinogens and toxic chemicals: studies with liver microsomes of 30 Japanese and 30 Caucasians. J Pharmacol Exp 1994; 70:414–423.

14. Riesenman C. Antidepressant drug interactions and the cytochrome P450 system: a critical appraisal. Pharmacotherapy 1995; 15:84S–99S.

15. Pollock BG. Recent developments in drug metabolism of relevance to psychiatrists. Harvard Rev Psychiatry 1994; 2:204–213.

16. Ereshefsky L, Riesenman C, Lam YWF. Antidepressant drug interactions and the cytochrome P450 system: the role of cytochrome P450 2D6. Clin Pharmacokinet 1995; 29:10–19.

17. Ketter TA, Callahan AM, Post RM. Nefazodone relief of alprazolam inter-

dose dysphoria: a potential therapeutic benefit of 3A3/4 inhibition. J Clin Psychiatry 1996; 57:307.

18. Nemeroff CB, O'Connor CM. Depression as a risk factor for cardiovascular and cerebrovascular disease: emerging data and clinical perspectives. Am Heart J 2000; 140:555–556.
19. Michelson D, Stratakis C, Reynolds J, Galliven E, Chrousos G, Gold P. Bone mineral density in women with depression. N Engl J Med 1996; 335: 664–666.
20. Akiskal HS. Factors associated with incomplete recovery in primary depressive illness. J Clin Psychiatry 1982; 43:266–271.
21. McDaniel JS, Musselman DL, Porter MR, Reed DA, Nemeroff CB. Depression in patients with cancer: diagnosis, biology, and treatment. Arch Gen Psychiatry 1995; 52:89–99.
22. Lynch ME. The assessment and prevalence of affective disorders in advanced cancer. J Palliat Care 1995; 11:10–18.
23. Spiegel D, Sands S, Koopman C. Pain and depression in patients with cancer. Cancer 1994; 74:2570–2578.
24. Emanuel EJ, Fairclough DL, Daniels ER, Clarridge BR. Euthanasia and physician-assisted suicide: attitudes and experiences of oncology patients, oncologists, and the public. Lancet 1996; 347:1805–1810.
25. Classen C, Butler LD, Koopman C, Miller E, DiMiceli S, Giese-Davis J, Fobair P, Carlson RW, Kraemer HC, Spiegel D. Supportive-expressive group therapy and distress in patients with metastatic breast cancer: a randomized clinical intervention trial. Arch Gen Psychiatry 2001; 58:494–501
26. Goodwin PJ, Leszcz M, Ennis M, Koopmans J, Vincent L, Guther H, Drysdale E, Hundleby M, Chochinov HM, Navarro M, Speca M, Hunter J. The effect of group psychosocial support on survival in metastatic breast cancer. N Engl J Med 2001; 345:1719–1726.
27. Wallace AE, Kofoed LL, West AN. Double-blind, placebo-controlled trial of methylphenidate in older, depressed, medically ill patients. Am J Psychiatry 1995; 152:929–931.
28. Breitbart W, Rosenfeld B, Kaim M, Funesti-Esch J. A randomized, double-blind, placebo-controlled trial of psychostimulants for the treatment of fatigue in ambulatory patients with human immunodeficiency virus disease. Arch Intern Med 2001; 161:411–420.
29. Grade C, Redford B, Chrostowski J, Toussaint L, Blackwell B. Methylphenidate in early poststroke recovery: a double-blind, placebo-controlled study. Arch Phys Med Rehabil 1998; 79:1047–1050.
30. Masand PS, Tesar GE. Use of stimulants in the medically ill. Psychiatr Clin North Am 1996; 19:515–547.
31. Anda R, Williamson D, Jones D, Macera C, Eaker E, Glassman A, Marks J. Depressed affect, hopelessness, and the risk of ischemic heart disease in a cohort of U.S. adults. Epidemiology 1993; 4:285–294.
32. Littman AB. Review of psychosomatic aspects of cardiovascular disease. Psychother Psychosom 1993; 60:148–167.

33. Shapiro PA. Psychiatric aspects of cardiovascular disease. Psychiatr Clin North Am 1996; 19:613–629.
34. Glassman AH, Shapiro PA. Depression and the course of coronary artery disease. Am J Psychiatry 1998; 155:4–11.
35. Nemeroff CB, Musselman DL. Are platelets the link between depression and ischemic heart disease? Am Heart J 2000; 140:S57–S62.
36. Frasure-Smith N, Lesperance F, Talajic M. Depression following myocardial infarction: impact on 6-month survival. JAMA 1993; 270:1819–1825.
37. Frasure-Smith N, Lesperance F, Talajic M. Depression and 18-month prognosis after myocardial infarction. Circulation 1995; 91:999–1005.
38. Carney RM, Freedland KE, Rich MW, Smith LJ, Jaffe AS. Ventricular tachycardia and psychiatric depression in patients with coronary artery disease. Am J Med 1993; 95:23–28.
39. Katon W, Sullivan M, Russo J, Dobie R, Sakai C. Depressive symptoms and measures of disability: a prospective study. J Affect Disord 1993; 27:245–254.
40. Glassman AH, Roose SP, Bigger JT Jr. The safety of tricyclic antidepressants in cardiac patients: risk-benefit reconsidered. JAMA 1993; 269:2673–2675.
41. Nelson JC, Kennedy JS, Pollock BG, Laghrissi-Thode F, Narayan M, Nobler MS, Robin DW, Gergel I, McCafferty J, Roose S. Treatment of major depression with nortriptyline and paroxetine in patients with ischemic heart disease. Am J Psychiatry 1999; 156:1024–1028.
42. Shapiro PA, Lesperance F, Frasure-Smith N, O'Connor CM, Baker B, Jiang JW, Dorian P, Harrison W, Glassman AH. An open-label preliminary trial of sertraline for the treatment of major depression after acute myocardial infarction (the SADHAT Trial). Sertraline Anti-Depressant Heart Attack Trial. Am Heart J 1999; 137:1100–1106.
43. Cardiac Arrhythmia Suppression Trial (CAST) Investigators. Preliminary report: effect of encainide and flecainide on mortality in a randomized trial of arrhythmia suppression after myocardial infarction. N Engl J Med 1989; 321:406–412.
44. Cardiac Arrhythmia Suppression Trial (CAST) II Investigators. Effect of the antiarrhythmic agent moricizine on survival after myocardial infarction. N Engl J Med 1992; 327:227.
45. Roose SP; Glassman AH. Antidepressant choice in the patient with cardiac disease: lessons from the cardiac arrhythmia suppression trial (CAST) studies. J Clin Psychiatry 1994; 55:83–87.
46. Roose SP, Glassman AH, Attia E, Woodring S. Comparative efficacy of selective serotonin reuptake inhibitors and tricyclics in the treatment of melancholia. Am J Psychiatry 1994; 151:1735–1739.
47. Stoudemire A. New antidepressant drugs and the treatment of depression in the medically ill patient. Psychiatr Clin North Am 1996; 19:495–514.
48. Ereshefsky L. Drug-drug interactions involving antidepressants: focus on venlafaxine. J Clin Psychopharmacol 1996; 16:37S–53S.
49. Krishnan KRR, Hays JC, Blazer DG. MRI-defined vascular depression. Am J Psychiatry 1997; 154:497–501.

50. Krishnan KRR. Depression as a contributing factor in cerebrovascular disease. Am Heart J 2000; 140:70–76.
51. Robinson RG. Psychiatric management of stroke. Psychiatr Ann 2002; 32:121–127.
52. Rosenstein DL, Nelson JC, Jacobs SC. Seizures associated with antidepressants: a review. J Clin Psychiatry 1993; 54:289–299.
53. Hoogendijk WJG, Sommer IEC, Tissingh G, Deeg DJH, Wolters EC. Depression in Parkinson's disease: the impact of symptom overlap on prevalence. Psychosomatics 1998; 39:416–421.
54. Cummings JL, Masterman DL. Depression in patients with Parkinson's disease. Int J Geriatr Psychiatry 1999;14:711–718.
55. Starkstein SE, Mayberg HS, Leiguarda R, Preziosi TJ, Robinson RG. A prospective longitudinal study of depression, cognitive decline, and physical impairments in patients with Parkinson's disease. J Neurol Neurosurg Psychiatry 1992; 55:377–382.
56. Liu CY, Wang SJ, Fuh JL, Lin CH, Yang YY, Liu HC. The correlation of depression with functional activity in Parkinson's disease. J Neurol 1997; 244:493–498.
57. Goetz CG, Tanner CM, Klawans HL. Bupropion in Parkinson's disease. Neurology 1984; 34:1092–1094.
58. Fink M. Electroshock: Restoring the Mind. New York: Oxford University Press, 1999.

17

A Population-Based Approach to Chronic Depression: Implications for Practice and Policy

Gregory E. Simon and Evette J. Ludman
Center for Health Studies
Group Health Cooperative
Seattle, Washington, U.S.A.

THE EPIDEMIOLOGICAL MAP OF CHRONIC AND RECURRENT DEPRESSION

Over 20 years ago, Goldberg and Huxley [1] described a model for the distribution of common mental disorders in the population. This model describes distinct levels of attention or care for depressive or anxiety disorders: those receiving no health services, those seen in primary care but not recognized, those recognized and treated in primary care, those seen in specialty care, and those seen in hospitals. These levels of care are separated by a series of "filters" which govern passage from one level to the next. For example, the first filter governs how and when a person with symptoms of depression or anxiety might appear in the primary care clinic, whereas the second filter governs how and why those symptoms might be recognized and treated by the primary care physician. In an ideal world, passage through these filters would depend solely on clinical need: For example, all patients with clinically significant symptoms would be recognized and treated, and all patients with persistent symptoms following initial primary care treatment would be referred to specialty care. Unfortunately, the level or intensity of treatment for depression is often strongly influenced by factors other than clinical need. Recognition of depression, initiation of treatment, or referral to specialty care may depend primarily on nonclinical factors (stigma, race, education, availability of insurance coverage) and those with greatest clinical need may go unrecognized or untreated.

The concept of filters described by Goldberg and Huxley [1] is a useful tool for understanding the cross-sectional epidemiology of depression. In general, patients with more severe or persistent depression will pass through the initial filters to reach specialty care. Not only will the prevalence of depression increase from one level to the next, but the mean severity of illness will increase as well. Patients who have passed through several filters to reach specialty or inpatient care, however, will also be exposed to progressively higher levels of treatment. Consequently, untreated depression may predominate in community or primary care samples, whereas specialty and inpatient samples will include many with persistent depression despite treatment. This distinction has important implications for efforts to improve treatment and reduce the burden of depression in the population.

To describe the course of depression over time, we must consider both the typical average course of depressive symptoms and the degree of fluctuation around that average. In most samples of patients treated for depression, depressive symptoms show a curvilinear pattern of improvement over time. Mean symptom levels decline rapidly over 2–4 months and then stabilize. These two phases of the recovery curve reflect a mixture of patients with rapid recovery and persistent symptoms. Approximately 20 years ago, VonKorff [2] proposed a mathematical model (the mixed exponential model) to describe this mixture of patients with good and poor prognoses. According to this model, the average course of depressive symptoms in any population reflects the combination of two different symptom trajectories. One group displays a rapid decline in symptoms to an equilibrium (or asymptote) near the zero point. The other displays a slow decline toward an equilibrium of significant residual symptoms. Differences in prognoses between samples of patients can be explained by the relative proportions of these favorable-prognosis and unfavorable-prognosis groups. Expressed in the language of Goldberg and Huxley [1], patients in the poor-prognosis group are more likely to pass through successive filters to reach higher levels of care. In the progression from community samples to primary care to specialty care, we should expect to see a progressively higher proportion of patients with minimal or partial recovery following acute-phase treatment.

Among patients treated for depression, persistence of significant symptoms following acute-phase treatment seems to be the most important predictor of long-term prognosis. For example, in a large sample of primary care patients treated for depression, approximately 40% reached remission by 6 months [3]. In this group of remitted patients, the probability of satisfying criteria for major depression at any time during the subsequent 18 months was only 20%. In contrast, another 40% of patients had significant residual symptoms after 6 months of primary care treatment. In this group, probability of major depression during long-term (i.e., 18-month) follow-up was more than three times as great as among those in remission at 6 months. This group with significant residual symptoms also accounted for over 75% of depressive episodes observed during long-term follow-up.

The economic and social burden of depression also concentrates in the minority of patients with persistent or chronic depression. Long-term findings from the National Institute of Mental Health (NIMH) Psychobiology of Depression study have documented the psychosocial impairment associated with persistent depression [4–5]. In the primary care sample described above [3], the 15% of patients with persistent depression 12 months after starting treatment accounted for 35% of disability days and 45% of health services costs over the next year.

The epidemiological findings described above have several important implications for practice and policy. First, the scenario of full remission of depression followed by relapse is actually relatively uncommon. Recurrence or relapse of depression is usually superimposed on a background of significant residual symptoms. Second, long-term prognosis of depression treatment is more strongly related to residual symptoms than to prior history of depression. In other words, the strongest risk factor for poor outcome is potentially modifiable by more appropriate and vigorous initial treatment. Third, the greatest opportunity for improving outcomes occurs where the filters described by Goldberg and Huxley [1] function poorly. When those filters function optimally, patients with persistent depression will be detected and "passed through" to the next level of care (e.g., patients with persistent depression after primary care treatment referred on to specialty care). When those filters function poorly, patients with persistent depression remain in a lower level of care—receiving either no treatment or treatment that has already been proven to be ineffective. This group of patients with inadequately treated chronic depression has the most to gain from systematic quality improvement efforts.

A GAP ANALYSIS OF CURRENT MANAGEMENT

The process of care for depressive disorders can be viewed as series of specific steps. The first of these is presentation to a health care provider— either a general medical provider or a specialty mental health provider. Recognition and diagnosis of depression is the next necessary step in the process toward appropriate treatment. Third, an efficacious treatment must be recommended by the provider and accepted by the patient. Fourth, adequate follow-up care is essential to assess response to treatment and make necessary adjustments.

A relatively small number of community residents with depressive disorders have no contacts with healthcare providers. In the Epidemiologic Catchment Area survey, over 75% of community residents with depressive disorder had some contact with a general medical provider over a 12-month period [6]. The more recent National Comorbidity Survey found that 83% had some healthcare contact [7]. Neither of these studies specifically examined use of health services among those with chronic or recurrent depression. It is reasonable to assume, however, that the likelihood of using health services is even higher among those with chronic depression. Abundant evidence demonstrates that depression is associated with increased use of medical services [8–9], and health service use is greatest among those with persistent depression [10].

Among patients with depressive disorders presenting to healthcare providers, a significant proportion go unrecognized. Among depressed patients presenting in primary care, up to half may go unrecognized by the treating physician [11]. Risk factors for nonrecognition include presentation with a somatic complaint [12,13] and the presence of comorbid medical condition [14]. Because recognition of depression is related to severity and persistence of depressive symptoms [15,16], however, it is likely that a smaller proportion of patients with chronic or recurrent depression go unrecognized. Nonrecognition is, of course, less of a concern in the specialty clinic where patients typically present with overt psychological symptoms.

Even when depression is recognized, patients may receive nonspecific treatment or treatments without demonstrated efficacy. In some settings (especially outside the United States), prescription of benzodiazepines or sedatives alone remains common [17,18]. Use of benzodiazepines is especially common among the elderly [19]. Among patients receiving psychotherapy, we cannot determine what proportion receive the specific and structured treatments that have been proven to be effective in randomized trials.

Among patients initiating antidepressant pharmacotherapy, premature discontinuation and inadequate dosing are common. Approximately 30% of patients initiating an episode of pharmacotherapy never refill the initial prescription (i.e., discontinue treatment within the first month) [20,21]. Among those who continue treatment, half or more may receive doses less than recommended by expert guidelines [18,20,21]. As a consequence, only approximately half of patients initiating antidepressant treatment in primary care or community psychiatric practice receive an adequate course of acute-phase pharmacotherapy [20,22].

Frequency and continuity of follow-up often fall short of minimal recommendations. As many as 30% of patients beginning pharmacotherapy (in primary care or psychiatric practice) do not make a single follow-up visit [22]. The limited data available suggest that premature discontinuation of psychotherapy is at least as great a problem as is premature discontinuation of pharmacotherapy [23]. In the U.S. National Comorbidity Survey, fewer than 30% of patients initiating care for depression had at least four treatment contacts over 12 months [24].

The most recent data suggest improvement in some of these areas and little change in others. Increases in overall rates of antidepressant treatment [25–27] suggest that efforts to educate patients and primary care physicians have led to increasing rates of recognition and initiation of treatment. The advent of serotonin reuptake inhibitors and other newer antidepressants has simplified antidepressant dosing. As an apparent consequence, more recent data suggest improvement in the adequacy of antidepressant newer medications [28]. Unfortunately, continuity of treatment and frequency of follow-up are still far from optimal. Based on data from 2000 patients, fewer than 60% of patients beginning antidepressant treatment receive at least 12 weeks of continuous pharmacotherapy (the criterion included in the National Commission for Quality Assurance Health Plan Employer Data and Information Set or HEDIS reporting system) [29,30]. A distressingly small 15–25% of patients met the HEDIS standard for follow-up care after a new antidepressant prescription—a criterion of only three visits in 90 days) [30]. For both measures, results were more disappointing for disadvantaged patients covered by Medicaid programs [31].

As a consequence of failures at each of these steps, few patients with chronic or recurrent depression receive treatment of sufficient intensity or duration. In a recent national survey, only 30% of respondents with probable depressive disorder had received some appropriate treatment during the last year [32]. In 1986, Keller and colleagues reported that patients entering the NIMH Collaborative Program longitudinal study had typically received only low levels of treatment (either pharmacotherapy or psychotherapy) prior to enrollment [33]. Ten years later, a disappointingly similar finding was reported in a sample of patients entering a treatment trial for chronic depression—fewer than 30% had ever had a truly adequate trial of pharmacotherapy [34]. A recent long-term follow up of the original Collaborative Program cohort [35] documented persistent undertreatment of recurrent depression despite increasing availability of proven effective treatments.

Although attention has focused on shortcomings in primary care management of depression, available evidence suggests similar difficulties in specialty practice. Patients initiating depression treatment with psychiatrists are only slightly more likely to receive adequate dose and duration of pharmacotherapy than are patients treated by primary care physicians [20–22]. Frequency of follow-up care is significantly greater in specialty practice, but still falls far short of minimal recommended levels [22]. The limited data available suggest that rates of improvement in specialty practice are only slightly greater than those in primary care [22]. These data call into question a common belief that shortcomings in primary care management are a consequence of primary care physicians' deficient knowledge, skill, or motivation. Psychiatrists (a group presumed to have significantly greater knowledge, skill, and motivation to treat depression) have similar difficulties maintaining treatment adherence and participation in follow-up care.

The evidence reviewed above helps to clarify the priority targets for improving depression care. For patients with more severe or chronic depression, failure to recognize depression is one of the less common failure points on the path to appropriate treatment. Use of inappropriate treatments (e.g., benzodiazepines) as well as underdosing of antidepressants both appear to be decreasing in frequency. These three steps in the treatment process (recognition, treatment selection, medication dosing) are all discrete decisions amenable to change by appropriate training. Improving performance in these areas suggests that recent efforts to improve providers' awareness and knowledge may have led to significant improvements in care. Unplanned treatment discontinuation and the absence of systematic follow-up, however, remain significant problems. In these problem areas, efforts to change providers' knowledge or attitudes are necessary but not sufficient. Even the most knowledgable or motivated provider will do little good for a patient who never appears in the office. Addressing unplanned treatment discontinuation will require reorganization of practice to improve treatment adherence and continuity of follow-up. The following section discusses the need for practice reorganization in order to provide effective care for chronic depression.

ESSENTIAL ELEMENTS OF EFFECTIVE CHRONIC ILLNESS MANAGEMENT

Shortcomings in the management of chronic or recurrent depression are quite similar to those seen in the management of other chronic psychiatric and general medical conditions [36–39]. Patient education is inconsistent and disorganized. Treatment is often discontinued prematurely, and treatment discontinuation is rarely planned. The quality or intensity of treatment is often inconsistent with expert guidelines. Follow-up care is erratic, and there is no systematic monitoring of treatment adherence or clinical outcomes. Although providers may be aware of evidence-based guidelines, guideline recommendations are not systematically implemented.

The gaps described above reflect fundamental problems in the organization of general medical and specialty mental healthcare. Traditional health care systems are too often reactive, responding to as-needed requests for symptom management. Long term needs—such as systematic follow-up and support for more effective patient self-management—are seldom given a higher priority than short-term treatment of acute illness episodes. Constant pressure to increase patient volume and reduce costs only exacerbates these difficulties. Providers feel overwhelmed by immediate needs and seldom contemplate longer term needs. Both patients and providers feel increasingly dissatisfied.

Wagner, VonKorff, and colleagues have described a model of chronic illness management applicable to a wide range of conditions [40,41]. This model describes four essential elements of effective chronic illness care:

> Information systems adequate to support organized practice. Examples range from sophisticated computerized registries tracking all aspects of treatment in large populations to simple index card "tickler" files to remind providers of expected follow-up dates.
>
> Practice reorganization to support active follow-up care. Assuring adequate follow-up care requires that specific member(s) of the healthcare team be given both the responsibility and the resources for monitoring follow-up visit frequency, outreach to patients "lost to follow-up," and systematic assessment of treatment adherence and outcomes.
>
> Ready access to evidence-based expertise. Depending on the clinical scenario, the appropriate expertise might be a well-documented, evidence-based treatment algorithm, telephone consultation with an expert colleague, or the ready availability of specialty/ subspecialty consultation.
>
> Strong support for patient self-management. Long-term management of any chronic illness requires sustained attention to self-monitoring, adherence to often complex treatments despite side effects, and regular practice of compensatory and rehabilitation strategies. In other words, the most important aspects of long-term management occur outside the healthcare provider's control (or even awareness). Effective care must foster patients' active self-management and promote effective collaboration between patients and providers.

APPLYING CHRONIC ILLNESS MANAGEMENT PRINCIPLES TO DEPRESSION

Providing effective treatment for chronic depression will require significant reorganization of everyday practice. Traditional medical and psychiatric practice are organized to respond to patients "complaints." Providers seldom consider the needs of those not presenting for care. Long-term management of chronic illness is too often lost among more urgent concerns. Systematic education to foster self-management is not typically a priority. Both the structure and culture of current practice are barriers to effective care for chronic depression or other chronic illnesses.

Isolated provider education or training efforts are likely to have little impact on the quality or outcomes of care for chronic depression. Over the last decade, several randomized trials and quasiexperimental studies have evaluated educational programs intended to improve depression management in primary care [42–46]. These programs all included proven elements of physician education programs such as use of evidence-based guidelines, academic detailing, and interactive skills training (practicing and role play). Results of these trials have been universally disappointing with respect to achieving important changes in care. Some studies have found changes in medication selection, but none has demonstrated differences in quality of care or treatment outcomes. Taken as a whole, these studies suggest that training is sufficient to affect specific physician decisions (such as medication selection) but not sufficient to influence complex ongoing activities (such as maintaining treatment adherence or adjusting treatment according to clinical response).

Supporting effective self-management will be a key element of any population-based care improvement effort. The concept of *self-management* in treatment of chronic illness refers to the fact that patients themselves, along with their families, are the primary "caregivers" in the day-to-day management of illnesses such as depression or dysthmia [41]. Self-care tasks important for the management of depression and dysthymia include interacting with healthcare providers, adhering to recommended treatment protocols, and engaging in activities that promote positive mood. Other self-care tasks important to managing depressive disorders include monitoring of symptoms and managing the effects of depression on relationships and the ability to function in work and family roles. Healthcare providers can support effective self-management in a variety of ways. For instance, providers can help enhance patients' hopefulness, motivation, and confidence in their ability to manage their depression by offering a variety of options for treatment, helping patients set targeted goals that are meaningful and important to them, and coaching patients to identify options and steps toward problem-solving life difficulties or barriers to adherence. Providers can help patients create incremental, realistic action plans for self-care tasks, anticipate and plan for obstacles, and provide ongoing supportive follow-up. Providers can also help patients' self-care by connecting patients with peer and community resources for themselves and their families, and by providing encouragement by sharing the "success stories" of others. In the management of chronic medical conditions, systematic efforts to increase patient involvement in decision making have been shown to improve both satisfaction and clinical outcomes [47]. Lorig and colleagues have developed and tested a generalizable group program to promote self-management of chronic illness [48–50]. Motivational interviewing techniques developed by Miller, Rollnick, and colleagues have been adapted to increase participation in and adherence to depression treatment [51,52].

Improving the frequency and continuity of follow-up care may require innovative alternatives to traditional in-person visits. As discussed above, fewer than 25% of patients treated for depression receive minimally adequate follow-up care [30]. Even if health insurers were prepared to support significant increases in follow-up contact, patients might not readily accept more frequent in-person visits. When the time costs of treatment are considered (i.e., patients' time spent in travel, waiting, and visit), the costs to patients for a typical medication management visit are as great or greater than the cost for providing the visit [53]. Several recent studies have included systematic telephone follow-up as an alternative or supplement to traditional in-person visits [54–57]. Participation in these telephone follow-up programs has been excellent, and two studies have demonstrated significant improvements in patient outcomes when telephone follow-up was added to usual primary care [55,56]. Incremental costs of telephone visits are also relatively low compared to traditional in-person assessments [55]. Fully automated monitoring systems—via computer or telephone—have the potential for both greatest convenience and lowest cost. Any fully automated system, however, would depend on patients' willingness and motivation to participate.

Several research models and demonstration projects have successfully applied these principles of effective illness management to acute-phase depression treatment in primary care. The Collaborative Care models developed and tested by Katon and colleagues [58–60] incorporate each of the core elements of chronic disease management described above (a disease registry, active follow-up, increased availability of specialty expertise, and education to support self management). Compared to usual primary care for depression, both the liaison psychiatrist and liaison psychologist versions of collaborative care significantly improve both quality of care and clinical outcomes [58–60]. The Depression Management Program for "high utilizers" of medical care described by Katzelnick and colleagues also adheres closely to the model of chronic illness care described by Wagner and VonKorff [54]. The large-scale Partners in Care study by Wells and colleagues has recently demonstrated that effective depression management programs can be implemented across a range of primary care settings serving diverse populations of patients [61]. Following these successful research models, the Breakthrough Series (a collaborative effort of the Institute for Healthcare Improvement and the Robert Wood Johnson Foundation Program on Improving Chronic Illness

Care) has trained 20 diverse primary healthcare teams in the development and implementation of systematic depression care programs.

These successful depression management programs suggest a new and more clearly defined role for specialists in the overall management of depression. With available and appropriate support from specialists, primary care physicians can provide adequate treatment for the majority of depressed patients presenting in primary care. In many of these cases, the role of the specialist may be limited to education and informal (or "curbside" consultation). In some cases, brief consultation or collaborative management (a period in which responsibility for care is shared by the specialist and primary care physician) is necessary. For a substantial minority of patients, primary care treatment will be inadequate, and referral to specialty care is necessary. In some cases (e.g., history of nonresponse to appropriate primary care treatment, high suicide risk, possible bipolar disorder), the need for specialty care may be obvious at the time of presentation. In other cases, the need for specialty care becomes apparent following the failure of appropriate primary care. Obviously, systematic monitoring of the outcomes of primary care treatment is necessary in order to identify all patients needing specialty care. In the language of Goldberg and Huxley, an ideal relationship between primary and specialty care would make the filter between them both more indistinct (i.e., fostering consultation and collaborative practice) and more efficient (i.e., use of specialty care depending on illness severity and response to treatment rather than nonclinical factors).

Two recent studies by Katon and colleagues [60,62] have important implications for extending systematic depression care programs from acute phase to chronic treatment. Both studies were organized around systematic monitoring of all primary care patients initiating antidepressant treatment for depression. In the first program [60], patients with significant residual symptoms after 8 weeks of primary care treatment were randomly assigned to either continued usual care or to a psychiatrist Collaborative Care intervention similar to that described above. Patients receiving Collaborative Care treatment were significantly more likely to receive adequate antidepressant treatment and had significantly better clinical outcomes. The advantages of collaborative care, however, declined between the 3-month and 6-month assessments (the period during which specialty intervention was tapering off). Furthermore, this decline in clinical effect over time was attributable to loss of intervention effect among the subgroup of patients with more severe and complicated depression [63]. In other words, patients with more severe and complicated depression (those at highest risk for a chronic course) require sustained intervention in order to maintain good outcomes. The second program [62] focused on patients who were substantially recovered after 8 weeks of primary care treatment but reported a high risk of relapse (i.e., long duration of index episode, history of multiple recurrences). These patients were randomly assigned to either continued usual care or to a brief relapse prevention intervention provided in primary care. The intervention included systematic education regarding recurrent depression and the benefits of long-term antidepressant treatment. Study therapists engaged participants in a motivation-enhancing shared decision-making exercise regarding long-term medication use. The two psychoeducational sessions also included brief cognitive-behavioral skills training. Although patients in the intervention group were significantly more likely to continue antidepressant treatment, clinical benefits of the intervention were modest. The primary reason for the relatively small clinical effect of the intervention was the good prognosis among patients continuing in usual care—only 10–15% met criteria for major depressive episode at each of the follow-up assessments. Taken together, these studies suggest the following regarding systematic efforts to improve care for chronic or recurrent depression: First, care improvement should focus on patients with persistent symptoms, as this group is at greatest risk for poor long-term outcomes. Second, sustained intervention is necessary to produce sustained results. Third, patients with more severe and complicated depression may require ongoing (rather than brief) specialty involvement.

Extension of the above-described systematic depression management programs from primary care to specialty practice is an obvious next step. As discussed above, the core problems encountered in primary care practice (high rates of unplanned treatment discontinuation, lack of systematic follow-up care) are also common in specialty practice. Strong evidence (described above) demonstrates that systematic depression management programs significantly improve process and outcomes of depression treatment in primary care. It seems reasonable that extension of those programs to specialty practice would yield similar benefits. One of the greatest barriers to such an effort would be the traditional culture of specialty mental health practice. Stigmatization of depression and other psychiatric disorders has led to heightened concern about privacy of mental health treatment information. Many mental health providers would be concerned about the privacy implications of systematic follow-up programs. In addition, many mental health providers have viewed treatment dropout as a manifestation of resistance rather than a failure on the part of the healthcare system. To those with this view, vigorous outreach efforts might seem inappropriate.

POLICY BARRIERS TO IMPROVING CARE FOR CHRONIC DEPRESSION

Actual implementation of effective care programs may require significant shifts in both public opinion and public policy. Stigmatization of depression and other psychiatric disorders is still an important barrier to treatment. Discriminatory attitudes are institutionalized in the coverage policies of health insurers and government payers.

Providing effective treatment for chronic depression will almost certainly increase the direct costs of depression treatment. Increasing frequency of follow-up care will certainly increase use of outpatient services. By definition, increasing long-term adherence to antidepressant medications will increase spending on prescription drugs. Arguments for improving the quality of mental health services have often proposed that increased spending on mental health care will actually reduce overall health care expenditures—a cost-offset effect. This argument was supported by observational data demonstrating markedly higher general medical expenditures for patients with depression and other psychiatric disorders. To date, however, randomized trials have not found that improving the quality of depression care reduces overall health services costs [64]. Although expenditures for outpatient depression treatment may be partially offset by decreases in use of other outpatient services, net outpatient utilization appears to increase modestly. Results to date suggest that the argument for improving depression care should be reframed in terms of value rather than cost savings. Support for increased investment in depression treatment will depend on the balance of benefits and costs. Focusing on the question of cost reduction alone appears to imply that improving outcomes of depression care has no significant value.

The greatest economic benefits of improved depression treatment are likely to occur outside the healthcare system. Depression is consistently associated with decreased likelihood of paid employment, increases in work missed due to illness, and reports of decreased performance at work [65]. The monetary value of lost work productivity associated with depression certainly exceeds the value of the "excess" healthcare associated with depression [66]. Strong evidence demonstrates synchrony of change between depression and measures of work participation and disability (i.e., improvement in depression is associated with increases work participation and decreases in work missed because of illness) [67–69]. Although randomized trials have only recently begun to examine work participation and lost work productivity as outcomes, early evidence suggests that improved depression treatment results in increased work participation [61]. If the added costs of improved depression treatment are offset by economic benefits, more of those benefits probably accrue to employers and family members than to health insurers. Consequently, the market demand and political support for improved depression treatment will likely come from individual, governmental, and corporate purchasers of healthcare rather than from insurers or managed care organizations.

In competitive health insurance markets such as in the United States, changes in insurance regulation may be necessary to reduce economic disincentives for effective chronic illness management. Adverse selection refers to the understandable tendency of people with predictable healthcare needs (such as chronic depression) to choose health insurers offering the most generous treatment programs. This migration of higher need members into one health plan often leads to increased expenses and may lead to higher insurance premiums. Premium increases discourage the enrollment of lower need members (i.e., those without chronic conditions), further punishing the health plan for acting in a socially responsible way. The potential for adverse selection may be greater for chronic depression (and other chronic psychiatric disorders) than for most chronic medical conditions. The early onset of most chronic psychiatric disorders means that young adults are better able to predict future need for psychiatric treatment than they can predict future treatment for cancer or heart disease. Mandated minimum benefit levels for mental healthcare is one traditional method for minimizing adverse selection. Unfortunately, mandated minimum benefit levels have little meaning in the presence of strict requirements for preauthorization and concurrent review. In reality, actual receipt of specialty mental healthcare is more limited by managed care mechanisms than by official coverage limits. Eliminating disincentives to provide appropriate care for chronic conditions will require new mechanisms to promote fair competition. Risk adjustment is one method for "leveling the playing field" by rewarding insurance plans that enroll sicker or higher need members [70,71].

Improved quality measures could help shift the focus of healthcare competition from minimizing cost to improving quality of treatment. In the current U.S. health insurance marketplace, competition between health plans has focused almost exclusively on cost. Employers and other insurance purchasers have little or no information regarding access to or quality of care. Absent information on quality of treatment, purchasers will make decisions based on price, and insurers will compete on that basis alone. Refocusing insurance competition on quality rather than price will require valid and unbiased quality measures to guide healthcare purchasing decisions [72]. The U.S. National Commission on Quality Assurance HEDIS system of measures is an early attempt at such a system of quality measures [31]. The first generation of HEDIS psychiatric measures (focused on quality of inpatient care for mood disorders) have been criticized for lack of relation to true quality of care [73]. A second generation of measures (focused on continuity of pharmacotherapy and frequency of outpatient follow-up) has recently been introduced [29]. Although these more recent measures have a stronger empirical basis, the true test of their utility will be their impact on healthcare purchasing decisions.

Traditional reimbursement mechanisms may be a significant barrier to implementation of innovative care programs. Fee-for-service reimbursement ties payment to the delivery of a particular clinical service. Such an approach may not fit well with some of the newer follow-up approaches described above. In the case of telephone follow-up care, the administrative costs of billing may approach or exceed the actual costs of providing the service (estimated at $15–$20 per telephone contact) [55]. Mail or telephone outreach programs typically involve more time and effort locating and reaching patients than time spent in direct patient care. Creating incentives, for vigorous outreach activities will require reimbursement mechanisms that reward time spent pursuing difficult-to-reach patients.

CONCLUSION

In the total population of people experiencing depressive episodes, approximately one third experience a chronic or frequently relapsing course. This subgroup with chronic or recurrent depression accounts for the bulk of long-term morbidity, disability, lost work productivity, and excess healthcare utilization attributable to depression. Although those with more chronic or recurrent depression are more likely to find their way to specialty care, a significant number remain in primary care or remain untreated in the community.

Gaps in the current management of depression are well documented. Among patients initiating depression treatment (either pharmacotherapy or psychotherapy), fewer than 30% receive treatment consistent with expert guidelines. Unfortunately, intensity of treatment is not related to severity or chronicity of illness. Studies specifically focused on chronic or recurrent depression also find a similar low proportion receiving appropriate care.

Providing appropriate treatment for chronic depression will require a significant reorganization of care. Simple physician education or screening efforts have been proven to be insufficient. Key elements of an effective chronic illness management program include information systems adequate to support organized treatment, practice reorganization to support active follow-up care, ready access to evidence-based expertise, and strong support for patient self-management. In this respect, management of chronic depression does not differ from management of other chronic health conditions.

Unfortunately, significant economic and political barriers may interfere with widespread implementation of high-quality care programs for chronic depression. Because improved treatment will probably lead to modest increases in healthcare expenditures, the argument for improved depression care must be made to employers and the larger society emphasizing the impact of depression on daily functioning and work productivity. Valid and transparent measures of treatment quality will be necessary to create incentives for healthcare systems to improve treatment quality—refocusing competitive forces away from cost reduction alone. Barring the advent of a single-payer health system, reforms to the insurance marketplace (such as accurate risk adjustment) will also be needed so that health systems are not punished for offering higher quality care.

ACKNOWLEDGMENT

This work was supported by National Institute of Mental Health Grant # MH51338.

REFERENCES

1. Goldberg D, Huxley P. Mental Illness in the Community: The Pathways to Psychiatric Care. New York: Tavistock, 1980.
2. VonKorff M, Parker R. The dynamics of the prevalence of chronic episodic disease. J Chronic Dis 1980; 33:79–85.
3. Simon G. Long-term prognosis of depression in primary care. Bull WHO 2000; 78:439–445.
4. Coryell W, Scheftner W, Keller M, Endicott J, Maser J, Klerman GL. The enduring psychosocial consequences of mania and depression. Am J Psychiatry 1993; 150:720–727.
5. Judd L, Akiskal H, Zeller P, Paulus M, Leon A, Maser J, Endicott J, Coryell W, Kunovac J, Mueller T, Rice J, Keller M. Psychosocial disability during the long-term course of unipolar major depressive disorder. Arch Gen Psychiatry 2000; 57:375–380.
6. Regier D, Narrow WE, Rae DS, Mandersheid RW, Locke BZ, Goodwin FK. The de facto US mental and addictive disorders service system: Epidemiologic catchment area prospective 1-year prevalence rates of disorders and services. Arch Gen Psychiatry 1993; 50:85–94.
7. Kessler R, Zhao S, Katz S, Kouzis A, Frank R, Edlund M, Leaf P. Past-year use of outpatient services for psychiatric problems in the National Comorbidity Survey. Am J Psychiatry 1999; 156:115–123.
8. Kessler LG, Burns BJ, Shapiro S, Tischler GI, George LK, Hough RL, Bodison D, Miller RH. Psychiatric diagnoses of medical service users: evidence from the Epidemiologic Catchment Area program. Am J Public Health 1987; 77:18–24.
9. Simon G, VonKorff M, Barlow W. Health care costs of primary care patients with recognized depression. Arch Gen Psychiatry 1995; 52:850–856.
10. Simon G, Revicki D, Heiligenstein J, Grothaus L, VonKorff M, Katon W, Hylan T. Recovery from depression, work productivity, and health care costs among primary care patients. Gen Hosp Psychiatry 2000; 22:153–162.

11. Goldman L, Nielsen N, Champion H. Awareness, diagnosis, and treatment of depression. J Gen Intern Med 1999; 14:569–580.
12. Kessler D, Lloyd K, Lewis G, Gray D. Cross sectional study of symptom attribution and recognition of depression and anxiety in primary care. BMJ 1999; 318:436–439.
13. Weich S, Lewis G, Donmall R, Mann A. Somatic presentation of psychiatric morbidity in general practice. Br J Gen Pract 1995; 45:143–147.
14. Tylee A, Freeling P, Kerry S. Why do general practitioners recognize major depression in one woman patient and yet miss it in another. Br J Gen Pract 1993; 43:327–330.
15. Simon G, VonKorff M. Recognition, management, and outcomes of depression in primary care. Arch Fam Med 1995; 4:99–105.
16. Coyne J, Schwenk TL, Fechner-Bates S. Non-detection of depression by primary care physicians reconsidered. Gen Hosp Psychiatry 1995; 17:3–12.
17. Linden M, Lecrubier YBC, Benkert O, Kisely S, Simon G. The prescribing of psychotropic drugs by primary care physicians: an international collaborative study. J Clin Psychopharmacol 1999; 132–140.
18. Wells K, Katon W, Rogers B, Camp P. Use of minor tranquilizers and antidepressant medications by depressed outpatients: Results from the Medical Outcomes Study. Am J Psychiatry 1994; 151:694–700.
19. Simon G, VonKorff M, Barlow W, Pabiniak C, Wagner E. Predictors of chronic benzodiazepine use in a health maintenance organization sample. J Clin Epidemiol 1996; 49:1067–1073.
20. Simon G, VonKorff M, Wagner EH, Barlow W. Patterns of antidepressant use in community practice. Gen Hosp Psychiatry 1993; 15:399–408.
21. Katzelnick D, Kobak K, Jefferson J, Greist JHH. Prescribing patterns of antidepressant medications for depression in an HMO. Formulary 1996; 31:374–388.
22. Simon G, Von Korff M, Rutter C, Peterson D. Treatment process and outcomes for managed care patients receiving new antidepressant prescriptions from psychiatrists and primary care physicians. Arch Gen Psychiatry 2001; 58:395–401.
23. Howard K, Cornille T, Lyons J, Vessey J, Lueger R, Saunders S. Patterns of mental health service utilization. Arch Gen Psychiatry 1996; 53:696–703.
24. Katz S, Kessler R, Lin E, Wells K. Medication management of depression in the United States and Canada. J Gen Intern Med 1998; 13:77–85.
25. McManus P, Mant A, Mitchell B, Montgomery W, Marley J, Auland M. Recent trends in the use of antidepressant drugs in Australia 1990–1998. Med J Aust 2000; 173:458–461.
26. Pincus H, Tanielian T, Marcus S, Olfson M, Zarin D, Thompson J, Zito J. Prescribing trends in psychotropic medications: primary care, psychiatry, and other medical specialties. JAMA 1998; 279:526–531.
27. Sclar D, Robinson L, Skaer T, Galin R. Trends in the prescribing of antidepressant pharmacotherapy: office-based visits, 1990–1995. Clin Ther 1998; 20:871–884.

28. Kerr E, McGlynn E, Van Vorst K, Wickstrom S. Measuring antidepressant prescribing practice in a health care system using administrative data: implications for quality measurement and improvement. Jt Comm J Qual Improv 2000; 26:203–216.

29. Coltin K, Beck A. The HEDIS Antidepressant Measure. Behavioral Healthcare Tomorrow 1999; June:40–47.

30. National Results for Selected 2000 HEDIS and HEDIS/CAHPS Measures [Web Page]. Available at http://www.ncqa.org/programs/hedis/antidepressant00.htm (Accessed 13 July 2001).

31. National Results for Selected 2000 HEDIS and HEDIS/CAHPS Measures [Web Page]. Available at http://www.ncqa.org/programs/hedis/medicaidantidepressant00.htm. (Accessed 13 July 2001).

32. Young A, Klapp R, Sherbourne C, Wells K. The quality of care for depressive and anxiety disorders in the United States. Arch Gen Psychiatry 2001; 58:55–61.

33. Keller MB, Lavori PW, Klerman GL, Andreasen NC, Endicott J, Coryell W, Fawcett J, Rice JP, Hirschfield RMA. Low levels and lack of predictors of somatotherapy and psychotherapy received by depressed patients. Arch Gen Psychiatry 1986; 43:458–466.

34. Keller M, Harrison W, Fawcett J, Gelenberg A, Hirschfeld R, Klein D, Kocsis J, McCullough J, Rush A, Schatzberg A. Treatment of chronic depression with sertraline or imipramine: preliminary blinded response rates and high rates of undertreatment in the community. Psychopharmacol Bull 1995; 31:205–212.

35. Dawson R, Lavori P, Coryell W, Endicott J, Keller M. Course of treatment received by depressed patients. J Psychiatry Res 1999; 33:233–242.

36. Stockwell D, Madhaven S, Cohen H, Gibson G, Alderman M. The determinants of hypertension awareness, treatment, and control in an insured population. Am J Public Health 1994; 84:1768–1774.

37. Kenny S, Smith P, Goldschmid M, Newman J, Herman W. Survey of physician proactive behaviors related to diabetes mellitus in the US: physician adherence to consensus recommendations. Diabetes Care 1993; 16:1507–1510.

38. Hirsch C, Winograd C. Clinic-based primary care of frail older patients in California. West J Med 1992; 156:385–391.

39. Andrews G. Should depression be managed as a chronic illness? BJM 2001; 322:419–421.

40. Wagner E, Austin B, VonKorff M. Organizing care for patients with chronic illness. Milbank Q 1996; 74:511–544.

41. VonKorff M, Gruman J, Schaefer J, Curry S, Wagner E. Collaborative management of chronic illness. Ann Intern Med 1997; 127:1097–1102.

42. Lin E, Katon W, Simon G, VonKorff M, Bush T, Rutter C, Saunders K, Walker E. Achieving guidelines for treatment of depression in primary care: Is physician education enough? Med Care 1997; 35:831–842.

43. Goldberg H, Wagner E, Fihn S, Martin D, Horowitz C, Christensen D, Cheadle A, Diehr P, Simon G. A randomized controlled trial of CQI teams and Academic Detailing: Can they alter compliance with guidelines? Jt Comm J Qual Impr 1998; 24:130–142.

44. Brown J, Shye D, McFarland B, Nichols G, Mullooly J, Johnson R. Controlled trials of CQI and academic detailing to implement a clinical practice guideline for depression. Jt Comm J Qual Improv 2000; 26:39–54.

45. Lin E, Simon G, Katzelnick D, Pearson S. Does physician education on depression management improve treatment in primary care? J Gen Intern Med 2001; 16:614–619.

46. Thompson C, Kinmonth A, Stevens L, Peveler R, Stevens A, Ostler K, Pickering R, Baker N, Henson A, Preece J, Cooper D, Campbell M. Effects of a clinical-practice guideline and practice-based education on detection and outcome of depression in primary care: Hampshire Depression Project randomised controlled trial. Lancet 2000; 15:185–191.

47. Clark N, Becker M, Janz N, Lorig KRW, Anderson L. Self-management of chronic disease by older adults: A review and questions for research. J Aging Health 1991; 3:3.

48. Lorig K, Seleznick M, Lubeck D, Ung E, Chastain R, Holman H. The beneficial outcomes of the arthritis self-management course are not adequately explained by behavior change. Arthritis Rheum 1989; 32:91–95.

49. Lorig K, Mazonson P, Holman H. Evidence suggesting that health education for self-management in patient with chronic arthritis has sustained health benefits while reducing health care costs. Arthritis Rheum 1993; 36: 439–446.

50. Lorig K, Sobel D, Stewart A, Brown B, Bandura A, Ritter P, Gonzalez V, Laurent D, Holman H. Evidence suggesting that a chronic disease self-management program can improve health status while reducing hospitalization: a randomized trial. Med Care 1999; 37:5–14.

51. Miller W, Rollnick S. Motivational Interviewing: Preparing People to Change Addictive Behavior. New York: Guilford Press, 1991.

52. Rollnick S, Miller W. What is motivational interviewing? Behav Cog Psychother 1995; 23:325–334.

53. Simon G, Manning W, Katzelnick D, Perarson S, Henk H, Helstad C. Cost-effectiveness of systematic depression treatment for high utilizers of general medical care. Arch Gen Psychiatry 2001; 58:181–187.

54. Katzelnick D, Simon G, Pearson S, Manning W, Helstad C, Henk H, Cole S, Lin E, Taylor L, Kobak K. Randomized trial of a depression management program in high utilizers of medical care. Arch Fam Med 2000; 9:345–351.

55. Simon G, VonKorff M, Rutter C, Wagner E. A randomized trial of monitoring, feedback, and management of care by telephone to improve depression treatment in primary care. BMJ 2000; 320:550–554.

56. Hunkeler E, Meresman J, Hargreaves W, Fireman B, Berman W, Kirsch A, Groebe J, Braden P, Getzell M, Feigenbaum P, Hurt W, Peng T, Salzer M. Efficacy of nurse telehealth care and peer support in augmenting treatment of depression in primary care. Arch Fam Med 2000; 9:700–708.

57. Tutty S, Simon G, Ludman E. Telephone counseling as an adjunct to antidepressant treatment in the primary care system: a pilot study. Effect Clin Pract 2000; 4:170–178.

58. Katon W, VonKorff M, Lin E, Walker E, Simon G, Bush T, Robinson P, Russo J. Collaborative management to achieve treatment guidelines: Impact on depression in primary care. JAMA 1995; 273:1026–1031.

59. Katon W, Robinson P, VonKorff M, Lin E, Bush T, Ludman E, Simon G, Walker E. A multifaceted intervention to improve treatment of depression in primary care. Arch Gen Psychiatry 1996; 53:924–932.

60. Katon W, Von Korff M, Lin E, Simon G, Walker G, Unutzer J, Bush T, Russo J, Ludman E. Stepped collaborative care for primary care patients with persistent symptoms of depression. Arch Gen Psychiatry 1999; 56: 1109–1115.

61. Wells K, Sherbourne C, Schoenbaum M, Duan N, Meredith L, Unutzer J, Miranda J, Carney M, Rubenstein L. Impact of disseminating quality improvement programs for depression in managed primary care: a randomized controlled trial. JAMA 2000; 283:212–230.

62. Katon W, Rutter C, Ludman E, Von Korff M, Lin E, Simon G, Bush T, Walker E, Unutzer J. A randomized trial of relapse prevention of depression in primary care. Arch Gen Psychiatry 2001; 58:241–247.

63. Walker E, Katon W, Russo J, Von Korff M, Lin E, Simon G, Bush T, Ludman E, Unutzer J. Predictors of outcome in a primary care depression trial. J Gen Intern Med 2000; 15:859–867.

64. Simon G, Katon W, Von Korff M, Unutzer J, Lin E, Walker E, Bush T, Rutter C, Ludman E. Cost-effectiveness of a collaborative care program for primary care patients with persistent depression. Am J Psychiatry. In press.

65. Simon G, Barber C, Birnbaum H, Frank R, Greenberg P, Rose R, Wang P, Kessler R. Depression and work productivity: the comparative costs of treatment versus nontreatment. J Occup Environ Med 2001; 43:2–9.

66. Greenberg P, Stiglin LE, Finkelstein SN, Berndt ER. The economic burden of depression in 1990. J Clin Psychiatry 1993; 54:405–418.

67. Simon G, Katon W, Rutter C, VonKorff M, Lin E, Robinson P, Bush T, Walker E, Ludman E, Russo J. Impact of improved depression treatment in primary care on daily functioning and disability. Psychol Med 1998; 28:693–701.

68. VonKorff M, Ormel J, Katon WJ, Lin EHB. Disability and depression among high utilizers of health care. Arch Gen Psychiatry 1992; 49:91–100.

69. Mintz J, Mintz LI, Arruda MJ, Hwang SS. Treatments of depression and the functional capacity to work. Arch Gen Psychiatry 1992; 49:761–768.

70. Pincus H, Zarin D, West J. Peering into the 'black box.' Measuring outcomes of managed care. Arch Gen Psychiatry 1996; 53:870–877.

71. Fowles J, Weiner J, Kutson D, Fowler E, Tucker A, Ireland M. Taking health status into account when setting capitation rates: a comparison of risk-adjustment models. JAMA 1996; 276:1316–1321.

72. Epstein A. Rolling down the runway: the challenges ahead for quality report cards. JAMA 1998; 279:1691–1696.

73. Druss B, Rosenheck R. Evaluation of the HEDIS measure of behavioral health care quality. Psychiatr Serv 1997; 48:71–75.

18

Improving Long-Term Adherence to Treatment in Major Depression

John Zajecka and Margaret Beeler
Rush Medical College
    and The Women's Board Depression Treatment
    and Research Center
Rush–Presbyterian–St. Luke's Medical Center
Chicago, Illinois, U.S.A.

INTRODUCTION

Over the last several decades, an increasing number of effective pharmacological and nonpharmacological treatments for depression have become available, including antidepressants, electroconvulsive therapy (ECT), time-limited psychotherapies, and investigational treatments. The efficacy of these treatment modalities, particularly the use of antidepressants, for the acute, continuation, and maintenance phases of treatment has been well established in the literature. When choosing a treatment for depression, the clinician must consider all factors (acute and long term) that will optimize efficacy, tolerability, safety, and adherence. Common factors that are frequently overlooked include dosing schedule (once per day vs twice or three times per day), the cost of treatment (for uninsured patients or those forced to pay "out-of-pocket"), and possible long-term side effects. The profile of the ideal antidepressant would include (1) efficacy in acute and long-term treatment,

(2) well tolerated during both acute and long-term treatment (clinicians must remain cognizant of the fact that side effects of some medications may occur later when the patient is feeling better), (3) acute and long-term safety (including treatment of comorbid illness), and any factors that the clinician believes could be individualized to the patient that may impact adherence to treatment.

Historically, the emphasis in treating depression has been on the acute phase of treatment, with a paucity of data on the continuation and maintenance phases of treatment. It is important for the clinician to establish the patient's baseline symptoms and any factors that may be attributed to side effects, or adherence, before treatment is initiated. It is more challenging for the clinician to attempt to collect this information later in treatment when the patient has responded to the medication. For example, a patient's perception of acute phase depressive symptoms may change once in long-term treatment. Physicians should be mindful of the fact that physicians treating this patient in the future need such information to make decisions later in treatment.

Physicians can best help patients by setting expectations for treatment outcome at a realistic level. For example, patients with major depression uncomplicated by other psychiatric or medical illness should expect full remission of and recovery from symptoms. For patients who have been chronically depressed, or those for whom there may be primary or secondary gains associated with their illness, the physician should explore concerns the patient may have about becoming "well." It is not uncommon for patients, especially those with chronic depressions, to fear what others will expect from them if they achieve symptomatic improvement (e.g., Will they be expected to return to a full-time work schedule for the first time in years? Will they be forced to confront issues that they may have dismissed as "secondary" to the depression?). It is most effective for physicians to address these concerns with the patient early in treatment.

Studies suggest that the risk of recurrent depressive episodes increases with each past episode, and that there is between a 50 and 90% chance of developing another episode following one or two depressive episodes, respectively [1–4]. Subsequent episodes often occur sooner, are of longer duration, are more severe, and are often less responsive to treatment [5–7]. In order to emphasize the importance of adherence to long-term treatment, clinicians should take the time to tailor a treatment program to fit the needs of the patient. Individualizing a patient's treatment promotes long-term adherence and, thus, efficacy of treatment. As there is increasing recognition and acceptance that depression may be a chronic or recurrent medical illness, a greater understanding of the importance of long-term treatment is still needed.

TREATMENT OF MAJOR DEPRESSION

In treating major depressive disorder, it is essential that all patients receive adequate treatment during the acute (12–16 weeks), continuation (4–9 months), and maintenance (1 year or more) phases [3]. Greater emphasis has been placed on long-term treatment, as all patients treated for depression require a continuation phase of treatment following an acute response. The specific duration of maintenance treatment should be individualized for each patient and may require "extended" or lifelong treatment for many patients [8]. Patients who should be considered for extended maintenance antidepressant treatment are those who have had two or more depressive episodes, chronic depression, double depression, severe depressive episodes (i.e., psychosis, suicidality), poor recovery between episodes, and other medical, psychiatric, or psychosocial variables that may exacerbate recurrence or relapse [7–11].

The goals of the acute phase of treatment should be to achieve a full remission of all symptoms and to optimize safety, side effects, and compliance. Maintaining remission leads to recovery during long-term treatment. Anything less than achieving remission and recovery is no different than failing to treat the depression at all. The goals of the long-term or continuation and maintenance phases of treatment should include reducing the likelihood of relapse and recurrence, restoring psychosocial function, and reducing the risk of suicide in addition to optimizing safety, side effects, and overall compliance. Additionally, it is important for clinicians to manage comorbid psychiatric or medical conditions that could impact long-term outcome of treatment.

It is important that a physician discuss long-term treatment with the patient early in the course of treatment and again after remission and recovery have been achieved. Relapse during long-term treatment has been cited as high as 57% [12] and may be the result of a number of overlapping factors: inadequate response during acute treatment, inadequate treatment, comorbid medical or psychiatric illness, psychosocial factors, and poor compliance. It has been found that failure to achieve a full remission of depressive symptoms during the acute phase of treatment may increase the likelihood of relapse [7,12,13]. Studies also suggest that long-term treatment should include maintaining the same dose of an antidepressant that was used to achieve remission during the acute treatment phase [3,14]. Further research is needed to assess treatment strategies in the continuation and maintenance phases with both psychotherapy and ECT. New-onset or undiagnosed comorbid medical and psychiatric illnesses should be considered in a patient who relapses during long-term antidepressant treatment. Some common comorbid or misdiagnosed psychiatric disorders include substance abuse disorders, bipolar disorders, anxiety disorders, psychotic disorders, eating disorders, and personality disorders. Finally, poor compliance with antidepressant treatment should be considered as a potential cause for a relapse during apparent antidepressant treatment.

ADHERENCE TO ANTIDEPRESSANT TREATMENT

Problems with adherence to antidepressant treatment remain the most common and significant obstacles in the treatment of both acute and long-term phases of major depression. Studies suggest that up to 70% of patients taking antidepressants are noncompliant either as a result of missed doses, premature discontinuation, or both [15,16]. Lin et al. [17] reported several common reasons why patients prematurely discontinued their antidepressant either early or later in treatment, with the most common reason being side effects in both early and late discontinuations. Patients also reported poor adherence to antidepressant treatment because they believed they no longer needed medication, felt "better," felt the medication was not working, or simply ran out of pills. Additionally, these patients reported that specific educational messages improved their compliance with antidepressant treatment. Patients were encouraged to take antidepressant medication daily, continue treatment for at least 2–4 weeks before expecting improvement, continue taking the antidepressant even if feeling better, and not stop taking medication without consulting the physician. Educational messages presented early in treatment were associated with better compliance overall with antidepressants [17].

Side Effects

Side effects attributed to antidepressant medications greatly impact treatment compliance and should be taken into consideration for all patients who are treated with antidepressants during acute and long-term depression. Discussion with patients and management of potential early (during acute treatment) and persistent or late-onset side effects should enhance compliance during all treatment phases. The recent development of the newer classes of antidepressants has presented safer and more tolerable treatment options for both acute and long-term depression. Early-onset side effects, such as nausea, anxiety, insomnia, and somnolence, associated with some of these newer antidepressants frequently abate within the first few weeks of treatment.

The recent recognition and management of persistent and late-onset antidepressant side effects has helped draw attention to the established need for long-term treatment. Insomnia, somnolence, weight gain, asthenia, and sexual side effects are common persistent and late-onset side effects associated with some of the newer antidepressants which may impact optimal long-term treatment outcome, including quality-of-life and adherence. Similar to early-onset antidepressant side effects, most persistent and/or late-onset side effects, if present, can be managed effectively. Even when using older antidepressant treatments (e.g., tricyclic antidepressants [TCAs], and monoamine oxidase inhibitors [MAOIs]), it is important to educate patients, manage side effects, and address any of the patient's concerns that may impair adherence.

Before classifying symptoms, it is important that physicians give a careful differential diagnosis to the etiology of new-onset side effects that appear later in the course of antidepressant treatment, as they may not be direct side effects of the medication. This differential diagnosis should include the consideration of symptom(s) as a residual symptom of the depression, reemergence of the depression, comorbid disorders (i.e., bipolar disorder, substance use disorders/withdrawal, other medical illnesses), other concomitant medication, and antidepressant discontinuation syndrome.

Antidepressant Discontinuation Syndrome

Antidepressant discontinuation syndrome can be a major cause of adverse events during the treatment of depression. Clinicians should be alerted to this phenomenon if a cluster of symptoms occur, especially after the acute phase of treatment. Antidepressant discontinuation syndrome can lead to a misdiagnosis of relapse or late-onset side effects and can be a sign of poor compliance, especially if it is repeated.

Antidepressant discontinuation syndrome can occur as a result of missed doses, abrupt dose reduction, and/or the discontinuation of some antidepressant medication [18]. Symptoms of antidepressant discontinuation syndrome can appear as early as 1 day after the medication is reduced or discontinued. These symptoms can be erroneously attributed to a side effect and/or reemergence of symptoms of the underlying illness. Common symptoms include anxiety, agitation, insomnia, light headedness, dizziness, vertigo, fatigue, nausea, flulike symptoms, myalgia, sensory disturbances (e.g., numbness/tingling), and the return of depressive symptoms. These symptoms can last for variable periods of time. Incidences of antidepressant discontinuation syndrome have been reported with TCAs, short half-life selective serotonin reuptake inhibitors (SSRIs), and venlafaxine [18]. There have been few, if any, cases of antidepressant discontinuation syndrome associated with bupropion, fluoxetine, mirtazapine, or nefazadone [18,19]. It is important that physicians consider potential antidepressant discontinuation syndrome when such symptoms emerge later in treatment.

STRATEGIES FOR IMPROVING COMPLIANCE TO ANTIDEPRESSANT TREATMENT

It is essential to tailor long-term treatment for depression to the specific needs of the individual patient. The patient should be educated as to what can be expected during different stages of treatment, as the perception of the patient often differs from that of the clinician. Keeping a patient informed, and an active participant in treatment, will encourage adherence to long-term care. Katon et al. [20] found that patients who were monitored closely and who made more frequent and more intensive visits for the treatment of their depression had greater adherence to their antidepressant treatment. These patients were also more likely to rate their quality of care highly and rate their antidepressant treatment as "good" or "excellent." Primary care physicians and psychiatrists working together can help encourage patients to adhere to antidepressant treatment. Physicians can also assist in improving medication compliance by surveying the availability and necessity of refills for antidepressant medications [20].

There have been many suggestions made for overcoming "barriers" in the long-term treatment of major depression. Emphasizing the importance of depression case management services in primary care fields can also help with adherence to the treatment of depression. Similarly, physicians can work together to achieve agreement on how long-term treatment could be managed. Following patients closely can encourage both patient compliance and patient involvement in treatment [21,22]. Clinicians should strive to establish a partnership with the patient early in treatment in order to promote better adherence to long-term treatment.

CONCLUSIONS

The majority of patients treated for major depression require some form of long-term antidepressant treatment. Many of these patients will need "extended" or lifelong treatment [22]. Optimizing efficacy while minimizing side effects is essential during both acute and long-term phases of antidepressant treatment. When choosing an antidepressant during the acute phase, it is essential to consider early-onset and persistent or late-onset side effects in addition to any other issues that may impact the patient's treatment over time. Early- and late-onset side effects can significantly impair adherence to antidepressant treatment and optimal recovery from depression. Patients should be educated early about what to expect during the different phases of their antidepressant treatment. This information should be reiterated during remission and then recovery when a patient's cognitive perception may have changed.

Adherence can be enhanced through early and ongoing educational messages to the patient regarding treatment issues such as side effects and the importance of sustaining illness remission. Keeping a patient well-informed about issues associated with long-term antidepressant treatment will encourage dialogue between the patient and clinician and will increase patient compliance. Additionally, this will allow for the clinician's differential diagnosis of new-onset symptoms during long-term treatment. This communication is essential and will allow for treatment to be tailored to the needs of each individual patient. Physicians should work together to follow patients closely, thus encouraging adherence to the treatment of the depression. After all, the patient's safety and optimal treatment should be considered above all else.

REFERENCES

1. Keller MB, Lavori PW, Lewis CE, et al. Predictors of relapse in major depressive disorder. JAMA 1983; 250:3299–3304.
2. Keller MB, Lavori PW, Mueller TI, et al. Time to recovery, chronicity and levels of psychopathology in major depression: a 5-year prospective follow-up of 431 subjects. Arch Gen Psychiatry 1992; 49:809–816.
3. Frank E, Kupfer DJ, Parel JM, et al. Three-year outcomes for maintenance therapies in recurrent depression. Arch Gen Psychiatry 1990; 47:1093–1099.
4. Thase ME, Sullivan LR. Relapse and recurrence of depression: a practical approach for prevention. CNS Drugs 1995; 4:261–277.
5. Keller MB, Klerman GL, Lavori PW, et al. Long-term outcome of episodes of major depression: clinical and public health significance. JAMA 1984; 252: 788–792.
6. Keller MB. Depression: underrecognition and undertreatment by psychiatrists and other health care professionals. Arch Intern Med 1990; 150:946–948.
7. Rush AJ, Thase ME. Strategies and tactics in the treatment of chronic depression. J Clin Psychiatry 1997; 58(suppl 13):14–22.
8. DJ Kupfer. J Clin Psychiatry 52(suppl):28–34, 1991; AHCPR Rockville, MD: U.S. Dept of Health and Human Services; 1993. Publication 93-0551.
9. Clinical Practice Guideline Number 5: Depression in Primary Care. vol 2. Treatment of Major Depression. Rockville, MD: U.S. Dept Health Human Services, Agency for Heath Care Policy and Research. AHCPR publication 93-0551, 1993.
10. Rush AJ, Hollon S, Beck AT, et al. Depression: must pharmacology fail for cognitive therapy to succeed? Cognitive Ther Res 1978; 2:199–206.
11. Bielski RJ, Friedel RO. Prediction of tricyclic antidepressant response: a critical review. Arch Gen Psychiatry 1976; 33:1479–1489.
12. Byrne SE, Rothschild AJ. Loss of antidepressant efficacy during maintenance therapy: possible mechanisms and treatment. J Clin Psychiatry 1998; 59:279–288.
13. Fawcett J. Antidepressants: partial response in chronic depression. Br J Psychiatry 1994; 26(suppl):37–41.
14. Thase ME, Sullivan LR. Relapse and recurrence of depression: a practical approach for prevention. CNS Drugs 1995; 4:261–277.
15. Katon W, von Korff M, Lin E, et al. Adequacy and duration of antidepressant treatment in primary care. Med Care 1992; 30:67–76.

16. Perel JM. Compliance during tricyclic antidepressant therapy: pharmaco-kinetic and analytical issues. Clin Chem 1988; 34:881–887.
17. Lin EH, von Korff M, Katon W, et al. The role of the primary care physician in patients' adherence to antidepressant therapy. Med Care 1995; 33:67–74.
18. Zajecka JM, Tracy KA, Mitchell S. Discontinuation symptoms after treatment with serotonin reuptake inhibitors: a literature review. J Clin Psychiatry 1997; 58:291–297.
19. JM Zajecka, W Miles, T Cobb, et al, The safety and abrupt discontinuation of nefazodone. In: New Research Program and Abstracts of the 151st annual Meeting of the American Psychiatric Association: June 4, 1998: Toronto, Ontario, Canada. Abstract NR716:262.
20. Katon W, von Korff M, Lin E, et al. Collaborative management to achieve treatment guidelines. Impact on depression in primary care. JAMA 1995; 273(13):1026–1031.
21. von Korff M, Katon W, Unutzer J, Wells K, Wagner EH. Improving depression care: barriers, solutions, and research needs. J Fam Pract 2001; 50(6):E1.
22. Zajecka JM. Clinical issues in long-term treatment with antidepressants. J Clin Psychiatry 2000; 61(suppl 2):20–25.

19

Management of Antidepressant-Induced Side Effects

Gustavo Kinrys

Cambridge Hospital and Harvard Medical School
Boston, Massachusetts, U.S.A.

**Naomi M. Simon, Frank J. Farach,
and Mark H. Pollack**

Massachusetts General Hospital
and Harvard Medical School
Boston, Massachusetts, U.S.A.

INTRODUCTION

The incidence of treatment-emergent side effects upon initiation and main-tenance of antidepressant therapy in clinical practice is difficult to estimate. Certainly, however, no currently available antidepressant is entirely free of side effects. Thus, the management of side effects is paramount in the treatment of mood and anxiety disorders, as medication tolerability may determine compliance and ultimately treatment effectiveness and the patient's resultant quality of life. Administration of adequate doses of antidepressants both during acute and maintenance treatment has been demonstrated as critical to achieve a sustained remission in depressed patients [1]. The high rate of relapse associated with treatment discontinuation suggests that many depressed patients may require long-term treatment with antidepressants [2]. Successful management of depression thus hinges, in part, on the patient's ability to tolerate full doses of antidepressants over extended periods of time. Critical to the effort to optimize treatment outcome and facilitate administration of medication at adequate doses over time are the availability of better tolerated antidepressants and the timely management of treatment-emergent adverse effects. Management of antidepressant-induced side effects, including patient education about such potential adverse effects, is critical to enhance patient compliance. Compliance with prescribed medication regimens clearly diminishes as the incidence and severity of side effects increase [3,4]. The prescription of suboptimal doses of antidepressants or the rapid abandonment of one agent to switch to another in response to the emergence of side effects can significantly prolong the period of untreated illness or promote relapse in patients who have responded to pharmacotherapy. Many depressed patients labeled as "treatment resistant" or with residual symptoms after initial pharmacotherapy respond to an increase in dosage [5]. Attention to treatment-emergent adverse side effects may facilitate the dose increases necessary for successful treatment of refractory patients. Furthermore, physician concern and frequent assessment of side effects along with prompt education and treatment of the affected patient enhances the therapeutic alliance and minimizes premature abandonment of treatment.

GENERAL PRINCIPLES (Table 1)

Patient Education and Compliance

Anticipation and open discussion of probable side effects at treatment initiation with reassuring explanations about their usual time course and potential management strategies can significantly improve patient communication with and confidence in the physician. This will also reduce feelings of anxiety and discouragement, as well as frank noncompliance when side effects do develop.

1. Review of the most common side effects (e.g., increased anxiety, gastrointestinal distress, sexual dysfunction, or sleep disturbance with selective serotonin reuptake inhibitors [SSRIs]), as well as any serious side effects that are particularly associated with a given medication or class of medication (e.g., risk of seizure with high doses of bupropion or priapism with trazodone) is recommended. Review of potential adverse effects and discussion of alternative strategies provides the patient with informed consent for the use of psychotropic medication and increases their sense of involvement in their care.

TABLE 1   General Strategies for Side Effects Management

Patient education and compliance
  Anticipate probable side effects.
  Provide reassurance that management strategies available in the event of
    side effects.
  Many side effects are time limited, and/or dose dependent.
  Most are reversible after drug reduction or discontinuation.
Optimization of drug selection
  Selecting a drug with more favorable side effects profile may prevent or
    minimize their emergence.
  Prefer newer agents for populations such as children, the elderly, the neuro-
    logically impaired, and the medically ill.
Minimal effective dosage
  Use the lowest effective dose at treatment initiation and gradually titrate up.
  Follow the maxim: "start low, and go slow".
Use of adjunctive agents
  Adding pharmacological antidotes rather than switching agents to manage
    side effects may prevent delay of therapeutic response.
  Allow time for adaptation or spontaneous improvement to develop.
Side effect emergence versus symptoms of illness
  Be aware that symptoms of underlying mood and anxiety disorders may be
    similar to medication side effects.
  Symptoms that begin after medication is initiated and worsen in a dose
    dependent fashion are more likely to be medication related.

2. Reassurance that management strategies are available to minimize
    emergent adverse effects, that many side effects may occur during
    periods of upward titration or are otherwise time limited, and that
    side effects are usually reversible after drug reduction or discontin-
    uation will facilitate patient compliance. Patients may be more
    willing to tolerate attempts to achieve therapeutic doses if they are
    prepared for the possibility of emergent side effects during periods
    of upward dose titration and anticipate that these adverse effects
    may subside, particularly if similar adaptation occurred at prior
    dose levels.

Optimizing Drug Selection

Appropriate selection of an antidepressant medication can prevent undesirable side effects (Table 2). For example, the newer antidepressants (e.g.,
SSRIs, bupropion, venlafaxine, nefazodone, mirtazapine) generally have a
more favorable side effect profile than older agents such as the tricyclic
antidepressants (TCAs) and monoamine oxidase inhibitors (MAOIs). The

TABLE 2 Adverse Effects of Antidepressants

	Orthostatic hypotensions	Cardiac conduction	Anticholinergic	Sedation	Weight gain	Nervousness/ insomia	GI distress	Sexual dysfunction
Tricyclics (TCAs)								
Amitriptyline	++++	++++	++++	++++	++++	++	++	++
Imipramine	++++	++++	+++	+++	+++	++	++	++
Doxepin	+++	++	+++	++++	++++	++	++	++
Clomipramine	+++	+++	++++	++++	+++	++	+++	+++
Desipramine	++	++	++	++	++	+++	+	++
Nortriptyline	++	++	+++	+++	++	++	+	++
Protriptyline	+++	+++	+++	++	++	+++	+	++
MAOIs								
Phenelzine	++++	+	++	+++	++++	++	++	++
Tranylcypromine	+++	+	+	++	++	+++	++	++
SSRIs								
Fluoxetine	+	+	+	+	+	++	+++	+++
Sertraline	+	+	+	+	+	++	+++	+++
Paroxeline	+	+	++	+++	+	+	+++	+++
Citalopram	+	+	+	++	+	++	+++	+++
Fluvoxamine	+	+	+	+	+	++	+++	+++
Others								
Bupropion	+	+	+	+	+	+++	++	+
Trazodone	+++	++	+	++++	+	+	++	+[a]
Nefazodone	++	+	+	++	+	+	++	+
Venlafaxine	+++	+	+	++	+	++	+++	++
Mirtazapine	++	+	+	+++	+++	+	+	+

[a] Priapism.

SSRIs, selective serotonin reuptake inhibitors; MAOIs, monoamine oxidase inhibitors.

Relative likelihood of adverse effects: + = none to minimal; ++ = low; +++ = moderate; ++++ = high.

Source: Ref. 5a., courtesy of The McGraw-Hill Companies.

newer agents are often better tolerated by patients with comorbid medical illnesses that may be exacerbated by adverse properties associated with the older antidepressants such as orthostatic hypotension or anticholinergic effects. Among the TCAs, secondary amines (e.g., desipramine and nortriptyline) are generally better tolerated than are the tertiary amines (e.g., amitriptyline, doxepin, or imipramine) .

Dosing

Although use of adequate amounts of pharmacotherapeutic agents is critical to achieving the goal of optimal outcome, use of the lowest effective dose may improve tolerability, and underscores the importance of regular monitoring and clinical assessment during dose titration. "Start low and go slow" is always good practice when administering agents such as antidepressants, particularly for patients with comorbid anxiety and agitation who are often quite sensitive to activating side effects such as jitteriness or nervousness early in treatment. As adverse effects are often dose dependent, gradual and slow dose titration is preferred, and will often minimize side effects early on while permitting eventual achievement of the therapeutic medication levels that can be critical to optimizing outcome for a given individual. This concept is especially important among special patient populations at risk for side effects (e. g., children, the elderly, the anxious, agitated or neurologically impaired, and the medically ill). These patients may not be able to tolerate usual doses of antidepressants, or they may require long periods of adaptation to a given dose. However, inadequate dosing or dose reduction during maintenance therapy below levels required to achieve remission will increase the risk of relapse, and should be avoided.

Use of Adjunctive Agents

An alternative to medication discontinuation that may alleviate and manage side effects without causing a delay or loss of therapeutic response is the use of adjunctive, ameliorative agents. Such an approach, particularly during medication initiation, may provide reassurance and a sufficient reduction in side effects to allow time for adaptation to occur, since side effects often subside over time.

Side Effects Versus Symptoms of Illness

Many side effects commonly attributed to an antidepressant trial may, in fact, represent preexisting or exacerbated symptoms of the patient's underlying affective disorders (e.g., insomnia, nausea, diarrhea, constipation, fatigue, anorexia) or other associated medical afflictions (e.g., irritable bowel syndrome, chronic fatigue syndrome, fibromyalgia). Symptoms that begin after medication is initiated and worsen in a dose-dependent fashion are more likely to be medication related.

In this chapter, we review side effects typically associated with antidepressant agents and discuss strategies for their management, with the goal of improving medication compliance, treatment outcome, and overall quality of life.

ANTIDEPRESSANT-INDUCED SIDE EFFECTS

Sexual Side Effects

Sexual dysfunction is a common problem reported with many antidepressants during acute and long-term treatment [6]. Impairment in sexual functioning and satisfaction should be frequently assessed, as it can contribute to noncompliance with treatment; frequently, sexual dysfunction can be managed successfully without medication discontinuation. The clinician should assess the patient's level of sexual function prior to antidepressant initiation (including inquiry about changes that may have occurred as a result of the patient's current illness) in order to establish a baseline against which subsequent changes can be compared and appropriately attributed. Patients should be educated about possible sexual side effects that may occur early or later during treatment, and they should be reassured that emergent effects may be treatable and are reversible with discontinuation of the antidepressant. Pretreatment assessment and education may facilitate the discussion of emergent sexual difficulties later, as well as aid in the accurate diagnosis of relevant factors influencing sexual difficulties at baseline and throughout treatment. A systematic approach that first defines the specific nature of the complaint (i.e., libido, arousal, ejaculation, and/or orgasm), and then attempts to determine potential causes will yield optimal results. Understanding the underlying physiology of sexual function and the potential disruptions caused by antidepressants can help guide selection of an appropriate management strategy for the specific type of sexual dysfunction.

Decreased Libido

Decreased libido may be a symptom of a mood or anxiety disorder, as well as secondary to antidepressant administration. In addition, the impact of antidepressants on arousal and orgasm over time may secondarily precipitate decreased libido. When diminished libido becomes persistent, or worsens after other symptoms of depression are relieved, an adverse medication effect should be suspected. The pathophysiology of decreased libido appears to involve multiple factors, including decreased dopamine activity in the meso-limbic system via 5-HT$_2$ receptor stimulation, and less commonly SSRI-associated increased prolactin legels [7,8].

Arousal Dysfunction

Sexual arousal appears to be mediated by both central and peripheral nervous system components. Centrally, dopamine in the mesolimbic system (similar to libido) may be interrupted by serotonin reuptake inhibition [9]. Periph-erally, sympathetic and parasympathetic activity (acetylcholine) mediates the spinal reflexes associated with erection and clitoral engorgement, which may also be modulated by serotonin; inhibition of these pathways results from serotonin reuptake inhibition [10]. Moreover, nitric oxide has been implicated in the regulation of arousal function at a peripheral level by affecting vascular changes necessary for erection [11]. Persistent inhibitory effects on libido and/or orgasmic function can have indirect negative effects over time on sexual arousal.

Another potential antidepressant-induced arousal dysfunction is pria-pism, a sustained and painful erection which can occur with a number of antidepressants, but has been reported to occur most frequently with tra-zodone (approximately 1 in 1000–10,000 men). Trazodone-related priapism usually occurs within the first 4 weeks of therapy, but has been reported as late as 18 months into treatment, and appears to be independent of dose [12]. Men prescribed trazodone should be warned about this potential side effect and instructed to discontinue the medication immediately if any unusual erectile or urinary symptoms occur. Priapism is a medical emer-gency that warrants precipitous evaluation by a urologist, Although con-servative medical management, including intracavernosal injection of alpha-adrenergic agonists (metaraminol) promoting venoconstriction and detumescence are commonly effective, surgical intervention may be neces-sary; this can result in permanent impotence.

Ejaculatory Dysfunction

Ejaculation and orgasm appear to be primarily regulated at the peripheral spinal level. Sympathetic and parasympathetic tone-mediating ejaculation and orgasm are regulated by norepinephrine and dopamine activity, which is influenced by the agonist action of increased serotonin availability on the 5-HT$_2$ receptor, secondarily decreasing norepinephrine and dopamine activ-ity required for orgasm and ejaculation [10,13]. Ejaculatory dysfunction associated with antidepressants includes delayed, retrograde, or painful ejaculation, as well as anhedonic or nonorgasmic ejaculation.

Anorgasmia and Delayed Orgasm

Delayed orgasm, or anorgasmia, has been associated with TCAs, MAOIs, SSRIs, and atypical antidepressants, and appears to be related to the serotonergic properties of these agents. This observation may explain the low incidence of orgasmic dysfunction with bupropion (whose mechanism is not serotonergic) or nefazodone, trazodone, and mirtazapine (which have direct 5-HT$_2$ antagonism). Occasionally, spontaneous orgasms while yawning have also been reported with the SSRIs, trazodone, and clomipramine. The pathophysiology of this effect is unclear.

Nonpharmacological Management Strategies

Selection of an agent with a low propensity to induce sexual dysfunction (e.g. bupropion, nefazodone, mirtazapine) is an important option for the prevention and management of antidepressant-induced sexual side effects, but should be considered in the context of other clinical considerations including efficacy, spectrum of activity, and other treatment-emergent adverse events. In the event of treatment-emergent sexual dysfunction, there are a number of general management strategies to consider. First, consider a period of observation to allow time enough for adaptation and tolerance to develop and to rule out other potential etiologies; a recent study suggests that if a sexual side effect does not subside after 4–6 months in the absence of intervention, it will likely persist [14]. Although the use of "drug holidays" has been recommended by some [15], particularly for patients on agents with relatively short half-lives, use of this intervention may be associated with relapse and emergent discontinuation symptoms and encourages noncompliance with treatment. Similarly, reduction of dose may be considered for sexual (and other) adverse effects, as antidepressant-induced sexual side effects appear for some patients to be dose related [16]; however, this option may also be associated with an elevated risk of relapse. Other options include the discussion of nonpharmacological attempts to improve sexual arousal and the use of pharmacological antidotes. The decision about which of these strategies is indicated depends on the patient's level of discomfort, the presence of other side effects, whether adequate response to the current agent has been achieved, relative contraindications to drug discontinuation (e.g., high risk of suicide prior to adequate treatment), and history of therapeutic response to other agents.

Pharmacological Interventions

Few controlled studies assess the safety, tolerability, and efficacy of pharmacological antidotes for treatment-emergent sexual dysfunction, and most of the available literature consists of case series or reports. When choosing an antidote, the clinician should utilize available knowledge regarding the pathophysiology of sexual dysfunction along with reports of effective strategies. Although prn "as needed" dosing of some of these interventions has been reported to be helpful, clinical experience suggests that most agents are more effective when used on a daily schedule, with the exception of sildenafil. Strategies that have been used successfully to treat the sexual side effects of antidepressants are discussed below (Table 3).

Sildenafil. Sildenafil's mechanism of action involves an increase in nitric oxide associated with phosphodiesterase inhibition, producing increased blood flow to the genital tissue and smooth muscle relaxation,

TABLE 3 Therapeutic Strategies for Antidepressant-Induced Sexual Dysfunction

Agent	Dose
Sildenafil	50–100 mg as needed
Bupropion	75–200 mg qd-bid
Yohimbine	5.4–16.2 mg bid-tid
Buspirone	10–20 mg bid-tid
Mirtazapine	7.5–45 mg qhs
Nefazodone	50–150 mg qd-bid
Dopaminergic agonists	
Amantadine	100 mg tid-qid
Pergolide	Start at 0.05 mg and titrate by 0.1 mg every 2–3 days up to 2–5 mg
Ropinirole	Start at 0.25 mg qhs and titrate up to 2–4 mg bid
Pramipexole	Start at 0.125 mg tid and titrate up to 0.5–1.5 mg tid
Stimulants	
Methyphenidate	5–20 mg bid
Dextroamphetamine	5–20 mg bid
Pemoline	18.75–112.5 mg qd
Modafinil	200–400 mg qd-bid
Cholinergic agents	
Bethanechol	10–30 mg qd-bid
Neostigmine	7.5–15.0 mg 30–60 min before sexual intercourse
Gingko biloba	60–80 mg tid
Cyproheptadine	4–8 mg qd-bid

which consequently improves erectile function. Although sildenafil (50–100 mg po 30–60 min prior to sexual activity) has been approved only for the treatment of erectile dysfunction in men, anecdotal reports suggest that it may be useful in counteracting sexual side effects of antidepressants manifested in all phases of the sexual cycle in both men and women [17], and controlled trials are underway. Unlike other pharmacological interventions for sexual dysfunction, sildenafil can be used on an as needed basis. However, potential side effects include hypotension, flushing, sweating, palpitations, and visual changes. Sildenafil is contraindicated for patients on nitrates or those with significant cardiac conditions.

Bupropion. Use of adjunctive bupropion (75–200 mg qd-bid) is frequently effective for relieving antidepressant-induced sexual dysfunction including libido, erectile, and orgasmic difficulties [18]; however, bupropion is contraindicated with MAOIs. Although SSRIs may decrease the metabolism of bupropion, raising serum levels and thus lowering the seizure threshold, this has not represented a clinically significant problem to date. However, adjunctive bupropion should be initiated at low doses to minimize adverse interactions, particularly with agents that may inhibit cytochrome P450 isoenzymes 3A4 and 2D6 such as paroxetine and fluoxetine. The probable mechanism for bupropion's effects on sexual function is an increase in both norepinephrine and dopamine activity [19]. Bupropion may be additionally useful as augmentation for patients with only a partial therapeutic antidepressant response.

Dopamine Agonists. Use of dopamine agonists may improve libido, as well as erectile, ejaculatory, and orgasmic dysfunction. Several case reports have suggested the efficacy of stimulants such as methylphenidate (5–10 mg qd-bid), pemoline (18.75–112.5 mg/day) and dextroamphetamine (5–10 mg qd-bid) for antidepressant-induced sexual dysfunction [20,21]. However, higher dosages may produce worsening of sexual functioning. Use of stimulants may be indicated when patients have concomitant sexual dysfunction, partial antidepressant response symptoms such as fatigue or apathy, or comorbid attention deficit disorder or concentration difficulties without comorbid substance abuse.

Amantadine (100 mg bid-tid) and pergolide (0.05 mg, titrated up by 0.1 mg every 2–3 days up to 2–5 mg per day in divided dosing) have been reported to be helpful, although a placebo-controlled trial with amantadine for SSRI-induced sexual dysfunction did not demonstrate significant efficacy for the active medication [22]. Ropinirole hydrochloride, a dopamine agonist (initiated at 0.25 mg qhs and titrated up to 2–4 mg bid) has been reported to be well tolerated and to ameliorate SSRI-induced sexual dysfunction in a case series [23]; similarly, pramipexole (initiate 0.125 mg tid, titrate up to 0.50–1.5

mg tid) may be helpful as well. Potential side effects include nausea, vomiting, drowsiness, and hallucinations. Dopaminergic agents should be used cautiously in patients with a prior history of psychosis.

Buspirone. Clinical experience as well as a placebo-controlled study [24] suggests that use of adjunctive buspirone (5–20 mg tid) may improve sexual dysfunction. This effect may be a result of buspirone's effects as a mixed agonist-antagonist on $5-HT_{1a}$ receptors, effects on the dopamine system, and the $alpha_2$ antagonism by one of its metabolites.

Postsynaptic Serotonin Antagonists. Nefazodone and mirtazapine appear to have minimal or no negative impact on sexual functioning despite their serotonergic properties. These antidepressants produce significant postsynaptic serotonin blockade ($5-HT_2$ receptors); in addition, mirtazapine is an $alpha_2$ antagonist, which may cause a consequent increase in norepinephrine activity and result in improvement of SSRI-induced sexual dysfunction. As with bupropion, use of these agents for augmentation may have a salutary effect on mood as well as reversing emergent sexual dysfunction [25].

Gingko Biloba. Ginkgo biloba may improve sexual function because of its ability, like that of sildenafil, to increase peripheral blood flow to the genital tissues. Ginkgo biloba (60–120 mg tid) has been reported to be helpful in improving libido [26]. As with any over-the-counter herbal preparation, ginkgo biloba should be used with caution given the lack of evidence supporting its safety and tolerability and the potential for as yet unknown drug interactions. It has established anticoagulant properties, and may cause headaches, flatulence, and other gastrointestinal side effects.

Yohimbine. Yohimbine, a presynaptic $alpha_2$-adrenergic antagonist, has been used clinically to improve libido, arousal, and orgasmic dysfunction associated with antidepressants [27]. Treatment is initiated at 2.7 mg qd and increased by 2.7 mg qd every 2–3 days up to 5.4–10.8 mg bid-qid if necessary. Use of 5.4 mg 1–2 hr prior to sexual activity has also been anecdotally reported as being effective for some patients [28]. The mechanism remains unclear, but it is likely related to the noradrenergic activity of yohimbine. Full response may take several weeks to develop, and potential side effects include anxiety, agitation, nausea, lightheadedness, sweating, and provocation of panic attacks, limiting its use. Yohimbine is contraindicated for patients treated with MAOIs.

Cyproheptadine. The use of cyproheptadine, an antihistamine with $5-HT_2$ antagonist properties, may relieve anorgasmia, improve libido, and reverse ejaculatory and erectile dysfunction induced by SSRIs [29], TCAs, and

MAOIs. Side effects include typical antihistaminergic effects such as sedation and weight gain. Serotonin antagonism associated with cyproheptadine administration has been anecdotally reported to interfere with or reverse antidepressant efficacy, which is a significant concern. Dosing begins at 2 mg qhs with dosing titrated against efficacy and sedation up to 4–8 mg/day in once-daily or twice-daily dosing.

Cholinergic Agonists. Use of cholinergic agonists such as bethanechol (10–30 mg/day bid) or neostigmine (7.5 – 15.0 mg) 30–60 min before sexual intercourse may enhance libido and improve erectile and ejaculatory function for men treated with anticholinergic agents such as TCAs [30]. However, experience with these agents is limited and potential not insignificant side effects include abdominal cramps, rhinorrhea, sialorrhea, diarrhea, and flushing.

Gastrointestinal Effects

Nausea and Dyspepsia

Nausea and dyspepsia may emerge during antidepressant therapy. For many patients, these symptoms are time limited, subsiding within days or weeks of treatment initiation or dose escalation. However, for some patients, symptoms may persist. Management strategies for gastrointestinal distress (Table 4) include instructing the patient to take their medication after meals, the use of divided dosing, or administration of adjunctive agents such as antacids (magnesium sulfate, aluminum hydroxide), bismuth subsalicylate, and H_2 blockers (famotidine 20–40 mg/day or ranitidine 150 mg qd-bid). Metoclopramide (5–10 mg qd-bid) has been used for antidepressant-induced dyspepsia and nausea, but should be limited to short-term use owing to the risk of extrapyramidal symptoms and even tardive dyskinesia as a result of its dopamine-blocking properties.

Diarrhea

Diarrhea may occur, particularly with administration of serotonergic antidepressants with minimal anticholinergic effects, including the SSRIs. As with nausea and dyspepsia, diarrhea is often transient, resolving over days to weeks; however, it may persist in some patients. Management strategies include the use of antidiarrheal agents such as loperamide (2–4 mg qd-qid max 16 mg/day), diphenoxylate hydrochloride (Lomotil 5 – 10 mg bid-qid), or attalpugite (Kaopectate 1.2 – 1.5 gr after each bowel movement, maximum 9 g/day). For SSRI-induced diarrhea, cyproheptadine (2–4 mg qd-bid), *Lactobacillus acidophilus* culture (one capsule with meals), and psyllium (1 tsp qd-tid) may be helpful for some patients.

TABLE 4   Therapeutic Strategies for Gastrointestinal Distress

Dyspepsia and Nausea	
Dose after meals:	
OTC antacids	
H_2 Blockers	
Famotidine	20–40 mg qd
Ranitidine	150 mg qd-bid
Nizatidine	15–30 mg qd
Metoclopramide	5–10 mg qd-bid
Bismuth subsalicylate	30 mL qd
Diarrhea	
Diphenoxylate HCL	5 mg bid qid
Loperamide	2–4 mg bid-qid
Cyproheptadine	4–8 mg qd-bid
Lactobacillus acidophilus	One capsule with meal
Psyllium	1 tbsp qd-tid
Kaopectate	1.2–1.5 g as needed, max 9.0 g/day
Constipation	
Increase physical activity	
Increase fluid & fiber intake	
Laxatives	
Psyllium	1–2 tbsp. qam
Docussate sodium	100 mg bid-tid
Milk of magnesia	30 mL qhs
Senna	8.6 mg qd-tid
Bethanechol	10–30 mg qd-tid

Constipation

Constipation may occur as a result of decreased motility of the gastro-intestinal tract due to the anticholinergic action of some antidepressants, particularly the TCAs, but can be seen with all agents. In elderly patients, severe obstipation and paralytic ileus may develop, posing serious risks, and requiring emergent medical consultation. Maintaining adequate hydration and intake of dietary bulk (vegetables, fruits, and whole grains), as well as physical activity, can prevent or relieve constipation. Bulk-forming laxatives (psyllium 1–2 tbsp. qam; Metamucil), stool softeners (docusate sodium 100 mg bid-tid; Colace), or senna (8.6 mg qd-qid) may be useful. The cholinergic agent bethanechol (10–30 mg qd-tid) relieves constipation due to anticholi-nergic antidepressants in some patients. Intermittent and short-term use of cathartic laxatives (milk of magnesia 30 mL qhs) can be effective, but chronic use may actually reduce intestinal motility and worsen constipation.

Cardiovascular Effects

Orthostatic Hypotension

Orthostatic hypotension is more common with the use of MAOIs, TCAs, and trazodone than with the newer antidepressants such as SSRIs, bupropion, mirtazapine, and venlafaxine. For TCAs, trazodone and nefazodone, orthostatic hypotension is most likely a result of alpha$_1$-adrenergic blockade [31]. Patients who complain of lightheadedness, dizziness, or near syncope should have orthostatic vital signs measured. Additional caution is recommended with elderly patients, those on concomitant antihypertensive medications that may prevent compensatory hemodynamic reflexes, and patients with cardiac or cerebrovascular disease. Orthostatic hypotension can be dose dependent, but tolerance to this effect may not develop. Clinicians should perform a thorough assessment of other factors that may exacerbate antidepressant-induced orthostasis such as a low-salt diet, restricted fluid intake, dehydration, hypoadrenalism, hypothyroidism, or concomitant use of antihypertensives. Identification of these factors and consequent modification or treatment may reduce or eliminate antidepressant-assoçiated orthostasis. Orthostatic hypotension that is more prominent during the day may be reduced by switching to bedtime or divided dosing. Alternatively, switching to or starting with an agent with a lower propensity for alpha$_1$ blockade such as the SSRIs, venlafaxine, or bupropion may prevent or reduce the incidence of orthostasis. Among the TCAs, nortriptyline has been reported to have the least propensity to induce orthostasic hypotension [32]. Clinical experience suggests that gradual dose titration or dose reduction of the newer antidepressants may minimize or prevent orthostasis. Nonpharmacological management includes adequate hydration and salt intake, education of patients regarding the possibility of orthostasis (especially during dosing adjustment), and instruction to rise slowly from a prone or sitting position and to sit or lie down if experiencing lightheadedness in order to avoid falls. For some patients, use of support hose and exercises to strengthen the calf muscles and prevent dependent fluid pooling maybe helpful. Pharmacological management strategies should be considered for patients who fail to respond to nonpharmacological interventions. One option is the use of fludrocortisone acetate (0.05–0.2 mg qd), a potent mineralocorticoid that increases fluid volume and may reverse hypotension in 1–2 weeks; however, patients should be monitored for the development of hypertension, edema, or electrolyte abnormalities [33]. Adjunctive thyroid hormone (triiodothyronine 25–50 µg/day or thyroxine 0.1–0.2 mg/day) may also be helpful. The successful administration of metoclopramide (10 mg tid) has been reported [34], although it carries a risk of extrapyramidal symptoms or tardive dyskinesia and should be reserved for severe, refractory cases only. For patients not on MAOIs, the use of stimulants (methylphenidate 10–40 mg/day or dextro-amphetamine 2.5–20.0 mg/day), or the use of the alpha$_2$ antagonist yohim-bine (2.7–10.8 mg qd-tid) are also options.

Hypertension

Venlafaxine has been reported to produce sustained blood pressure increases in a dose-dependent fashion. Sustained hypertension (defined as treatment-emergent supine diastolic blood pressure > 90 mm Hg and ≥ 10 mm Hg above baseline for three consecutive visits) has been reported for 3% of patients at doses of < 100 mg/day, but for up to 13% of patients at doses of > 300 mg/day [35]. Elevations usually do not exceed 10–15 mm Hg and generally emerge within 1–2 months of treatment, although some cases manifest later. A recent meta-analysis suggested that the effects of venlafaxine on blood pressure are dose dependent and only significant in dosages above 300 mg/day; thus, blood pressure concerns should not deter first-line use of venlafaxine for patients with cardiovascular disease [36].

Baseline blood pressure does not generally predict treatment-related hypertension, although patients with preexisting hypertension should be monitored closely. Patients receiving higher doses of venlafaxine should have periodic blood pressure monitoring (i.e., every 1–2 weeks for the first month and then at regular follow-up visits thereafter). Management of clinically significant hypertension consists of dose reduction, switching to an alternative agent, or adjunctive use of an antihypertensive.

Hypertensive Crisis

Hypertensive crisis may occur in patients on MAOIs (phenelzine, tranyl-cypromine) who ingest sympathomimetic drugs or consume dietary tyramine (Tables 5 and 6). There have also been reports of spontaneous hypertensive reactions in diet compliant patients on MAOIs [37]. The hyper-tensive crisis may occur minutes to hours following the ingestion of tyramine-containing foods or sympathomimetic drugs, and may include severe occipital headache, stiff neck, flushing, palpitations, retro-orbital pain, nausea, and sweating. Extreme elevations of blood pressure can lead to intracerebral bleeding. Prevention is the most important management intervention for this potentially fatal adverse effect. Patients should be provided with a compre-hensive list of contraindicated foods and medications and instructed to maintain copies at multiple locations and to carry them for reference. They should be instructed to seek immediate medical assistance if symptoms of a hypertensive reaction occur. Historically, some clinicians used to provide one

TABLE 5 Relative Restriction of Foods and Beverages with MAOI Use

Absolute (Contraindication)	Moderate (Avoid large quantities)	Unnecessary (Generally safe)
Beef and chicken liver	Bottled or canned beer	Bananas
Aged or pickled meats	White or red wine	Peanuts
(pepperoni, salami,	Vodka, gin	Raisins
bologna), poultry, and	Meat tenderizers	Raspberries
fish (herring, caviar)	Caffeine and	Soy milk
Cured or dried fish	dark chocolate	Fresh gravy
Aged cheeses		Beef/chicken bouillon
Overripe fruits (including		Yeast powder used
avocados)		in baking
Canned figs		Fresh and mild
Yeast extracts		cheeses (ricotta,
(marmite, bovril)		cottage, cream,
Broad (fava) bean pods		farmer)
Banana peel		Fresh meat, poultry,
Sauerkraut		or fish
Soy sauce or		
soybean condiments		
Chianti wine		
Tap beer		

Source: Adapted from Ref. 36a.

or two 10-mg capsules of nifedipine for patients to carry and take sublingually on the way to an emergency room if they developed symptoms of a hypertensive crisis. However, this strategy has been recently considered to be controversial and abandoned owing to reports of severe hypotension, reflex tachycardia, syncopal episodes, acute myocardial infarction, and sudden death when nifedipine was used to treat malignant hypertensive emergencies [38]. Sodium nitroprusside or phentolamine are the treatments of choice in an emergency room or intensive care setting to maintain blood pressure control. Beta-blockers are contraindicated. When a hypertensive reaction occurs owing to a dietary indiscretion, continued MAOI treatment should be reconsidered.

Disturbances of Rate and Rhythm

Sinus tachycardia may occur in patients on TCAs, MAOIs, venlafaxine, or bupropion; however, it is rarely clinically significant. A decrease in heart rate is occasionally observed in patients on nefazodone or SSRIs; however, with the exception of patients with underlying sinoatrial (SA) or atrioventricular (AV) node dysfunction, it rarely requires medical attention.

TABLE 6   Important MAOI Drug Interactions

Hypertensive crisis
  Amphetamines
  Bupropion
  Buspirone
  Cocaine
  Cyclobenzaprine
  Dexamphetamine
  Ephedrine
  Guanethidine
  Isometheptene
  Isoproterenol
  Levodopa
  Metaraminol
  α-Methyldopa
  Methylphenidate
  Pemoline
  Phencyclidine
  Phentermine
  Phenylephrine
  Phenylpropanolomine
  Pseudoephedrine
  Reserpine
  Tricyclics

Serotonin syndrome
  Clomipramine
  Dexfenfluramine
  Dextromethorphan
  Fenfluramine
  Meperidine
  Mirtazapine
  Nefazodone
  Rizatriptan
  Sibutramine
  SSRI antidepressants
  Sumatriptan
  Tramadol
  Tricyclics
  L-tryptophan
  Venlafaxine
  Zolmitriptan

Enhanced hypoglycemic effects
  Oral hypoglycermics

Delirium
  Disulfiram

For some patients, underlying conduction defects and arrhythmias may be exacerbated by TCAs or trazodone. Toxic levels of TCAs, underlying conduction disease (especially multifascicular block), and the postmyocardial infarction (MI) period are risk factors for TCA-related arrhythmias. Patients over the age of 40 years and those with a history of cardiac disease should have a baseline electrocardiogram to rule out QTc prolongation or other manifestations of conduction system disease. High doses or overdoses of trazodone have also been associated with ventricular arrhythmias in patients with preexisting cardiac disease [39]. In general, the newer antidepressants (SSRIs, nefazodone, venlafaxine, and bupropion) have a relative low risk of cardiotoxicity and should be prescribed preferentially for patients with a history of cardiac disease.

Anticholinergic Effects

The blockade of muscarinic cholinergic receptors is responsible for adverse medication effects such as dry mouth, blurred vision, urinary retention, constipation (see section B on gastrointestinal effect above), and confusion. Anticholinergic activity varies substantially among antidepressants [31]. The SSRIs, venlafaxine, bupropion, nefazodone, and trazodone have far less anticholinergic action than secondary amine TCAs such as desipramine and nortriptyline, which themselves are less anticholinergic than tertiary amine TCAs such as imipramine, amitriptyline, and doxepin. Selection of agents with low muscarinic receptor binding is the first step in minimizing anticholinergic side effects. Nonetheless, for many patients, tolerance to anticholinergic side effects develops with ongoing antidepressant therapy.

Dry Mouth (Xerostomia)

Decreased salivation may result in the development of stomatitis, halitosis, and dental caries. Use of sugarless hard candy or gum may stimulate salivation without producing dental caries or weight gain. Patients should also be advised to avoid caffeinated beverages, tobacco, and alcohol, as they tend to dry out the mouth. Artificial saliva preparations may also be helpful (Saliva Substitute, Salivart, Salix, Optimoist). Preparations containing cholinergic agents (1% Pilocarpine solution tid-qid or as needed, prepared by mixing a 4% pilocarpine solution and water in 1:3 ratio) may be useful topically as a mouth rinse.

Bethanechol (10–30 mg qd-tid) is another option in the treatment of clinically significant anticholinergic side effects including xerostomia. However, cholinergic agents should not be used in patients with asthma, because they may promote bronchoconstriction. Clinical experience suggests that even elderly patients tolerate bethanecol dosages up to 10 mg tid [40]. Dosing should start low with gradual upward titration until relief of symptoms or emergent adverse reactions to bethanecol (i.e., abdominal cramping, rhinorrhea, diarrhea, flushing, tearing, or sialorrhea).

Blurred Vision

Blurred vision due to anticholinergic-induced pupillary dilation tends to remit within a few weeks of treatment initiation. For patients with persistent visual disturbances, use of 1% pilocarpine drops (1 drop tid) or bethanecol orally (10–30 mg qd-tid) may improve symptoms [41,42]. However, anticholinergic antidepressants may increase intraocular pressure, precipitating acute glaucoma, and should be avoided in patients with a history of narrow-angle glaucoma. Opthalmological evaluation of patients at risk for glaucoma is warranted prior to initiation of anticholinergic antidepressants.

Urinary Hesitancy and Retention

Anticholinergic antidepressants may cause urinary hesitancy, retention, atonic bladder with stasis, secondary urinary tract infections, and rarely hydronephrosis. Elderly patients, particularly those with mechanical outflow obstruction (i.e., prostate hypertrophy) are at risk to develop these complications. Clinical experience suggests that bethanecol (10–30 mg qd-tid) can be safely used for patients without mechanical obstruction [43]. However, bladder damage may occur in patients with prostatic hypertrophy administered cholinergic agents owing to the induction of forceful bladder contraction against a fixed obstruction; consequently, cholinergic agents are contraindicated for these patients. Significant urinary retention warrants an emergent urological consultation, discontinuation of the antidepressant agent, and use of a less anticholinergic agent. Despite a lack of significant anticholinergic activity, urinary hesitancy and retention have occasionally been anecdotally reported in patients on SSRIs, bupropion, trazodone, and MAOIs.

Central Anticholinergic Toxicity

Excessive cholinergic blockade in the central nervous system (CNS) can result in agitation, confusion, myoclonic jerks, and psychotic symptoms, and may occur independently of other systemic anticholinergic symptoms (flushing, pupillary dilation, dry mouth and skin, constipation, urinary retention, and increased temperature). Patients may present with central anticholinergic toxicity following accidental or purposeful overdoses with TCAs or after therapeutic dosages, particularly in populations more susceptible to anticholinergic toxicity such as children, the elderly, or brain-injured patients. Management strategies include prompt discontinuation of the antidepressant, supportive and symptomatic treatment (i.e., agitation and psychosis may require low doses of high potency or atypical antipsychotics). In an emergency room or hospital setting, physostigmine (1–2 mg slow IV push over 2 mins repeated every 30 mins as needed or 1–2 mg IM every hour) can be administered. Physostigmine should only be administered under close monitoring, as its administration may cause bronchoconstriction, hypotension, and seizures [44].

Dermatologic Effects

Maculopapular Rash

Erythematous maculopapular rashes are the most common cutaneous reactions to antidepressants. They tend to occur shortly after initiation of treatment, and are usually time limited regardless of antidepressant continuation [45]. For patients with pruritus, use of antihistamines such as diphenhydramine (25–50 mg qd-tid), fexofenadine (60–90 mg bid), or cetirizine (5–20 mg qd), or 1% hydrocortisone cream applied topically may provide relief. The level of patient discomfort and history of response to prior antidepressants are important aspects of the decision whether to continue the medication or switch to alternatives. However, signs of systemic involvement such as fever, altered liver function tests, or leukocytosis suggest a generalized immune reaction, and require immediate discontinuation of the antidepressant agent. In order to minimize the possibility of cross reactivity, an antidepressant from a different class is the preferred switching/substitution strategy for these patients. Although uncommon, severe reactions including generalized urticaria, erythema multiforme, or toxic epidermal necrolysis have been reported. Cutaneous erythematous plaques with atypical lymphoid infiltrates or pseudolymphomas have been reported in some patients on SSRIs and benzodiazepines [46].

Lamotrigine, an anticonvulsant that is used for treatment of bipolar depression and refractory unipolar depression, has been associated with rash including severe reactions such as Stevens-Johnson's syndrome [47]. The use of a gradual titration strategy such as initiating at 25 mg a day with increases of no more than 25 mg per week has appeared to reduce the incidence of severe cutaneous reactions to lamotrigine, and is highly recommended. Patients should be instructed to report any lamotrigine-associated rashes promptly. In general, the development of severe or atypical dermatological reactions should prompt medication discontinuation of the offending agent and consideration of dermatologic consultation.

Hyperpigmentation

Antidepressant-induced hyperpigmentation has been described rarely with long-term use of imipramine and amitriptyline. It occurs in a photodistribution fashion on the face, arms, and back of the hands. Laser treatment has been reported as being effective for imipramine-induced hyperpigmentation [48].

Hair Loss (Alopecia)

Medication-induced alopecia is an occasional side effect of many psychotropic agents, including valproate. However, SSRIs, tricyclic antidepressants, maprotiline, trazodone, and other new antidepressants have been reported more rarely to lead to alopecia [49–52]. Drug-induced alopecia generally lessens or remits entirely after dose reduction or drug discontinuation. Other potential common underlying causes of alopecia should be considered and include trichotillomania, female hormonal abnormalities, hypothyroidism, and polycystic ovary disease. Although the mechanism of antidepressant-induced alopecia remains unknown in most cases, multivitamins containing supplemental selenium and zinc have been reported to be helpful for some patients. The therapeutic value of mineral supplements remains unclear.

Central Nervous System Effects

Tremors

Fine and rapid tremors of the extremities can occur as a side effect of antidepressants and may be exacerbated by anxiety or caffeine use. Anxiolytic interventions and limitation of caffeine intake can be helpful. Pharmacological strategies include the use of beta-blockers (e.g., propranolol 10–20 mg bid-tid or atenolol 25–100 mg qd) or low doses of benzodiazepines (e.g., lorazepam 1–2 mg bid-qid or clonazepam 0.5–2.0 mg qd-bid). Gabapentin (300–5600 mg/day) may also be useful.

Headaches

Headaches are among the most common side effects of SSRIs. Patients with preexisting tension headaches and/or migraines appear to be more susceptible and may experience exacerbations. Conversely, SSRIs as well as TCAs have also been reported to alleviate tension headaches, and are used clinically to treat migraines [53,54]. This may indicate that some headaches are a manifestation of a depressive or anxiety disorder, and suggests that dysregulation in serotonin or other neurotransmitters may underlie both conditions. Clinical experience suggests that adaptation to this adverse effect may occur over time.

Management strategies include switching to another antidepressant class or symptomatic treatment with conventional pain relievers including acetaminophen or ibuprofen (400–800 mg as needed). For migraines, use of triptans (i.e., sumatriptan 25–50 mg orally or 6 mg SC as needed) may be useful. In addition, anecdotal reports suggest agents such as valproate (250–500 mg qd-bid), low-dose nortriptyline or amitriptyline (25–50 mg qd), or gabapentin 300–5400 mg/day may be useful for headache prophylaxis.

Jitteriness and Restlessness

Jitteriness and increased anxiety are commonly seen with the initiation or dose escalation of TCAs, SSRIs, venlafaxine, and bupropion, particularly in patients with preexisting anxiety. For example, jitteriness can occur in up to 30% of patients initiated on SSRIs [55]. In general, jitteriness usually remits within a few days to weeks and can be minimized by initiation of treatment at low doses (i.e., imipramine 10–25 mg or fluoxetine 5–10 mg) and with a slow upward titration to allow for adaptation. Concomitant use of benzodiazepines (e.g., clonazepam 0.5 mg qd-bid) or gabapentin (300–5400 mg/day) at treatment initiation can prevent initial jitteriness or anxiety exacerbation. Some patients on serotonergic agents may experience an akathisialike motor restlessness which may respond to the addition of propranolol (20–40 mg bid-qid), benzodiazepines (e.g., clonazepam 0.5 mg qd-bid), or gabapentin (300–5400 mg/day). Dosage reduction may also be helpful if clinically indicated.

Fatigue and Sedation

The differential diagnosis of somnolence or fatigue during antidepressant therapy should include the underlying mood or anxiety disorder itself, residual symptoms of depression, a comorbid medical illness, concomitant medications, a primary sleep disorder (e.g., obstructive sleep apnea), altered sleep cycle, and substance-use disorders. The presentation of fatigue may be complicated by the presence of SSRI-associated apathy (see section on apathy and indifference) below. Management strategies (Table 7) for sedation and fatigue include switching most or all doses of a sedating agent to evenings or bedtime, increasing caffeine intake, use of hypnotic agents at night to minimize daytime naps and normalize the sleep cycle, modafinil 200–400 mg qd, psychostimulants (methylphenidate 10–40 mg qd-bid, dextroamphetamine, pemoline 18.75–112.5 mg qd), or use of low doses of a stimulating antidepressant such as desipramine (25–50 mg qd), or bupropion (75–100 mg qd-bid). For patients on MAOIs, use of psychostimulants or concomitant antidepressants is complicated by the risk of a hypertensive crisis. Tricyclic levels may increase when these agents are coadministered with SSRIs so plasma levels should be monitored and dose titration made gradually. Mirtazapine induced daytime somnolence maybe alleviated by

TABLE 7 Therapeutic Stategies for Antidepressant-Associated
Fatigue and Sedation

Correct sleep disturbance (e.g., bedtime hypnotic)
Bedtime dosing
Lower dose
Caffeine
Adjunctive activating antidepressant (SSRIs)
  Desipramine (25–50 mg/d)
  Bupropion (75–200 mg qd-bid)
Stimulants (SSRIs)
  Methylphenidate (10–40 mg/d
  Dextroamphetamine (10–20 mg/d)
  Magnesium pemoline (18.75–112.5 mg/d)
  Modafanil 100–200 mg bid
Dopaminergic agonists (SSRI and MAOI)
  Amantadine (100 mg tid-qid)
  Pergolide (start at 0.05 mg and titrate by 0.1 mg every 2–3 days up to 2–5 mg)
  Ropinirole (start dose at 0.25 mg qhs and titrate up to 2–4 mg bid)
  Pramipexole (start dose at 0.125 mg tid and titrate up to 0.5–1.5 mg tid)
Thyroid supplementation (SSRIs and MAOIs)
  T_3 25–50 mg/d

---

increasing the dose or initiating mirtazapine at 30 mg qd, as lower dosages have been associated with stronger antihistaminergic action and higher doses with greater noradrenergic effects [56]. Other adjunctive strategies that have been useful in clinical practice for fatigue associated with antidepressants include addition of dopaminergic agents such as amantadine (100 mg tid-qid), ropinirole (2–4 mg bid), pramipexole (0.5–1.5 mg tid), or pergolide (2–5 mg/day in divided doses) and addition of thyroid hormone (i.e., T_3 25–50 µg qd).

Sleep Disturbances, Vivid Dreams, and Nightmares

Antidepressants may produce disturbed sleep, nightmares, and hypnagogic or hypnopompic activity (abnormal perceptions including hallucinations while falling asleep or awakening). For TCA-treated patients, these effects may be secondary to medication-induced decreases in rapid eye movement (REM) and increased stages 3 and 4 sleep [57]. SSRIs can have detrimental effects on sleep architecture by reducing REM sleep, increasing its latency, and decreasing slow-wave sleep. It has been proposed that SSRI-induced reduction of slow-wave sleep is due to its lack of 5-HT_2 antagonism [58]. Of note, nefazodone has not been associated with abnormal sleep architecture [59]. Potentially effective strategies for medication-induced insomnia include improved sleep hygiene and stimulus control measures including avoiding caffeine intake, particularly proximate to bedtime, limiting fluid intake before bedtime, restricting physical, mental and sexual activities prior to sleep, and avoiding daytime naps. Switching antidepressant dosing to earlier in the day or decreasing the dose are also possible interventions, but impact on the response of the primary psychiatric disorder under treatment should be monitored. Adjunctive use of pharmacological antidotes such as trazodone (50–300 mg qhs), mirtazapine (7.5–30 mg qhs excluding patients on MAOIs), benzodiazepines, zolpidem (5–10 mg qhs), zaleplon (10–20 mg qhs), gabapentin (300–5400 mg qhs), topiramate (25–200 mg qhs), and sedating antihistamines (e.g. diphenhydramine 25–100 mg qhs) are potentially effective strategies. However, tolerance may develop to their efficacy, and these interventions do not correct abnormalities in sleep architecture.

Myoclonus

Brief and sudden jerking or twitching movements of the extremities may be seen in up to 40% of patients on TCAs [60]. Nocturnal myoclonus or symptoms resembling restless legs syndrome may be seen occasionally with MAOIs, SSRIs, and other serotonergic agents as well [61]. Nocturnal myoclonus may also represent a periodic limb movement disorder and is likely due to increased serotonergic tone and secondary dopamine blockade [62]. Myoclonus may be relieved by dosage reduction, medication discontinuation, changing dosing away from bedtime (for nocturnal myoclonus), and use of anticholinergic agents or dopamine agonists such as pramipexole (0.5–1.5 mg qd-tid), ropinirole (2 – 4 mg bid), and bupropion [63]. Beta-blockers such as propranolol (10–20 mg bid-tid) and clonazepam 0.5–2.0 mg qhs may also alleviate nocturnal myoclonus. Anecdotal reports also suggest the potential benefit of trazodone (50–300 mg qd), cyproheptadine (4–16 mg qd), valproate or carbamazepine (at therapeutic levels), and gabapentin (300–5400 mg/d).

Bruxism

Bruxism (teeth grinding) may be mechanistically related to other extrapyramidal side effects of antidepressants (e.g., tremors, acute dystonic reactions) that involve decreased dopaminergic activity secondary to increased serotonergic tone; among antidepressants, bruxism is most commonly seen with more serotonergic agents. Nonpharmacological strategies include the use of a mouth guard device for the protection of teeth and the temporomandibular joint. Antidepressant dosage reduction, diazepam (5–30 mg qd), gabapentin (300–5400 mg gd),and buspirone (10–30 mg tid) and dopaminergic agents have been reported helpful as well [64–66].

Paresthesias

Numbness, tingling, or pinprick sensations may occur with antidepressant use and have been associated most frequently with MAOIs. MAOIs interfere with the absorption of vitamin B_6 (pyridoxine) [67], and this may be causative in some cases; supplemental pyridoxine 50–150 mg qhs maybe helpful. Alternatively, use of low doses of a benzodiazepine (e.g., clonazepam 0.5–2.0 mg qd-bid) may be symptomatically helpful.

Apathy or Amotivational Syndrome

Indifference and apathy have been described in patients treated over time with antidepressants, particularly the SSRIs and MAOIs. In general, apathy or a sense of "grayness" occurs insidiously, independent of sedation, and appears in some cases to be dose-dependent, with decreases in dosage leading to improvement. Although the mechanism remains unclear, some hypothesize apathy and amotivation to be secondary to serotonergically mediated inhibition of dopamine function [68,69]. The apparent efficacy of dopaminergic agents to treat apathy or amotivation is consistent with this hypothesis. Management strategies include switching to a different antidepressant class or adding a stimulant or other agents with dopaminergic action such as bupropion (75–300 mg qd-bid), amantadine (100 mg tid-qid), ropinirole (1–2 mg bid), pramipexole (0.5–1.5 mg tid), modafinil (100–200 mg bid), or pergolide (2–5 mg/day in divided doses).

Serotonin Syndrome

The use of SSRIs have been associated with the emergence of the potentially life-threatening manifestation of excessive serotonergic activity, the "serotonin syndrome," characterized by mental status changes, myoclonus, restlessness, hyperreflexia, hyperthermia, hemodynamic instability, and ataxia. In most cases, serotonin syndrome is seen in the context of increased serotonin availability arrived at through a variety of mechanisms. Use of combined SSRIs, MAOIs, or TCAs have been implicated [70, 71]. Concomitant use of SSRIs and tryptophan or hypericum (St. John's wort) have also been described as being responsible for serotonin syndrome [72]. The use of serotonergic medications (e.g., SSRIs) or narcotics (especially meperidine and dextromethorphan) in combination with an MAOI is contraindicated and may result in a serotonin syndrome. In order to prevent the emergence of serotonin syndrome, at least a 2-week washout period is recommended for most SSRIs (5 weeks for fluoxetine because of its long half-life) prior to switching to an MAOI. When switching to an SSRI, 2 weeks are required after discontinuation of a MAOI to allow resynthesis of the monoamine oxidase enzyme.

Hematological Effects

Serotonin is involved in the regulation of platelet function. Several case reports suggest that patients treated with SSRIs or other antidepressants with serotonergic activity may develop bleeding abnormalities, such as petechiae or bruising [73,74]. One case report found a reduction in SSRI-induced bleeding with the administration of vitamin C [75].

Agranulocytosis

Agranulocytosis is a blood dyscrasia that has been rarely associated with the use of antidepressants including TCAs, MAOIs, SSRIs, and other new agents [76,77]. The presence of agranulocytosis requires prompt hematological consultation and medication discontinuation.

Other Effects

Syndrome of Inappropriate Secretion of Antidiuretic Hormone

Hyponatremia (serum sodium concentration less than 135 mmol/L) due to the syndrome of inappropriate secretion of antidiuretic hormone (SIADH) is an increasingly recognized, although apparently relatively uncommon, adverse effect associated with SSRIs and other antidepressants. The actual incidence of antidepressant-induced SIADH is difficult to determine owing to confounding factors such as the presence of concurrent medications and medical conditions; in addition, not all cases of hyponatremia represent SIADH. Although hyponatremia has been reported with all SSRIs, tricyclics, venlafaxine, and recently with reboxetine [78,79], most studies of the issue are either individual case reports or are small, retrospective, and limited by confounding variables. Recent studies suggest that risk factors for developing hyponatremia while on an SSRI include age, female gender, prior history of hyponatremia, and concomitant use of other medications known to induce hyponatremia [80,81]. Data from the World Health Organization database for spontaneous reporting of adverse drug reactions suggest that the risk of antidepressant-associated hyponatremia is higher in women, in the elderly, during the summer, and during the first weeks of treatment [82]. For the majority of patients with SSRI-associated hyponatremia, the sodium concentration returns to normal within days to weeks of SSRI discontinuation. [80]. Common symptoms of hyponatremia range from fatigue and weakness to mental status changes, including frank delirium. Treatment strategies include fluid restriction, supportive measures, and, symptomatic treatment. Clinicians should be aware of the possibility of this insidious, frequently serious, and potentially life-threatening complication. It is reasonable to check serum sodium concentrations before initiating any antidepressant agent in elderly patients and periodically to reassess them during the first 2–4 weeks of treatment.

Weight Gain

Weight gain may be a frequent cause of medication noncompliance and has been commonly associated with TCAs (especially the tertiary amines such as amitriptyline, imipramine, and doxepin), MAOIs (especially phenelzine), and variably with the SSRIs [83]. Weight gain may be related to the antihistaminic and serotonergic properties of these agents and has been frequently reported with the newer antidepressant mirtazapine [84]. Bupropion, venlafaxine, and nefazodone may be less likely to cause weight gain [85,86] and should be considered in patients with preexisting obesity or body image and weight preoccupations. Although the mechanism of weight gain remains unclear, both histamine and serotonin promote satiety [87]; hence, their antagonism may produce overeating and in some patients intense carbohydrate craving. However, many patients experience significant weight gain without changes in appetite or food intake. If weight gain occurs during antidepressant administration, dietary modification and increased exercise should be recommended. Patients should avoid the use of high-calorie beverages to treat dry mouth. Behavioral modification and weight control programs should be considered if necessary. Low doses of agents that have both antidepressant and anorectic effects (e.g., methylphenidate, bupropion) can be added to a non-MAOI antidepressant to limit weight gain. In fact, bupropion has been associated with weight loss in several depression clinical trials [88,89], and a recent study in obese patients suggested that bupropion may be an effective strategy to achieve weight loss [90]. Switching to an antidepressant less likely to produce weight gain may deter further weight changes. In the rare patient whose weight gain is attributable to accumulation of fluid and/or edema, support stockings, leg elevation, or judicious use of a diuretic such as hydrochlorothiazide (12.5–25 mg qd) or amiloride (5–10 mg gd) maybe helpful. Recent reports of the efficacy of topiramate (25–100 mg qd-bid) as a weight-control strategy may indicate a future role of topiramate for the management of weight gain in SSRI-treated patients [91–93], but topiramate's use is limited by side effects such as sedation and cognitive dysfunction. Other potentially valuable options to control weight gain include adjunctive treatment with sibutramine (5–15 mg qd) and modafinil (200–400 mg qd) [94]. Case reports suggest potential efficacy of histamine H_2 receptor antagonists (nizatidine 15–300 mg/day, famotidine 20–40 mg qd) [95] and dopaminergic agents (e.g., amantadine 100 mg tid-qid; pramipexole 0.5–1.5 mg tid) [96] for control of weight gain.

Excessive Sweating

Hyperhidrosis or excessive sweating may occur with all antidepressants. Nonpharmacological measures such as daily showering the application of cornstarch or talcum powder may provide relief. Antiperspirants and astringent solutions, some of which are available over-the-counter, such as aluminum acetate or aluminum sulfate, applied to the commonly affected areas (axillae, feet, or hands), and other aluminum-containing preparations, such as 6% aluminum chloride in alcohol or 20% aluminum chloride hexahydrate (i.e., Drysol) may also be helpful. However, these preparations may be irritating to the skin, and consequently should be limited to use once a day or less frequently, and they should be applied only to the affected skin when dry and intact. Pharmacological strategies include topical and systemic agents that have significant anticholinergic action such as benztropine, a potent anticholinergic, which has been reported to be effective for night sweats (0.5–1.0 mg qd-bid) [84]. Glycopyrrolate (1–2 mg qd-tid orally or topical cream preparation), dosed according to the severity of the sweating, has been reported to be effective for hyperhidrosis [97,98]. In addition, there are reports that alpha$_1$-adrenergic antagonists such as terazosin, doxazosin (1–2 mg qhs), and clonidine (0.1–0.25 mg qd-qid) may be helpful to reduce antidepressant-induced sweating [99]. Dosing should be initiated at low doses and titrated up gradually to minimize the risk of hypotension. Oxybutynin, an agent often used in the treatment of bladder spasms and overactive bladder, and propantheline bromide, used for bladder spasms, are also clinically effective therapeutic approaches; however, multiple daily dosing (up to five times/day) is required. A relatively new treatment approach is the use of botulinum toxin for patients who have hyperhidrosis restricted to axillary and palmar areas [100]. It is, however, an often painful and expensive remedy. It is important to note this approach has not been clinically tested for antidepressant-induced sweating.

Hypomania and Mania

Hypomania or mania may occur during treatment with all antidepressants including in patients without a known history of bipolar disorder. In patients with unipolar depression, the manic switch rate has been reported to be less than 1% [101,102]. Patients with a history of bipolar disorder who are not on mood stabilizers are at much higher risk—up to 24% of patients in one study [103]. Limited data, mostly from retrospective studies, suggest that among antidepressants, TCAs are the most likely cause of a manic switch, followed by SSRIs, and with lower rates being observed for bupropion and MAOIs [104]. A recent meta-analysis suggested that paroxetine may have a lower switch rate than other SSRIs [105]. Management of antidepressant-induced manic states generally includes reduction or discontinuation of the antidepressant and treatment of the manic episode. Mild hypomania may remit with dose reduction or discontinuation of the antidepressant alone, but more severe presentations may require treatment with a mood stabilizer, benzodiazepine, and/or a antipsychotic.

Suicidal Ideation

Suicidal ideation has been reported to be a rare adverse effect of antidepressant treatment, but does not appear to be associated with any specific agent. Suicidal ideation in patients on antidepressants may be primarily attributable to the underlying psychiatric disorder requiring treatment such as depression or borderline personality disorder. However, rarely patients may have a paradoxical reaction to antidepressant administration. Although the potential mechanisms for this effect remain uncertain, hypotheses include antidepressant-induced overstimulation, particularly in anxious or agitated patients, causing dysphoria, and also akathisia-like motor restlessness causing intense distress [106]. Antidepressant-induced mania can also increase the risk of self-harm. If preexisting suicidality is exacerbated or new-onset suicidal ideation develops after the initiation of antidepressant treatment, the clinician should consider the possible contribution of the antidepressant therapy and evaluate for treatment-emergent akathisia, hypomania, or agitation. In such cases, antidepressant discontinuation or using of adjunctive beta-blockers or benzodiazepines may be effective. Initiating antidepressant treatment at low doses with slow upward titration may reduce the risk of such effects; dosage reduction, antidepressant class switch, or discontinuation are potential management approaches.

Discontinuation Syndrome and Withdrawal Phenomena

Abrupt cessation of a TCA may result in a withdrawal syndrome including flulike symptoms such as nausea, vomiting, diarrhea, malaise, fatigue, myalgias, cold sweats, chills, insomnia and anorexia, and symptoms of cholinergic rebound. Vivid dreams or nightmares are also common. Abrupt discontinuation of SSRIs, nefazodone, venlafaxine, and mirtazapine can also produce flulike symptoms similar to the tricyclic withdrawal syndrome with the addition of characteristic neurological symptoms such as dizziness or vertigo, unsteady gait, tremulousness, and dysesthesias [107]. Abrupt discontinuation of higher doses, particularly of shorter acting agents, elevates the risk for a discontinuation syndrome. Symptoms may manifest hours to day following discontinuation. For TCAs, much of the withdrawal symptomatology has been attributed to cholinergic rebound [108]; however, the description of discontinuation-related distress associated with SSRIs suggests a potential role for serotonergic mechanisms. The withdrawal syndrome can be minimized by patient education about the need to avoid abrupt discontinuation and use of a gradual taper schedule that has been adjusted and individualized according to the patient's response. For some patients, substitution of a longer acting antidepressant such as fluoxetine for a shorter acting agent may facilitate discontinuation [109]. Recent work suggests that cognitive-behavioral therapy may also decrease discontinuation-related distress [110]. Symptomatic treatment, including analgesics for aches and benzodiazepines or gabapentin for sleep disturbance or increased anxiety, may also improve patient comfort. Patients should be reassured of the generally transient and benign nature of withdrawal-related symptoms, and instructed that prompt resumption of the medication should provide relief.

CONCLUSION

The management of antidepressant side effects is a complex task that requires knowledge of the principles of psychopharmacology, good communication skills and patient rapport, and, in many instances, creativity. Although the newer antidepressants are generally associated with fewer side effects than older agents, proper management of all side effects will enhance patient compliance and consequently promote the clinical effectiveness of antidepressant pharmacotherapy.

REFERENCES

1.   E Frank, DJ Kupfer, JM Perel, C Comes, DB Jarrett, AG Mallinger, ME Thase, AB McEachran, VJ Grochocinski. Three-year outcomes for maintenance therapies in recurrent depression. Arch Gen Psychiatry 47:1093–1099, 1990
2.   ME Thase. Relapse and recurrence in unipolar major depression: short-term and long-term approaches. J Clin Psychiatry 1990; 51(suppl):51–57.
3.   DB Christensen. Drug taking compliance: a review and synthesis. Health Serv Res 13:171–187, 1978
4.   EE Madden Jr. Evaluation of outpatient pharmacy patient counseling. J Am Pharm Assoc 13:437–443, 1973
5.   M Fava, JF Rosenbaum, L Cohen, S Reiter, M McCarthy, R Steingard, K Clancy. High-dose fluoxetine in the treatment of depressed patients not responsive to a standard dose of Fluoxetine. J Affect Disord 25:229–234, 1992.
5a. J Smoller, MH Pollack, D Lee. Management of antidepressant-induced side effects. In: T Stern, J Herman, P Slavin, eds. The MGH Guide to Psychiatry in Primary Care. New York: McGraw Hill, 1998.
6.   JM Zajecka. Clinical issues in long-term treatment with antidepressants. J Clin Psychiatry 61:20–25, 2000.
7.   HY Meltzer, M Young, J Metz, VS Fang, PM Schyve, RC Arora.

Extrapyramidal side effects and increased serum prolactin following fluoxetine, a new antidepressant. J Neural Transm 45:165–175, 1979.

8. RJ Baldessarini, E Marsh. Fluoxetine and side effects. Arch Gen Psychiatry 47:191–192, 1990.

9. RT Segraves. Effects of psychotropic drugs on human erection and ejaculation. Arch Gen Psychiatry 46:275–284, 1989.

10. MH Pollack, S Reiter, P Hammerness. Genitourinary and sexual adverse effects of psychotropic medication. Int J Psychiatry Med 22:305–327, 1992.

11. MS Finkel, F Laghrissi-Thode, BG Pollock, J Rong. Paroxetine is a novel nitric oxide synthase inhibitor. Psychopharmacol Bull 32:653–658, 1996.

12. JW Thompson Jr, MR Ware, RK Blashfield. Psychotropic medication and priapism: a comprehensive review. J Clin Psychiatry 51:430–433, 1990.

13. J Zajecka, J Fawcett, M Schaff, H Jeffriess, C Guy. The role of serotonin in sexual dysfunction: fluoxetine-associated orgasm dysfunction. J Clin Psychiatry 52:66–68, 1991.

14. AL Montejo-Gonzalez, G Llorca, JA Izquierdo, A Ledesma, M Bousono, A Calcedo, JL Carrasco, J Ciudad, E Daniel, J de la Gandara, J Derecho, M Franco, MJ Gomez, JA Macias, T Martin, V Perez, JM Sanchez, S Sanchez, E Vicens. SSRI-induced sexual dysfunction: fluoxetine, paroxetine, sertraline, and fluvoxatnine in a prospective, multicenter, and descriptive clinical study of 344 patients. J Sex Marital Ther 23:176–194, 1997.

15. AJ Rothschild. Selective serotonin reuptake inhibitor-induced sexual dysfunction: efficacy of a drug holiday. Am J Psychiatry 152:1514–1516, 1995.

16. J Zajecka, S Mitchell, J Fawcett. Treatment-emergent changes in sexual function with selective serotonin reuptake inhibitors as measured with the Rush Sexual Inventory. Psychopharmacol Bull 33:755–760, 1997.

17. SH Kennedy, SM McCann, M Masellis, RS McIntyre, J Raskin, G McKay, GB Baker. Combining bupropion SR with venlafaxine, paroxetine, or fluoxetine: a preliminary report on pharmacokinetic, therapeutic, and sexual dysfunction effects. J Clin Psychiatry 63:181–186, 2002.

18. M Fava, MA Rankin, JE Alpert, AA Nierenberg, JJ Worthington. An open trial of oral sildenafilin antidepressant-induced sexual dysfunction. Psychother Psychosom 67:328–331, 1998.

19. MJ Gitlin, R Suri, L Altshuler, J Zuckerbrow-Miller, L Fairbanks. Bupropion-sustained release as a treatment for SSRI-induced sexual side effects. J Sex Marital Ther 28:131–138, 2002.

20. BD Bartlik, P Kaplan, HS Kaplan. Psychostimulants apparently reverse sexual dysfunction secondary to selective serotonin re-uptake inhibitors. J Sex Marital Ther 21:264–271, 1995.

21. MJ Gitlin. Treatment of sexual side effects with dopaminergic agents. J Clin Psychiatry 56:124, 1995.

22. D Michelson, J Bancroft, S Targum, Y Kim, R Tepner. Female sexual dysfunction associated with antidepressant administration: a randomized, placebo-controlled study of pharmacologic intervention. Am J Psychiatry 157:239–240, 2000.

23. JJ Worthington, NM Simon, NB Korbly, RH Perlis, JF Rosenbaum, MH Pollack. Ropinirole for SSRI-induced sexual dysfunction. Paper presented at the American Psychiatric Association Annual Meeting, New Orleans, May 5–10, 2001.

24. M Landen, G Bjorling, H Agren, T Fahlen. A randomized, double-blind, placebo-controlled trial of buspirone in combination with an SSRI in patients with treatment-refractory depression. J Clin Psychiatry 59:664–668, 1998.

25. RD Reynolds. Sertraline-induced anorgasmia treated with intermittent nefazodone. J Clin Psychiatry 58:89, 1997.

26. AK Ashton, K Ahrens, S Gupta, PS Masand. Antidepressant-induced sexual dysfunction and Ginkgo biloba. Am J Psychiatry 157:836–837, 2000.

27. HJ Vogt, P Brandl, G Kockott, JR Schmitz, MH Wiegand, J Schadrack, M Gierend. Double-blind, placebo-controlled safety and efficacy trial with yohimbine hydrochloride in the treatment of nonorganic erectile dysfunction. Int J Impot Res 9:155–161, 1997.

28. E Hollander, A McCarley. Yohimbine treatment of sexual side effects induced by serotonin reuptake blockers. J Clin Psychiatry 53:207–209, 1992.

29. D Aizenberg, Z Zemishlany, A Weizman. Cyproheptadine treatment of sexual dysfunction induced by serotonin reuptake inhibitors. Clin Neuropharmacol 18:320–324, 1995.

30. MJ Gitlin. Psychotropic medications and their effects on sexual function: diagnosis, biology, and treatment approaches. J Clin Psychiatry 55:406–413, 1994.

31. E Richelson. Pharmacology of antidepressants–characteristics of the ideal drug. Mayo Clin Proc 69:1069–1081, 1994.

32. SP Roose, AH Glassman, SG Siris, BT Walsh, RL Bruno, LB Wright. Comparison of imipramine- and nortriptyline- induced orthostatic hypotension: a meaningful difference. J Clin Psychopharmacol 1:316–319, 1981.

33. M Simonson. Controlling MAO inhibitor hypotension. Am J Psychiatry 5:1118–1119, 1964.

34. JF Patterson. Metoclopramide therapy of MAOI orthostatic hypotension. J Clin Psychopharmacol 7:112–113, 1987.

35. RL Rudolph, AT Derivan. The safety and tolerability of venlafaxine hydrochloride: analysis of the clinical trials database. J Clin Psychopharmacol 16:54S–59S; discussion 59S–61S, 1996.

36. ME Thase. Effects of venlafaxine on blood pressure: a meta analysis of original data from 3744 depressed patients. J Clin Psychiatry 59:502–508, 1998.

36a. DM Gardner, KI Shulman, SE Walker, SAN Tailor. The making of a user-friendly MAOI diet. J Clin Psychiatry 57:99–104, 1996.

37. PE Keck Jr., A Vuckovic, HG Pope Jr., AA Nierenberg, GW Gribble, K White. Acute cardiovascular response to monoamine oxidase inhibitors: a prospective assessment. J Clin Psychopharmacol 9:203–206, 1989.

38. E Grossman, FH Messerli, T Grodzicki, P Kowey. Should a moratorium be placed on sublingual nifedipine capsules given for hypertensive emergencies and pseudoemergencies? JAMA 276:1328–1331, 1996.

39. M Haria, A Fitton, D McTavish. Trazodone. A review of its pharmacology, therapeutic use in depression and therapeutic potential in other disorders. Drugs Aging 4:331–355, 1994.

40. J Rosen, BG Pollock, LP Altieri, EA Jonas. Treatment of nortriptyline's side effects in elderly patients: a double blind study of bethanechol. Am J Psychiatry 150:1249–1251, 1993.

41. DF Klein, R Gittelman, F Quitkin, A Rifkin. Diagnostic and Drug Treatment of Psychiatric Disorders: Adults and Children. 2d ed. Baltimore: Williams & Wilkins, 1980.

42. J Bernstein. Drug Therapy in Psychiatry. Boston: J Wright, 1983.

43. HC Everett. The use of bethanechol chloride with tricyclic antidepressants. Am J Psychiatry 132:1202–1204, 1975.

44. BH Rumack. Anticholinergic poisoning: treatment with physostigmine. Pediatrics 52:449–451, 1973.

45. J Biederman, E Gonzalez, B Bronstein, H De Monaco, V Wright. Desipramine and cutaneous reactions in pediatric outpatients. J Clin Psychiatry 49:178–183, 1988.

46. AN Crowson, CM Magro. Antidepressant therapy. A possible cause of atypical cutaneous lymphoid hyperplasia. Arch Dermatol 131:925–929, 1995.

47. AH Guberman, FM Besag, MJ Brodie, JM Dooley, MS Duchowny, JM Pellock, A Richens, RS Stern, E Trevathan. Lamotrigine associated rash: risk/benefit considerations in adults and children. Epilepsia 40:985–991, 1999.

48. DH Atkin, RE Fitzpatrick. Laser treatment of imipramine induced hyperpigmentation. J Am Acad Dermatol 43:77–84, 2000.

49. JK Warnock, K Sieg, D Willsie, EK Stevenson, T Kestenbaum. Drug-related alopecia in patients treated with tricyclic antidepressants. J Nerv Ment Dis 179:441–442, 1991.

50. AD Ogilvie. Hair loss during fluoxetine treatment. Lancet 342:1423, 1993.

51. JA Bourgeois. Two cases of hair loss after sertraline use. J Clin Psychopharmacol 16:91–92, 1996.

52. G Zalsman, J Sever, H Munitz. Hair loss associated with paroxetine treatment: a case report. Clin Neuropharmacol 22:246–247, 1999.

53. GE Tomkins, JL Jackson, PG O'Malley, E Balden, JE Santoro. Treatment of chronic headache with antidepressants: a meta-analysis. Am J Med 111:54–63, 2001.

54. KA Holroyd, FJ O'Donnell, M Stensland, GL Lipchik, GE Cordingley, BW Carlson. Management of chronic tension-type headache with tricyclic antidepressant medication, stress management therapy, and their combination: a randomized controlled trial. JAMA 285:2208–2215, 2001.

55. JD Amsterdam, M Hornig-Rohan, G Maislin. Efficacy of alprazolam in reducing fluoxetine-induced jitteriness in patients with major depression. J Clin Psychiatry 55:394–400, 1994.

56. J Fawcett, RL Barkin. Review of the results from clinical studies on the efficacy, safety and tolerability of mirtazapine for the treatment of patients with major depression. J Affect Disord 51:267–285, 1998.

57. A Flemenbaum. Pavor nocturnus: a complication of single daily tricyclic or neuroleptic dosage. Am J Psychiatry 133:570–572, 1976.

58. AL Sharpley, PJ Cowen. Effect of pharmacologic treatments on the sleepof depressed patients. Biol Psychiatry 37:85–98, 1995.

59. AL Sharpley, DJ Williamson, ME Attenburrow, G Pearson, P Sargent, PJ Cowen. The effects of paroxetine and nefazodone on sleep: a placebo controlled trial. Psychopharmacology (Berl) 126:50–54, 1996.

60. MJ Garvey, GD Tollefson. Occurrence of myoclonus in patients treated with cyclic antidepressants. Arch Gen Psychiatry 44:269–272, 1987.

61. M Dauer. Severe myoclonus produced by fluvoxamine. J Clin Psychiatry 56:589–590, 1995.

62. CM Dorsey, SE Lukas, SL Cunningham. Fluoxetine-induced sleep disturbance in depressed patients. Neuropsychopharmacology 14:437–442, 1996.

63. EA Nofzinger, A Fasiczka, S Berman, ME Thase. Bupropion SR reduces periodic limb movements associated with arousals from sleep in depressed patients with periodic limb movement disorder. J Clin Psychiatry 61:858–862, 2000.

64. MS Jaffee, JM Bostwick. Buspirone as an antidote to venlafaxine-induced bruxism. Psychosomatics 41:535–536, 2000.

65. ES Brown, SC Hong. Antidepressant-induced bruxism successfully treated with gabapentin. J Am Dent Assoc 130:1467–1469, 1999.

66. F Lobbezoo, GJ Lavigne, R Tanguay, JY Montplaisir. The effect of catecholamine precursor L-dopa on sleep bruxism: a controlled clinical trial. Mov Disord 12:73–78, 1997.

67. JW Stewart, W Harrison, F Quitkin, MR Liebowitz. Phenelzine-induced pyridoxine deficiency. J Clin Psychopharmacol 4:225–226, 1984.

68. R Hoehn-Saric, JR Lipsey, DR McLeod. Apathy and indifference in patients on fluvoxamine and fluoxetine. J Clin Psychopharmacol 10:343–345, 1990.

69. JM Zajecka. Clinical issues in long-term treatment with antidepressants. J Clin Psychiatry 61:20–25, 2000.

70. R Lane, D Baldwin. Selective serotonin reuptake inhibitor-induced serotonin syndrome: review. J Clin Psychopharmacol 17:208–221, 1997.

71. KA Sporer. The serotonin syndrome. Implicated drugs, pathophysiology and management. Drug Saf 13:94–104, 1995.

72. AA Izzo, E Ernst. Interactions between herbal medicines and prescribed drugs: a systematic review. Drugs 61:2163–2175, 2001.

73. DW Gunzberger, D Martinez. Adverse vascular effects associated with fluoxetine. Am J Psychiatry 149:1751, 1992.

74. JP Ottervanger, BH Stricker, J Huls, JN Weeda. Bleeding attributed to the intake of paroxetine. Am J Psychiatry 151:781–782, 1994.

75. JA Tielens. Vitamin C for paroxetine- and fluvoxamine-associated bleeding. Am J Psychiatry 154:883–884, 1997.

76. GM Levin, CL DeVane. A review of cyclic antidepressant-induced blood dyscrasias. Ann Pharmacother 26:378–383, 1992.

77. C Trescoli-Serrano, NK Smith. Sertraline-induced agranulocytosis. Postgrad Med J 72:446, 1996.
78. O Spigset, K Hedenmalm. Hyponatraemia and the syndrome of inappropriate antidiuretic hormone secretion (SIADH) induced by psychotropic drugs. Drug Saf 12:209–225, 1995.
79. P Ranieri, S Franzoni, M Trabucchi. Reboxetine and hyponatremia. N Engl J Med 342:215–216, 2000.
80. D Kirby, D Ames. Hyponatraemia and selective serotonin re-uptake inhibitors in elderly patients. Int J Geriatr Psychiatry 16:484–493, 2001.
81. Liu BA, Mittmann N, Knowles SR, Shear NH. Hyponatrernia and the syndrome of inappropriate secretion of antidiuretic hormone associated with the use of selective serotonin reuptake inhibitors: a review of spontaneous reports. Can Med Assoc J. 155:519–527, 1996.
82. O Spigset, K Hedenmalm. Hyponatremia in relation to treatment with antidepressants: a survey of reports in the World Health Organization data base for spontaneous reporting of adverse drug reactions. Pharmacotherapy 17:348–352, 1997.
83. M Fava. Weight gain and antidepressants. J Clin Psychiatry 61:37–41, 2000.
84. E Leinonen, J Skarstein, K Behnke, H Agren, JT Helsdingen. Efficacy and tolerability of mirtazapine versus citalopram: a double-blind, randomized study in patients with major depressive disorder. Nordic Antidepressant Study Group. Int Clin Psychopharmacol 14:329–337, 1999.
85. PH Silverstone, A Ravindran. Once-daily venlafaxine extended release (XR) compared with fluoxetine in outpatients with depression and anxiety. Venlafaxine XR 360 Study Group. J Clin Psychiatry 60:22–28, 1999.
86. N Sussman, DL Ginsberg, J Bikoff. Effects of nefazodone on body weight: a pooled analysis of selective serotonin reuptake inhibitor- and imipramine-controlled trials. J Clin Psychiatry 62:256–260, 2001.
87. JE Blundell, AJ Hill. Serotoninergic modulation of the pattern of eating and the profile of hunger-satiety in humans. Int J Obes 11:141–155, 1987.
88. N Harto-Truax, WC Stern, LL Miller, TL Sato, AE Cato. Effects of bupropion on body weight. J Clin Psychiatry 44:183–186, 1983.
89. J Feighner, G Hendrickson, L Miller, W Stem. Double-blind comparison of doxepin versus bupropion in outpatients with a major depressive disorder. J Clin Psychopharmacol 6:27–32, 1986.
90. KM Gadde, CB Parker, LG Maner, HR Wagner 2nd, EJ Logue, MK Drezner, KR Krishnan. Bupropion for weight loss: an investigation of efficacy and tolerability in overweight and obese women. Obes Res 9:544–551, 2001.
91. A Gordon, LH Price. Mood stabilization and weight loss with topiramate. Am J Psychiatry 156:968–969, 1999.
92. CJ Teter, JJ Early, CM Gibbs. Treatment of affective disorder and obesity with topiramate. Ann Pharmacother 34:1262–1265, 2000.
93. M van Ameringen, C Mancini, B Pipe, PG Farvolden. Topiramate for weight control in SSRI treated anxiety Disorder. Paper presented at the American Psychiatric Association Annual Meeting. New Orleans, May 5–10, 2001.

94. E Sacchetti, L Guarneri, D Bravi. H(2) antagonist nizatidine may control olanzapine-associated weight gain in schizophrenic patients. Biol Psychiatry 48:167–168, 2000.

95. M Floris, J Lejeune, W Deberdt. Effect of amantadine on weight gain during olanzapine treatment. Eur Neuropsychopharmacol 11:181–182, 2001.

96. JM Pierre, BH Guze. Benztropine for venlafaxine-induced night sweats. J Clin Psychopharmacol 20:269, 2000.

97. SL Atkin, PM Brown. Treatment of diabetic gustatory sweating with topical glycopyrrolate cream. Diabet Med 13:493–494, 1996.

98. LL Hays, AJ Novack, JC Worsham. The Frey syndrome: a simple, effective treatment. Otolaryngol Head Neck Surg 90:419–425, 1982.

99. MM Butt. Managing antidepressant-induced sweating. J Clin Psychiatry 50:146–147, 1989.

100. IR Odderson. Axillary hyperhidrosis: treatment with botulinum toxin A. Arch Phys Med Rehabil 79:350–352, 1998.

101. M Peet. Induction of mania with selective serotonin re-uptake inhibitors and tricyclic antidepressants. Br J Psychiatry 164:549–550, 1994.

102. RH Howland. Induction of mania with serotonin reuptake inhibitors. J Clin Psychopharmacol 16:425–427, 1996.

103. C Henry, F Sorbara, J Lacoste, C Gindre, M Leboyer. Antidepressant-induced mania in bipolar patients: identification of risk factors. J Clin Psychiatry 62:249–255, 2001.

104. AL Stoll, PV Mayer, M Kolbrener, E Goldstein, B Suplit, J Lucier, BM Cohen, M Tohen. Antidepressant-associated mania: a controlled comparison with spontaneous mania. Am J Psychiatry 151:1642–1645, 1994.

105. JR Calabrese, DJ Rapport, SE Kimmel, MD Shelton. Controlled trials in bipolar I depression: focus on switch rates and efficacy. Eur Neuropsychopharmacol 1999; 4(suppl 9):S109–S112.

106. JF Lipinski Jr., G Mallya, P Zimmerman, HG Pope Jr. Fluoxetine-induced akathisia: clinical and theoretical implications. J Clin Psychiatry 50:339–342, 1989.

107. AF Schatzberg, P Haddad, EM Kaplan, M Lejoyeux, JF Rosenbaum, AH Young, J Zajecka. Serotonin reuptake inhibitor discontinuation syndrome: a hypothetical definition. Discontinuation Consensus Panel. J Clin Psychiatry 58:5–10, 1997.

108. SC Dilsaver, JF Greden, RM Snider. Antidepressant withdrawal syndromes: phenomenology and pathophysiology. Int Clin Psychopharmacol 2:1–19,1987.

109. JF Rosenbaum, M Fava, SL Hoog, RC Ascroft, WB Krebs. Selective serotonin reuptake inhibitor discontinuation syndrome: a randomized clinical trial. Biol Psychiatry 44:77–87, 1998.

110. MW Otto, MH Pollack, GS Sachs, SR Reiter, S Meltzer-Brody, JF Rosenbaum. Discontinuation of benzodiazepine treatment: efficacy of cognitive-behavioral therapy for patients with panic disorder. Am J Psychiatry 150:1485–1490, 1993.

Index

About the Editors

JONATHAN E. ALPERT is Associate Director of the Depression Clinical and Research Program and Chair of the Institutional Review Board, Massachusetts General Hospital, Boston, and Assistant Professor of Psychiatry, Harvard Medical School, Boston, Massachusetts. The author of more than 75 professional publications, he received the M.D. degree (1986) from Yale University School of Medicine, New Haven, Connecticut, and the Ph.D. degree (1987) in behavioral pharmacology from Cambridge University, England.

MAURIZIO FAVA is Director of the Depression Clinical and Research Program and Associate Chief of Psychiatry for Clinical Research, Massachusetts General Hospital, Boston, and Professor of Psychiatry, Harvard Medical School, Boston, Massachusetts. The author of more than 200 journal articles and several books, he is a member of the American College of Neuropsychopharmacology and the European College of Neuropsychopharmacology, among other organizations. He received the M.D. degree (1982) from the University of Padua School of Medicine, Italy.

ISBN 0-8247-4046-7